PRACTITIONER'S GUIDE TO THE NEUROPSYCHIATRY OF HIV/AIDS

Practitioner's Guide to the Neuropsychiatry of HIV/AIDS

Edited by

WILFRED G. van GORP
and
STEPHAN L. BUCKINGHAM

THE GUILFORD PRESS
New York   London

© 1998 The Guilford Press
A Division of Guilford Publications, Inc.
72 Spring Street, New York, NY 10012
http://www.guilford.com

Printed in the United States of America

This book is printed on acid-free paper.

Last digit is print number: 9 8 7 6 5 4 3 2 1

Library of Congress Cataloging-in-Publication Data

Practitioner's guide to the neuropsychiatry of HIV/AIDS / editors,
    Wilfred G. van Gorp and Stephan L. Buckingham.
        p.   cm.
    Includes bibliographical references and index.
    ISBN 1-57230-309-3 (hard cover: alk. paper)
    1. AIDS dementia complex.   I. van Gorp, W. G. (Wilfred G.)
    II. Buckingham, Stephan L.
    [DNLM: 1. AIDS Dementia Complex.   2. HIV Infections—psychology.
WC 503.5 M549 1998]
RC359.5.M46 1998
616.97′92—DC21
DNLM/DLC
for Library of Congress   97-42478
                                                                    CIP

Contributors

J. Hampton Atkinson, MD, HIV Neurobehavioral Research Center (HNRC), University of California at San Diego, San Diego, California

Carla Back, PhD, UCLA Alzheimer's Disease Center, UCLA Medical Center, Los Angeles, California

Rae-Lynn Benson-Duffy, OTR, Private consultant, Torrance, California; Faculty, Mount St. Mary's College Hope Center, Occupational Therapy Assistant Program, Los Angeles, California

Stephan L. Buckingham, MSSW, ACSW, Consultant and psychotherapist, New York, New York

Steven A. Castellon, PhD, Department of Psychiatry and Biobehavioral Sciences, UCLA School of Medicine, Los Angeles, California

Josepha A. Cheong, MD, Department of Psychiatry, University of Florida Medical Center, Gainesville, Florida

Jeffrey Cummings, MD, Departments of Neurology and Psychiatry, UCLA Medical Center, Los Angles, California

Dwight L. Evans, MD, Department of Psychiatry, University of Florida Medical Center, Gainesville, Florida

Igor Grant, MD, HIV Neurobehavioral Research Center (HNRC), University of California at San Diego, San Diego, California

Charles H. Hinkin, PhD, ABPP, Department of Psychiatry and Biobehavioral Sciences, UCLA School of Medicine; Director, Neuropsychology Assessment Laboratory, West Los Angeles Veterans Affairs Medical Center, Los Angeles, California

Susan Leavenworth, MA, JD, Doctoral student in psychology at the University of Louisville, Louisville, Kentucky; practicing attorney; and Certified Psychological Associate at Frazier Rehabilitation Center, Louisville, Kentucky

Robert G. Meyer, PhD, Department of Psychology, University of Louisville, Louisville, Kentucky

Bruce Miller, MD, Department of Neurology, Harbor–UCLA Medical Center, Torrance, California

Paul Satz, PhD, ABPP, Department of Psychiatry and Biobehavioral Sciences, UCLA School of Medicine, Los Angeles, California

Judith M. Saunders, RN, DNSc, FAAN, Consultant, Pasadena, California

Frederick A. Schmitt, PhD, Department of Neurology, University of Kentucky Medical Center, Lexington, Kentucky

Andrés Sciolla, MD, Department of Psychiatry, University of California at San Diego, San Diego, California

Jill Shapira, RN, C, MN, ANP, Department of Nursing, West Los Angeles Veterans Affairs Medical Center, Los Angeles, California

Michael Shernoff, MSW, Graduate School of Social Work (Adjunct), Hunter College, City University of New York, New York; private practice, New York, New York

Elyse J. Singer, MD, Department of Neurology, UCLA School of Medicine, Los Angeles, California; Department of Neurology, West Los Angeles Veterans Affairs Medical Center, Los Angeles, California

Ian Stulberg, LCSW, AIDS Service Center, Pasadena, California

Sharon M. Valente, RNCS, ANP, PhD, FAAN, Department of Nursing, University of Southern California Center for Health Professions, Los Angeles, California

Wilfred G. van Gorp, PhD, ABPP, Associate Professor of Psychology in Psychiatry and Director, Neuropsychology Assessment Service, Department of Psychiatry, Cornell University Medical College, New York, New York

Mary M. C. Wetherby, PhD, Private practice, Texarkana, Texas; Department of Psychology (Adjunct), Texas A & M University–Texarkana, Texarkana, Texas

Preface

Two years after the initial case report appeared of unusual cognitive symptoms associated with immunosuppression in a group of gay men, scientific papers began to refer to "mental status changes" in these patients. The Centers for Disease Control and Prevention (then known as the Centers for Disease Control) established diagnostic criteria for "HIV-related encephalopathy," qualifying an otherwise asymptomatic individual with dementia for an AIDS diagnosis, and hence for disability benefits. Subsequent research has investigated the degree and predominant location of brain changes in persons with HIV/AIDS, the response to various antiretroviral and protease inhibitor agents in persons with HIV-associated dementia, and the neuropsychological characteristics of these cognitive changes.

In light of this accumulated knowledge, there is a need for a sourcebook for mental health clinicians who work with HIV-infected clients, but who do not necessarily have training in neuropsychology, neuropsychiatry, or neurology.

This book is geared to the non-neurologically trained mental health clinician who nevertheless works with HIV-infected patients, some of whom have neurologic disease. Few mental health clinicians have training in identification of neurologically related mental status disturbances, or in psychotherapeutic work with and management of these individuals and their families and loved ones. Finally, the ethical and legal issues involved in treating patients with a higher prevalence of dementia than that encountered by most mental health clinicians in their practices must also be mastered. It is our hope that this book will aid the mental health clinician in understanding the neurologic, neuropsychiatric, and neuropsychological features associated with HIV infection, as well as the associated medicolegal and psychosocial issues encountered when working with neurologically impaired HIV-infected individuals.

WILFRED G. VAN GORP, PHD, ABPP
STEPHAN L. BUCKINGHAM, MSSW, ACSW

Contents

1. **Neuropsychological Features of HIV Disease**   1
   Charles H. Hinkin, Steven A. Castellon, Wilfred
   G. van Gorp, and Paul Satz

2. **Neurobiological Basis of Behavioral Changes in**   42
   HIV-1 Encephalopathy
   Carla Back, Bruce Miller, and Jeffrey Cummings

3. **Differential Diagnosis of HIV-1 Neurological**   65
   Disease
   Elyse J. Singer

4. **Neuropsychiatric Features of HIV Disease**   106
   Andrés Sciolla, J. Hampton Atkinson, and Igor
   Grant

5. **Pharmacological Interventions for**   201
   Neuropsychiatric Symptoms of HIV Disease
   Mary M. C. Wetherby, Josepha A. Cheong,
   Dwight L. Evans, and Frederick A. Schmitt

6. **Psychosocial Interventions in Persons with**   228
   HIV-Associated Neuropsychiatric Compromise
   Stephan L. Buckingham and Michael Shernoff

7. **Issues for Caregivers, Families, and Significant**   241
   Others
   Ian Stulberg and Jill Shapira

8. **Suicide and HIV Disease**   263
   Sharon M. Valente and Judith M. Saunders

 9. *Enhancing Adaptive Function in HIV-Associated Dementia*   294
    Rae Lynn Benson-Duffy

10. *HIV/AIDS and Mental Capacity: Legal and Ethical Issues*   311
    Robert G. Meyer and Susan Leavenworth

Index   333

1

Neuropsychological Features of HIV Disease

CHARLES H. HINKIN
STEVEN A. CASTELLON
WILFRED G. VAN GORP
PAUL SATZ

INTRODUCTION

In the last decade, a tremendous amount of research effort and clinical care has been devoted to understanding the neuropsychological changes associated with HIV-1 infection. From the first case reports of unexpected cognitive decline in AIDS (Navia, Cho, Petito, & Price, 1986b) to the impressively large studies of hundreds and thousands of infected patients that were ultimately performed (Miller et al., 1990; Heaton et al., 1995), our knowledge of the natural history of HIV-1-related dementia, our ability to accurately evaluate and diagnose HIV-infected patients, and (encouragingly) our increasing ability to treat neuropsychological deficits in patients with AIDS have all increased significantly.

Given the prevalence of HIV-1-associated cognitive impairment, neuropsychological evaluation is frequently a critical part of the diagnosis and treatment of HIV-1-infected individuals. Making decisions on important issues related to differential diagnosis (e.g., "worried well" status vs. subclinical cognitive decline; depression vs. dementia), and tracking medication response over time, are but two of the important roles the clinical neuropsychologist is called upon to play. This chapter provides an overview of the typical cognitive and behavioral sequelae of HIV-1 infection; it also covers such issues as the epidemiology of HIV-associated dementia, neuroimaging findings, the relationship between cognition and depression, and the accuracy of patients' self-reported cognitive status.

CASE STUDY

The following is a case study of an individual who exemplifies the characteristic cognitive and behavioral deficits seen in HIV-1-associated dementia complex. It should be noted that although this is not an uncommon presentation, many HIV-infected individuals do not develop neuropsychological deficits of the severity of those affecting this patient. We refer to this relatively prototypical case to illustrate various issues throughout the chapter.

> Mr. Smith, a 42-year-old, partnered white male with 16 years of education, presented for neuropsychological evaluation with complaints of trouble concentrating, forgetfulness, and difficulty doing two things at a time. His partner, who accompanied him, added that Mr. Smith was also increasingly apathetic and occasionally overly irritable. Medically, the patient was first diagnosed HIV-1-seropositive 8 years ago. Two years ago he suffered an episode of Pneumocystis carinii pneumonia (PCP), thus meeting diagnostic criteria for AIDS. His current CD4 T-cell count was 50. Current medications included zidovudine and saquinavir, 2′-deoxy-3′-thiacytidine, as well as a number of anti-opportunistic-infection agents. The patient was administered a comprehensive battery of neuropsychological tests, which revealed the following profile of strengths and deficits. On the Wechsler Adult Intelligence Scale—Revised (WAIS-R), Mr. Smith's Full Scale IQ was 110, with his Verbal IQ slightly higher than his Performance IQ. He encountered greatest difficulty on WAIS-R subtests sensitive to attentional difficulty, such as Digit Span and Arithmetic, as well as on timed measures such as the Digit Symbol subtest. In contrast, his best performances were on the Vocabulary and Information subtests—two WAIS-R tasks that are relatively resistant to the deleterious effects of HIV. Other areas of cognitive impairment observed on neuropsychological testing included (1) poor divided attention; (2) memory impairment for both verbal and nonverbal material that was "forgetful" in nature;

and (3) psychomotor slowing, seen as a difficulty in performing speeded tasks where thought is wedded to action. In addition, Mr. Smith also reported a significant degree of depressive symptomatology, as measured by both the Beck Depression Inventory (BDI) and the Minnesota Multiphasic Personality Inventory–2 (MMPI-2). In contrast, Mr. Smith performed well within normal limits on measures of language, visual–spatial ability, praxis, and calculation. Although aware of his difficulties, Mr. Smith reported that they had not yet had adverse impact upon his ability to perform most activities of daily living. However, because he was now having difficulty with the most demanding of his job responsibilities, he decided to go on disability leave from his job as a public accountant. (See Table 1.1 for a summary of Mr. Smith's neuropsychological test scores.)

TERMINOLOGY AND DIAGNOSTIC CRITERIA

There remains considerable confusion among both mental health professionals and the lay public about the appropriate terminology to use in describing the cognitive changes attendant upon HIV-1 infection. A number of different diagnostic labels have been employed over the years, including "AIDS dementia complex," which was first introduced by Navia, Jordan, and Price (1986b) to identify the constellation of cognitive, behavioral, and motor symptoms that can occur alone or in combination in HIV-affected individuals. Soon thereafter, Price and Brew (1988) proposed a scaling system in which the severity of AIDS dementia complex could be graded (e.g., stage 0 = absent, stage 1 = mild, stage 3 = severe), to capture the sometimes obvious differences in degree of cognitive impairment seen in HIV-infected individuals. Following these earliest attempts at developing meaningful nomenclature, labels such as "HIV-related encephalopathy," "HIV-1-associated cognitive/motor complex," and "dementia due to HIV disease" have also been used to describe essentially the same syndrome.

Some of the historically most important attempts to codify criteria for the diagnosis of HIV-related cognitive impairment are reviewed below.

Centers for Disease Control

In 1987 the Centers for Disease Control (CDC) published diagnostic criteria for HIV-related encephalopathy, which in some ways closely resembled Navia et al.'s (1986b) description of AIDS dementia complex. HIV-related encephalopathy was considered a condition that

TABLE 1.1. Neuropsychological Data for Mr. Smith

Age: 42	*Education:* 16 years
Presenting concerns:	Concentration difficulty, forgetfulness, trouble "doing two things at once"; more apathetic and irritable (according to informant)
CD4 count: 50	*History of opportunistic infections: Pneumocystis carinii* pneumonia (one bout 2 years ago)
Current medications:	Zidovudine, 2'-deoxy-3'-thiacytidine, saquinavir

Wechsler Adult Intelligence Scale–Revised:
　　　　Full Scale IQ: 110, Verbal IQ: 112, Performance IQ: 105
　　　　Best subtests: Vocabulary (91st percentile), Information
　　　　　　(91st percentile)
　　　　Worst subtests: Digit Span (16th percentile), Digit Symbol
　　　　　　(9th percentile)
Attention: Simple attn.: Intact, although digits backward somewhat low
　　　　Divided attn.: Poor (Auditory Consonant Trigrams: 4th percentile)
Memory: California Verbal Learning Test: Immediate Recall: 7/16
　　　　　　　　　　　　　　　　　　　Delayed Recall: 6/16
　　　　　　　　　　　　　　　　　　　Immediate Cued Recall: 10/16
　　　　　　　　　　　　　　　　　　　Delayed Recognition: 14/16
　　　　Wechsler Memory Scale–Revised: Logical Memory I: 50th percentile
　　　　　　　　　　　　　　　　　　Logical Memory II: 23rd percentile
　　　　　　　　　　　　　　　　　　Visual Reproduction I: 43rd percentile
　　　　　　　　　　　　　　　　　　Visual Reproduction II: 20th percentile

Other test data:
　Trail Making Test, Part B: 4th percentile: Suggestive of psychomotor slowing
　Stroop task, Part A: 13th percentile: Also suggestive of psychomotor slowing
　Wisconsin Card Sorting Test: 6/6 categories but higher than usual number of
　　perseverative errors
　Finger Tapping Test: Dominant hand, 35th percentile; nondominant hand,
　　29th percentile
　Beck Depression Inventory: 19 (suggestive of moderate level of depressive
　　symptomatology)
　Minnesota Multiphasic Personality Inventory–2: Scale 2 (Depression)
　　elevated ($T = 75$)

could qualify an otherwise asymptomatic person for a diagnosis of AIDS and was defined as follows:

Clinical findings of disabling cognitive and/or motor dysfunction interfering with occupation or activities of daily living, or loss of behavioral developmental milestones affecting a child, progressing over weeks to months, in the absence of a concurrent illness or other condition than HIV infection that could explain the findings. Methods to rule out such concurrent illness and conditions must include cerebrospinal fluid examination and either brain imaging (computed tomography or magnetic resonance) or autopsy.

Although this definition represented a significant step forward by providing a consensual definition and label for an HIV-related encephalopathy or dementia, it was nonetheless criticized as being ambiguous and imprecise, with certain key terms not adequately defined (e.g., "clinical findings," "disabling cognitive and/or motor dysfunction").

The CDC, also in 1987, developed the first system for HIV disease staging, primarily for the purposes of surveillance and classification. This earliest staging system consisted of four main groups. Group I included people with time-limited medical symptoms appearing at or shortly following initial seroconversion; group II included individuals who were medically asymptomatic; group III contained those with progressive generalized lymphadenopathy (enlarged lymph nodes), but without any other notable symptoms of infection; and group IV included people with AIDS or AIDS-related complex, including people with symptoms of constitutional disease (persistent fever, weight loss, and diarrhea). This staging system emphasized individuals with AIDS, the last stage of the disease, and was eventually criticized on that grounds as being insufficient for predicting disease progression prior to the appearance of AIDS.

In 1993, the CDC published a revised classification system for HIV infection, which is currently widely used for describing the stage of HIV infection in a given patient (Mapou & Law, 1994). This two-factor staging system groups patients on the basis of type and degree of physical symptoms present (asymptomatic, mildly symptomatic, or AIDS-defining opportunistic infection), as well as on the basis of degree of immunosuppression present (CD4 count of >500 cells/mm^3, 200–499 cells/mm^3, or <200 cells/mm^3). This revised staging system responded to the important observation that a high CD4 count can occur in medically symptomatic patients and a low count can occur in asymptomatic patients. The CDC 1993 classification system is shown in Table 1.2.

American Academy of Neurology

An AIDS Task Force from the American Academy of Neurology (AAN, 1991) attempted to further clarify and define diagnostic criteria for AIDS-related dementia and to make these criteria more objective. The AAN criteria recognize that cognitively impaired HIV-infected individuals may present with either a full-blown dementia syndrome or more mild and selective cognitive abnormalities. For this reason, HIV-1-associated cognitive/motor complex has been divided into two subgroups: HIV-1-associated dementia complex and HIV-1-associated minor cognitive/motor disorder. In HIV-1-associated minor cogni-

TABLE 1.2. Centers for Disease Control and Prevention (CDC) 1993 Revised Classification System for HIV Infection, and Expanded AIDS Surveillance Case Definition for Adolescents and Adults

	Clinical categories		
CD4+ T-cell categories	(A) Asymptomatic, acute (primary) HIV or PGL	(B) Symptomatic, not (A) or (C) conditions	(C) AIDS indicator conditions
(1) ≥500/L	A1	B1	C1
(2) 200–499/L	A2	B2	C2
(3) <200/L (AIDS indicator T-cell count)	A3	B3	C3

Note. Clinical categories C1–C3, B3, and A3 constitute the expanded AIDS surveillance case definition.

Category C: AIDS-defining illnesses or infections

(1) PCP (*Pneumocystis carinii* pneumonia)
(2) Cryptosporidium
(3) Tuberculosis
(4) Coccidiomycosis
(5) Recurrent pneumonia in the past year (other than PCP)
(6) Candidiasis (only pulmonary, esophageal, or bronchial)
(7) Wasting syndrome—diarrhea with loss of 15 lbs. or greater than 10% of body weight
(8) CMV (cytomegalovirus)
(9) Cryptococcus
(10) K.S. (Kaposi's sarcoma) or lymphoma
(11) Dementia due to HIV disease
(12) MAC (*Mycobacterium avium* complex)
(13) PML (progressive multifocal leukoencephalopathy)

Category B: Symptomatic non-AIDS conditions

(1) Oral candidiasis
(2) Vulvovaginal candidiasis
(3) Cervical dysplasia, moderate or severe
(4) Severe unexplained diarrhea, fever for over 1 month
(5) Oral hairy leukoplakia
(6) Herpes zoster (two distinct episodes or more than one site)
(7) Idiopathic thrombocytopenic purpura
(8) Pelvic inflammatory disease, severe

Category A: Asymptomatic

(1) PGL (persistent generalized lymphadenopathy)
(2) No symptoms

Note. From CDC (1992).

tive/motor disorder, activities of daily living and occupational performance are less severely impaired than in HIV-1-associated dementia complex, with the individual able to perform all but the most demanding aspects of work or activities of daily living. Table 1.3 provides the AAN criteria for HIV-1-associated cognitive/motor complex.

TABLE 1.3. American Academy of Neurology (AAN) Criteria for HIV-1-Associated Cognitive/Motor Complex

All of the following diagnoses require laboratory evidence for systemic HIV-1 infection (enzyme-linked immunosorbent assay [ELISA] test confirmed by Western blot, polymerase chain recreation, or culture).

I. Sufficient for diagnosis of AIDS

HIV-1-Associated Dementia Complex[*]

Probable (must have each of the following):

1. Acquired abnormality in at least *two* of the following cognitive abilities (present for at least 1 month): attention/concentration, speed of information processing, abstraction/reasoning, visuospatial skill, memory/learning, and speech/language.
    a) The decline should be verified by reliable history and mental status examination. In all cases, when possible, history should be obtained from an informant, and examination should be supplemented by neuropsychological testing.
    b) Cognitive dysfunction causing impairment of work or activities of daily living. The impairment should not be attributable solely to severe systemic illness.
2. At least one of the following:
    a) Acquired abnormality in motor function or performance verified by clinical examination (e.g., slowed rapid movements, abnormal gait, limb in coordination, hyperreflexia, hypertonia, or weakness), neuropsychological test (e.g., fine motor speed, manual dexterity, perceptual–motor skills), or both.
    b) Decline in motivation or emotional control or change in social behavior. This may be characterized by any of the following changes in personality such as apathy, inertia, irritability, emotional liability, or new onset of impaired judgment characterized by socially inappropriate behavior or disinhibition.
3. Absence of clouding of consciousness (delirium) during a period long enough to establish the presence of #1.
4. Evidence of another etiology, including active CNS opportunistic infection or malignancy, psychiatric disorders (e.g., depressive disorder), active alcohol or substance use, or acute or chronic substance withdrawal, must be sought from history, physical and psychiatric examination, and appropriate laboratory and radiological investigation (e.g., lumbar puncture, neuroimaging). If another potential etiology (e.g., major depressive disorder) is present, it is not the cause of the above cognitive, motor, or behavioral symptoms and signs.

Possible (must have one of the following):

1. Other potential etiology present (must have each of the following):
    a) As above (see **Probable**) #1, 2, and 3.
    b) Other potential etiology is present but the cause of #1 above is uncertain.
2. Incomplete clinical evaluation (must have each of the following):
    a) As above (see **Probable**) #1, 2, 3.
    b) Etiology cannot be determined (appropriate laboratory or radiological investigations not performed).

(continued)

TABLE 1.3. *(cont.)*

I. Not sufficient for diagnosis of AIDS

HIV-1-Associated Minor Cognitive/Motor Disorder

Probable (must have each of the following):

1. At least two of the following acquired cognitive, motor, or behavioral symptoms (present for at least 1 month) verified by reliable history (when possible, from an informant):

    a) Impaired attention or concentration

    b) Mental slowing

    c) Impaired memory

    d) Slowed movements

    e) Incoordination

    f) Personality change, or irritability or emotional liability

    Acquired cognitive/motor abnormality verified by clinical neurological examination or neuropsychological testing (e.g., fine motor speed, manual dexterity, perceptual–motor skills, attention/concentration, speed of processing of information, abstraction/reasoning, visuospatial skills, memory/learning, or speech/language).

2. Disturbance from cognitive/motor/behavioral abnormalities (see #1) causes mild impairment of work or activities of daily living (objectively verifiable or by report of a key informant.)

3. Does not meet criteria for HIV-1-associated dementia complex or HIV-1-associated myelopathy.

4. No evidence of another etiology, including active CNS opportunistic infection or malignancy, or severe systemic illness determined by appropriate history, physical examination, and laboratory and radiological investigation (e.g., lumbar puncture, neuroimaging). The above features should not be attributable solely to the effects of active alcohol or substance use, acute or chronic substance withdrawal, adjustment disorder, or other psychiatric disorders.

Note. From AAN (1991). Copyright 1991 by the American Academy of Neurology. Reprinted by permission.

*For research purposes, HIV-1-associated dementia complex can be coded to describe the major features:

    HIV-1-associated dementia complex requires criteria 1, 2a, 2b, 3, and 4.

    HIV-1-associated dementia complex (motor) requires criteria 1, 2a, 3, and 4.

    HIV-1-associated dementia complex (behavior) requires criteria 1, 2b, 3, and 4.

American Psychiatric Association

Finally, the fourth edition of the *Diagnostic and Statistical Manual of Mental Disorders* (DSM-IV; American Psychiatric Association, 1994) has for the first time included dementia due to HIV disease in the psychiatric nosology. As detailed in Table 1.4, to meet DSM-IV diagnostic criteria for dementia due to HIV disease, patients must have memory impairment as well as impairment in at least one other neuropsychological domain, such as language or executive function.

Furthermore, these deficits cannot occur solely in the context of a delirium and must be of sufficient severity to result in a decrement in occupational or social functioning.

Comment

Although arguments can be made in favor of any of these diagnostic schemes, it is our opinion that the AAN criteria best capture the neuropsychological sequelae of HIV infection, whereas the CDC classification is best for staging the physical status of infected patients. The CDC criteria would be applied as follows to Mr. Smith: Since he had already contracted an AIDS-defining opportunistic infection and had a CD4 count of less than $200/mm^3$, his physical status would be staged as CDC category C3. Neuropsychological testing documented the presence of moderate memory impairment, psychomotor slowing, poor divided attention, mild executive dysfunction, and depressed and irritable mood—deficits that led Mr. Smith to take disability leave from his job. Although relatively mild, these symptoms would nonetheless warrant a DSM-IV diagnosis of dementia due to HIV disease. Since his cognitive symptoms had only affected the more demanding aspects of

---

TABLE 1.4. American Psychiatric Association Criteria for Dementia Due to HIV Disease

A. The development of multiple cognitive deficits manifested by both:

(1) memory impairment (impaired ability to learn new information or to recall previously learned information)

(2) one (or more) of the following cognitive disturbances:
   (a) aphasia (language disturbance)
   (b) apraxia (impaired ability to carry out motor activities despite intact motor function)
   (c) agnosia (failure to recognize or identify objects despite intact sensory information)
   (d) disturbance in executive functioning (i.e., planning, organizing, sequencing, abstracting)

B. The cognitive deficits in Criteria A1 and A2 each cause significant impairment in social or occupational functioning and represents a significant decline from a previous level of functioning.

C. There is evidence from the history, physical examination, or laboratory findings that the disturbance is the direct physiological consequence of HIV infection.

D. The deficits do not occur exclusively during the course of a delirium.

Coding note: Also code 043.1 HIV infection affecting central nervous system on Axis III.

Note. Reprinted with permission from the *Diagnostic and Statistical Manual of Mental Disorders,* Fourth Edition. Copyright 1994 American Psychiatric Association.

his daily life, he would meet AAN criteria for HIV-1-associated minor cognitive/motor disorder.

INCIDENCE/PREVALENCE

HIV/AIDS

The CDC report that through December of 1996, approximately 580,000 cases of AIDS had been diagnosed in the United States, and more than one million individuals in the United States were HIV seropositive. Provisional data provided by the CDC in September 1997 showed a decline in AIDS incidence during 1996 compared with 1995 and a continued decline (23% drop) in the number of AIDS deaths. These figures reflect increased success with the medical care of HIV/AIDS including the development and increased utilization of antiretroviral combination therapy regimens.

While surveillance data are beginning to show encouraging trends, HIV infection remains one of the leading causes of death in the United States among persons aged 15 to 44 (Ventura, Peters, Martin, & Maurer, 1997). Additionally, ethnic minorities and women are being especially hard hit by HIV/AIDS in the U.S. (Green, Karon, & Nwanyanwu, 1992; Kalichman & Sikkema, 1994). For example, while the overall incidence of AIDS opportunistic infections among Black and Latino men and among Black women who had heterosexual risk factors (CDC, 1997).

Neuropsychological Deficits in HIV-1 Infection

Cognitive impairment is a frequent concomitant of HIV infection. This impairment, in its most severe form, presents as a dementia syndrome with symptoms severe enough to cause severe occupational impairment and to disrupt even the most basic activities of daily living. The annual incidence of HIV-associated dementia following the development of AIDS was recently estimated at 7% (McArthur et al., 1993), but it can vary considerably, depending on the referral population studied and the selection criteria used. Estimates of the prevalence of HIV-associated dementia range from 6% to 66%, with a consensus building that between 10% and 30% of patients with AIDS will eventually develop dementia (McArthur et al., 1993; Maj et al., 1994; Heaton et al., 1995). The survival times of patients who develop HIV-associated dementia can vary markedly, with one study estimating the median time of survival following a diagnosis of dementia at 6 months (McArthur et al., 1993).

The prevalence rates of less severe but significant cognitive impairment in medically symptomatic patients (those in CDC categories B and C) vary widely, again seemingly in part because of population characteristics and the impairment criteria used. The literature shows prevalence rates ranging from 12% (Miller et al., 1990) to 86% (Grant et al., 1987), with a recent well-done, large-scale study showing approximately 55% of all AIDS (CDC category C) patients and 44% of all mildly symptomatic (CDC category B) patients showing some degree of cognitive impairment (Heaton et al., 1995). Among symptomatic HIV-seropositive patients, cognitive deficits have been reported in almost all neuropsychological domains, including memory (Lunn et al., 1991; McKegney et al., 1990; Poutiainen, Iivanainen, Elovaara, Valle, & Lahdevirta, 1988), motor speed and control (Bornstein et al., 1991; Dunbar, Perdices, Grunseit, & Cooper, 1992; Lunn et al., 1991), abstraction ability (McKegney et al., 1990), verbal fluency (Stern et al., 1991), and self-regulation (Krikorian, Wrobel, Meinecke, Liang, & Kay, 1990).

At one point there was considerable debate about the frequency and degree of cognitive impairment in medically asymptomatic HIV-seropositive individuals. An early study of a small sample of asymptomatic subjects reported neuropsychological abnormalities in 44% of these patients, relative to HIV-seronegative controls (Grant et al., 1987). This study received widespread attention and led to suggestions that patients with early, asymptomatic HIV infection should not be allowed to perform certain government sector jobs. However, in a much larger study of neuropsychological functioning in asymptomatic individuals, Miller et al. (1990) found that asymptomatic subjects performed no worse than noninfected controls when matched for age and level of education. In fact, a number of cross-sectional and longitudinal studies have concluded that HIV-1-seropositive asymptomatic patients do not differ neuropsychologically from HIV-1-seronegative controls (Boccellari et al., 1993; Franzblau et al., 1991; Mauri et al., 1993; McAllister et al., 1992). On the other hand, some investigators *have* found differences on a group level between asymptomatic and control subjects (Bornstein et al., 1992; McKegney et al., 1990), or have found a higher frequency of neuropsychologically "abnormal" patients among asymptomatic patients relative to seronegative controls (Lunn et al., 1991; Wilkie, Eisdorfer, Morgan, Loewenstein, & Szapocznik, 1990). Capturing the inconsistency of the findings regarding cognitive impairment in asymptomatic HIV-infected patients, White, Heaton, Monsch, and the HNRC Group (1995) reviewed 75 neuropsychological studies of such subjects. They found that 32% of these studies showed significant neuropsychological differences between asymptomatic HIV-positive subjects and controls, whereas 47% of the studies found no significant group differences. In a well-done study using both a large sample and a thorough neuropsychological assessment battery, Heaton et al. (1995) found approximately that 30% of their asymptomatic subjects showed some evidence of cognitive impairment. Bornstein et al. (1992) found that approximately 10–20% of asymptomatic patients suffered from neuropsychological impairment to a degree that influenced their daily lives.

In conclusion, there is a steady increase in cognitive abnormalities as the disease progresses into the symptomatic stages, with the prevalence rate of significant neuropsychological impairment increasing markedly as a patient begins to show symptoms of AIDS (Heaton et al., 1995). Neuropsychological impairment is less obvious and prevalent in asymptomatic HIV infection, but there is a subset of patients who will show at least mild cognitive compromise. Research to date suggests that it is more the exception than the rule to see severe functional disruption in the earliest stages of HIV infection.

SECONDARY NEUROLOGICAL ILLNESSES IN HIV INFECTION

It is clear that HIV can be detected in the central nervous system (CNS) of infected patients (Navia et al., 1986a). Nearly half of all seropositive but asymptomatic individuals show evidence of HIV in their cerebrospinal fluid (Resnick et al., 1985) and nearly 90% of all patients who die of AIDS show evidence of neuropathological abnormalities of the CNS on autopsy (Collier, Gayle, & Bahls, 1987; Navia et al., 1986a).

Because opportunistic infections of the CNS occur frequently in immunosuppressed patients, when a patient is being evaluated for HIV-related dementia, the presence of secondary neurological illnesses must first be ruled out. In the United States, the most frequent CNS opportunistic infections leading to neuropsychological deterioration are cerebral toxoplasmosis, cryptococcal meningitis, and progressive multifocal leukoencephalopathy (PML) (McArthur, Selnes, Glass, Hoover, & Bacellar, 1994).

Cerebral toxoplasmosis is the most common HIV-related opportunistic neurological illness, affecting approximately 10–15% of all HIV-infected patients. Necrotic abscesses appear that are often multifocal and scattered throughout the cerebral hemispheres, with an affinity for the basal ganglia and frontal lobes (McArthur et al., 1994). Structural neuroimaging depicts toxoplasmosis as ring-enhancing mass lesions that may be difficult to differentiate from CNS lymphoma (as discussed below). Because it can produce one or more cerebral lesions, toxoplasmosis frequently has a focal presentation with neurobehavioral sequelae, dependent on the site(s) of lesion(s). Cerebral toxoplasmosis is often responsive to treatment, with approximately 80% of cases responding clinically within 1–4 weeks following initiation of pyrimethamine and sulfadiazine treatment (McArthur et al., 1994).

CNS lymphomas are another leading cause of secondary neurological illness in HIV-infected individuals. Like toxoplasmosis, a primary lymphoma often begins with a focal presentation, with one or more cortical regions differentially affected. Specific neurobehavioral syndromes (such as aphasia, agraphia, and ataxia) may be seen, depending on the site of the lesion, and focal neurological signs will develop in approximately 40% of all cases (McArthur et al., 1994). The typical presentation of CNS lymphomas includes a slowly progressive neurological deterioration, with death usually occurring within 3–4 months.

PML results from a papovavirus infection, which leads to a demyelinating disorder that affects the hemispheric white matter and causes patchy foci of demyelination. Typically, subcortical areas are the first sites of involvement, but the gray matter may also be affected—occasionally before any subcortical lesions are evident (McArthur et al., 1994). The cognitive changes associated with PML are typically related to the specific, often multiple brain regions affected by the virus. As with the CNS lymphomas, specific focal neurobehavioral syndromes may be present in the early stages of PML. Aphasia, apraxia, hemiparesis, hemineglect, and visual-field defects are commonly seen in PML. Following the diagnosis of PML, the patient usually deteriorates rapidly, with death often occurring within weeks to months after initial diagnosis.

NEUROIMAGING AND HIV INFECTION

Structural Neuroimaging

Computerized tomography (CT) studies in HIV-1 infection reveal generalized cerebral atrophy, with widened cortical sulci and enlarged ventricles, in the majority of patients with AIDS. Structural abnormality is much more frequently found in the later stages of HIV infection, with nearly 70% of all patients with AIDS showing some degree of atrophy (Raininko et al., 1992). Regardless of the stage of infection, central and cortical atrophy is the most frequently reported finding when CT is used.

Magnetic resonance imaging (MRI) is assuming an increasingly important role in the diagnostic workup of HIV-infected patients, with

T$_2$-weighted images most sensitive in detecting the brain abnormalities associated with HIV. MRI is better than CT for assessing the white matter pathology often found in HIV infection. MRI scans indicate that in addition to sulcal widening and ventricle enlargement, the white matter, particularly the periventricular white matter, is often abnormal in HIV-infected patients (McArthur et al., 1989; Elovaara et al., 1990).

Interestingly, most studies using structural neuroimaging techniques have failed to find a convincing association between degree of CT or MRI abnormality and neuropsychological deficit. (However, see Hall, Whaley, Robertson, & Hamby, 1996). A sizeable minority of HIV-infected patients show normal CT and MRI scans well into the middle and even late stages of HIV infection.

In conclusion, because structural neuroimaging yields largely non-specific findings and is not strongly associated with behavioral change, it is perhaps most useful in ruling out the presence of focal lesions due to secondary opportunistic infection.

Functional Neuroimaging

Functional neuroimaging employs techniques such as positron emission tomography (PET), single-photon emission computerized tomography (SPECT), and functional MRI (fMRI). Unlike structural imaging techniques such as X-rays, CT, and MRI, which provide a picture of the brain's structure, these newer techniques provide a picture of the brain's function—that is, which parts of the brain are working normally and which parts are not. Several studies (Hinkin et al., 1995a; Rottenberg et al., 1987; van Gorp et al., 1992) have employed PET scans using fluorodeoxyglucose, a radioactively labeled sugar that the brain uses as fuel. Those parts of the brain that are most active utilize the most glucose; the brain structures that are least active use less. This glucose metabolism can then be imaged. We have published two PET studies of cerebral metabolic abnormalities in HIV infection. Our first study (van Gorp et al., 1992) compared patients with AIDS to uninfected controls and found that the patients with AIDS demonstrated basal ganglia *hyper*metabolism (i.e., the subcortical structures that control psychomotor function, among other behaviors, were overly active in these patients). We also found that the subjects who were most demented had decreased metabolism of the temporal lobes, the brain area that is actively involved in memory. In an effort to understand how cerebral metabolism changes over time, we next looked at these patients' PET scans 6 months later (Hinkin et al., 1995a). As shown in Figure 1.1, we found that the subjects with AIDS demonstrated even greater hypermetabolism of the basal ganglia—a finding that may reflect increased effort expended by the brain in order to maintain its neuropsychological integrity.

NATURAL HISTORY AND CLINICAL COURSE

There is considerable individual variability in the clinical course of HIV-associated cognitive/motor complex. Although it is not possible to predict the exact course of illness in any one HIV-infected person, we are increasingly able to suggest a *typical* course of cognitive deterioration, from the first signs of CNS involvement to end-stage dementia. Some (but not all) patients report experiencing headaches, photophobia, and flu-like symptoms within the first few weeks of initial infection, similar to an aseptic meningitis. After these symptoms abate, the clinical course is frequently characterized by months or even years of latent, asymptomatic infection. The asymptomatic stage may last an average of 10 years before overt symptoms arise. Changes in cognitive functioning are often first observed concurrently with the appearance

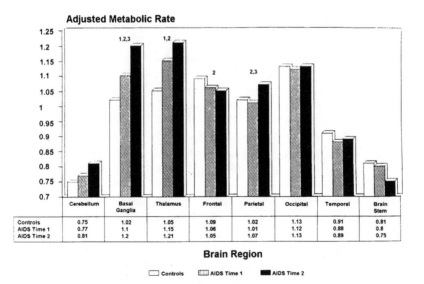

	Cerebellum	Basal Ganglia	Thalamus	Frontal	Parietal	Occipital	Temporal	Brain Stem
Controls	0.75	1.02	1.05	1.09	1.02	1.13	0.91	0.81
AIDS Time 1	0.77	1.1	1.15	1.06	1.01	1.12	0.88	0.8
AIDS Time 2	0.81	1.2	1.21	1.05	1.07	1.13	0.89	0.75

Brain Region

☐ Controls   ▨ AIDS Time 1   ■ AIDS Time 2

FIGURE 1.1. Ratios of local cerebral metabolic activity to whole-brain metabolic activity in the seronegative control subjects at time 1 and the AIDS group at time 1 and time 2. 1, significant difference, AIDS time 1 versus control subjects; 2, significant difference, AIDS time 2 versus control subjects; 3, significant difference, AIDS time 1 versus time 2. From Hinkin et al. (1995a). Copyright 1995 by the American Psychiatric Press. Reprinted by permission.

of constitutional symptoms. A recent study found relatively little cognitive decline prior to the onset of an AIDS-defining illness unless an overt dementia was present. Following onset of an AIDS-defining illness, cognitive decline was most pronounced in the area of fine motor skills, but relatively mild in other cognitive domains (Selnes et al., 1995). Other commonly observed cognitive changes include difficulty concentrating and paying attention (e.g., losing one's train of thought), as well as psychomotor slowing.

Although most clinicians have assumed that patients with HIV-related dementia will show a relatively steady decline in mental status once the initial cognitive signs are present, it appears that some patients instead have relatively stable periods of plateau, which are later followed by a more precipitous drop in intellectual functioning. Still others never evidence any overt signs of cognitive decline. The modal clinical course in HIV-1 infection, however, is generally believed to progress gradually through the following stages of cognitive impairment, which are based in part upon the AAN staging scheme for an AIDS-related dementia.

• *Subclinical.* Patients report decreased concentration, attention problems and loss of their train of thought. Mild forgetfulness, such as "double booking" of appointments, may also be seen. Work, unless especially demanding, may not be affected; commonly, basic activities of daily living are unimpaired. It is important to consider whether dysphoria or clinical depression is contributing to (or is even primarily responsible for) the self-reports of cognitive inefficiency.

• *Mild.* Individuals may report more pronounced cognitive changes, including psychomotor slowing, forgetfulness, and a decline in work performance. Modest changes in the more challenging activities of daily living are present, including personal finances (e.g., balancing checkbook, keeping track of bills). Also, patients often report experiencing difficulty keeping track of multiple appointments.

• *Moderate.* By this stage, patients are frequently unable to work at any but the most basic of occupational tasks, and may be unable to perform rapid psychomotor tasks such as driving. Memory is now impaired. Patients may need assistance with more demanding activities of daily living, such as housecleaning and cooking.

• *Severe.* At this stage, patients need assistance with most or all activities of daily living and are totally dependent upon others. Global cognitive impairment is present and obvious.

• *End-stage.* Patients are mute, bed-bound, incontinent, and globally cognitively impaired.

NEUROPSYCHOLOGICAL PERFORMANCE
BY DOMAIN IN HIV INFECTION

Numerous research studies have described how HIV-infected persons perform on neuropsychological testing (for reviews, see Grant & Martin, 1994; Kelly et al., 1997; Hinkin, van Gorp, & Satz, 1995b; van Gorp et al., 1993). Although some debate remains, a general consensus has been reached regarding which neuropsychological functions appear particularly susceptible to the effects of HIV infection (Butters et al., 1990; Bornstein, 1994). Once again, we need to stress that many infected patients never experience any significant cognitive impairment, and that generally the patients with more advanced illness (patients diagnosed with AIDS, with a CD4 count less than $200/mm^3$) are particularly likely to develop cognitive impairment (Grant et al., 1993; Heaton et al., 1995; Stern et al., 1995). Below, we describe which cognitive domains are most likely to decline and which tests of those behaviors appear best suited to detect such decline. Table 1.5 summarizes the findings regarding the domains.

Mental Status/Intelligence

Mental status screening tests usually consist of a brief series of questions that can be asked of a patient at bedside and that do not require any test materials other than paper and pencil. Patients are asked to engage in activities such as providing the date and the season, counting backward by 7's, repeating phrases such as "No ifs, ands, or buts," and remembering several words for a brief period of time.

Although of great utility in the examination of cortical dementias such as Alzheimer's disease, mental status screening examinations such as the Mini-Mental State Exam (MMSE; Folstein, Folstein, & McHugh, 1975), the Blessed Dementia Rating Scale (Blessed, Tomlinson, & Roth, 1968), and the Neurobehavioral Cognitive Status Examination (Schwamm et al., 1987) are of limited usefulness in detecting early signs of HIV-associated cognitive decline (Grant & Atkinson, 1995; Hinkin et al., 1995b). Generally, it is not until the moderate stage of HIV-associated dementia that patients score below suggested cutoff scores (e.g., MMSE ≤ 24).

Intelligence, as operationalized by the IQ and as assessed by the WAIS-R (Wechsler, 1981), is commonly affected in HIV-1 infection. This is particularly true for the Performance subtests of the WAIS-R, in which subjects receive bonus points for rapid completion of tasks such as the Block Design, Object Assembly, and Digit Symbol tests (Hinkin et al., 1995b). Digit Symbol is perhaps the most sensitive of all

TABLE 1.5. Neuropsychological Effects of HIV-1 Infection by Stage of Infection

Neuropsychological deficit/domain	Early, middle: Affected?	Late (dementia): Affected?	End-stage: Affected?
Abstraction	No	+/–	+/–
Agraphia	No	No	+/–
Calculation	No	+/–	Yes
Concentration	+/–	Yes	Yes
Digit span	No	+/–	Yes
Divided attention	+/–	Yes	Yes
Executive/frontal system functions	+/–	Yes	Yes
Expressive language	No	No	+/–
Judgment	No	+/–	+/–
Motoric functions	+/–	+/–	Yes
Mood			
Agitation	No	+/–	+/–
Anxiety	+/–	+/–	+/–
Depression	+/–	+/–	+/–
Mania	No	No	No
Naming	No	No	Yes
Psychomotor speed	+/–	Yes	Yes
Recent memory	+/–	Yes	Yes
Receptive language	No	No	+/–
Remote memory	No	No	No
Sensory functions	No	+/–	+/–
Verbal fluency	No	Yes	Yes
Visual construction	No	+/–	Yes
Visual perception	No	No	+/–

the WAIS-R subtests to the effects of HIV infection (Hinkin et al., 1995b). Because the Verbal subtests are largely untimed, HIV-1-infected subjects tend to perform better on these tasks. Of WAIS-R Verbal subtests, HIV-infected patients frequently have the greatest difficulty on the digits backward portion of Digit Span and Arithmetic, two measures sensitive to attentional disruption. Generally, patients perform adequately on the Vocabulary and Information subtests.

In addition to providing a measure of global intelligence and information regarding component cognitive processes such as visual construction or attention, the WAIS-R can also be of some assistance in detecting a focal opportunistic infection of the CNS. Should clinicians note more than a 15- to 20-point discrepancy between Verbal and Performance IQs, follow-up neuropsychological testing and referral for neurological testing and/or neuroimaging are indicated.

Attention/Concentration

Adequate attention is a requisite basis for virtually every higher-level cognitive function, since if patients are unable to pay attention, they will certainly have difficulty engaging in any additional cognitive processing. Accordingly, careful assessment of attention and concentration in the workup of HIV-1-infected patients is critical, especially given the myriad potential causes of diminished attention in HIV-infected patients. The detrimental effects of acute physical illness and/or chronic debilitation on attentional functioning must be considered. Along these lines, poor attention may also be caused by the effects of medication, prescribed or otherwise, and/or psychiatric distress.

One common cause of pronounced attentional impairment is delirium, also known as "acute confusional state." Delirium is a relatively common condition in HIV-infected patients, with published studies suggesting that nearly half of hospitalized HIV-infected patients sustain a delirium at some point during their inpatient hospitalization. Acute confusional state has many causes, including toxic or metabolic disorders, adverse medication response, hypoxia, systemic infection, or focal CNS opportunistic infections and neoplasms. Because delirium can reflect a potentially life-threatening underlying disease, it is crucial that immediate referral for medical care be initiated.

The clinical assessment of attention and concentration commonly includes evaluation of simple attention, sustained concentration, and divided attention. Of these, divided attention is most likely to be impaired in HIV-1 infection (E. M. Martin et al. 1995; Law et al., 1994; Sorenson, Martin, & Robertson, 1994). From a clinical perspective, two tasks have proven to be sensitive measures of divided attention: (1) the Auditory Consonant Trigrams (ACT) test, also known as the Brown–Peterson procedure, and (2) the Paced Auditory Serial Addition Task (PASAT). Both tests require patients to allocate attentional focus simultaneously to two activities. On the ACT, patients are provided with consonant triplets, and then must engage in an "interference" task, counting backward by 3's for varying periods of time (usually 3, 9, 18, and 36 seconds). Following completion of this interference task, the subject must then recall the original three letters. The PASAT requires patients to add the last two numbers from a continuous string of numbers presented at increasingly rapid rates. Trouble engaging in two such activities at the same time is one of the more common complaints of HIV-infected patients.

Difficulties with sustained concentration may underlie patients' complaints of trouble reading, despite an absence of actual reading

impairment. Alternatively (or conjunctively), fatigue or affective disturbance may account for subjective complaints of reading difficulty (van
Gorp et al., 1991). Although computerized measures of sustained
attention such as a continuous-performance test are best suited to
detect such impairment, clinical measures requiring patients to engage
continuously in a behavior can also be employed. Our group has found
that Parts A and B of the Stroop task, which require subjects to read
and/or name 100-item lists of either color words (e.g., "red," "blue,"
"green") or color blocks, assess this domain adequately. In general,
HIV-infected individuals as a group perform as well as seronegative
control subjects on tasks of sustained attention (Stern et al., 1991).

Finally, simple attention is generally within normal limits in early
HIV-associated dementia (Heaton et al., 1995). Usually only the most
demented, delirious, or acutely physically ill patients will demonstrate
severely impaired basic attention. As such, mental control tasks such
as counting backward or saying the alphabet are usually unimpaired.
On the WAIS-R Digit Span subtest and other digit span tests (also
putative measures of simple attention), most HIV-infected subjects
perform within normal limits, especially on digits forward (Grant et al.,
1987; Tross et al., 1988; van Gorp, Miller, Satz, & Visscher, 1989). When
patients are required to repeat strings of digits in the reverse direction
(i.e., digits backward), they are more likely to show slightly depressed
performance (Stern et al., 1991).

Speech and Language

Speech, which can be conceptualized as the mechanical production of
language, is frequently affected by HIV infection. Diminished volume
of speech, or "hypophonia," is common, as is "dysarthria" or reduced
intelligibility of speech. Not infrequently, speech is slowed among
HIV-infected patients when compared to premorbid levels.

In contrast, language is generally spared in HIV infection unless
individuals are severely demented, delirious, or suffering from a focal
CNS opportunistic infection affecting language areas of the brain. Both
expressive and receptive language abilities, as well as repetition, are
usually normal. Although patients frequently complain of difficulty
reading, this is almost always secondary to impaired concentration
rather than to alexia per se. Similarly, although many patients complain
of word-finding difficulty, performance on confrontation naming tests—
for example, the Boston Naming Test, in which patients must provide
the names for pen-and-ink drawings—is usually within normal limits
(Heaton et al., 1995; Janssen et al., 1989; Stern, Sano, Williams, &
Gorman, 1989; van Gorp et al., 1989). Writing, however, may be

adversely affected because of poorer penmanship. Among the typical neuropsychological tests of language, measures of verbal fluency are the only tasks on which HIV-infected individuals encounter difficulty (Hinkin et al., 1995b; Saykin et al., 1988). An example of a verbal fluency task is the Controlled Oral Word Association Test (Benton & Hamsher, 1989), in which patients must rapidly name as many words as possible that begin with certain letters of the alphabet. If HIV-infected patients demonstrate symptoms consistent with a frank aphasia, such as an inability to repeat, paraphasic errors, or an inability to produce or understand speech, this is almost always a cause for alarm; prompt medical treatment of the underlying cause (often a CNS opportunistic infection) is required.

Visual–Spatial Function

Visual–spatial abilities include such behaviors as visual construction, visual perception, visual scanning/tracking, and geographic/topographic orientation. Although early studies suggested that symptomatic subjects performed more poorly on neuropsychological tests of visual–spatial ability, such as the WAIS-R Block Design subtest (van Gorp et al., 1989; Tross et al., 1988), most researchers and clinicians now agree that visual–spatial abilities are largely spared in HIV infection (Poutiainen et al., 1988; Saykin et al., 1988; Stern et al., 1991). However, since many neuropsychological tests of visual–spatial ability (e.g., the Block Design subtest) are timed, psychomotor slowing may lead to a lowered score because patients do not receive bonus points for speed. Completion of complicated, unstructured visual–constructive tasks, such as the Copy portion of the Rey–Osterrieth Complex Figure Test, can also be affected. This is generally secondary to poor planning and problem solving rather than to visual–spatial impairment.

Memory

Impaired memory is common in HIV infection and is in fact required for the DSM-IV diagnosis of dementia due to HIV disease. The memory deficit in HIV infection is primarily one of retrieval rather than encoding or storage, although these stages can also be affected (Bornstein et al., 1993a; Hinkin et al., 1995b). Patients with AIDS may have difficulty with free recall (e.g., recall of story details or word lists), but when they are provided with cues or multiple-choice options, their performance often improves dramatically. Learning of new information may also be affected in HIV disease, but this generally does not resemble the amnestic quality of Alzheimer's disease. Frequently, because of attentional difficulty, patients have difficulty attending to and thus encoding new material to be learned; moreover, because of executive dysfunction, they may employ ineffective strategies to guide the encoding process.

In assessing infected patients' memory function, one should test both verbal memory (e.g., memory for word lists) and nonverbal memory (e.g., memory for designs). Verbal and nonverbal memory are equally susceptible to the effects of HIV infection (Stern et al., 1991); although several early studies suggested that nonverbal memory was perhaps more sensitive to the effects of HIV infection, this apparent sensitivity was more likely to have been due to the increased difficulty of typical nonverbal tasks.

Typically, neuropsychology has focused on "declarative memory," or memory for "knowing that." Another type of memory process has been termed "procedural memory," or "knowing how," and is exemplified by such activities as typing, playing a musical instrument, or riding a bike. The ability to learn new procedures, though commonly affected in other subcortical diseases such as Huntington's disease, appears to be affected in only a subgroup of patients with AIDS. Dr. Alex Martin and his colleagues (A. Martin et al., 1992) demonstrated that although on a group level patients with AIDS performed as well as seronegative controls did on a measure of procedural learning/memory, there was a subgroup of patients who clearly performed much worse. Interestingly, these researchers found that this subgroup of poor performers also evidenced higher levels of an excitatory neurotoxin (quinolinic acid) in their cerebrospinal fluid (A. Martin et al., 1992), strengthening the conclusion that impaired procedural learning is associated with CNS disease in patients with AIDS.

Working memory is that aspect of cognition that controls the simultaneous processing and active manipulation of information. For example, a working memory task might require subjects to complete a string of simple mental arithmetic problems (e.g., $5 + 3 =$ __, $9 - 4 =$ __, $6 + 7 =$ __, etc.) while simultaneously asking them to remember the last digit of each problem (in the example above, 3, 4, 7). There is compelling evidence suggesting that working memory is mediated by prefrontal structures and circuits that are intimately connected with subcortical regions (Baddeley, Della Sala, Papagno, & Spinnler, 1997; Gabrieli, Singh, Stebbins, & Goetz, 1996; Goldman-Rakic & Friedman, 1991). Recent studies of working memory in HIV-1 infection have shown that at least a subgroup of seropositive individuals show working memory deficits (Bartok et al., 1997; Sahakian et al., 1995; Stout et al., 1995).

Executive Functions

"Executive functions," or "frontal systems functions," are that behaviors which monitor, direct, and control other behaviors; they include such skills as problem solving, sequencing, judgment, inhibition, and divided attention. Although a clear consensus has yet to be reached (Claypoole et al., 1990; Stern et al., 1989; Poutiainen et al., 1988; Grant et al., 1987; Rubinow, Berettini, Brouwers, & Lane, 1988), it appears that only certain executive functions are significantly affected by HIV (see Sahakian et al., 1995). One such area of impairment is the ability to engage simultaneously in several tasks at once. An example of this is driving while talking on a car phone or engaging in conversation while watching television. In a minority of patients with AIDS, difficulties with inhibition and judgment also arise (Saykin et al., 1988). In such cases, patients may underestimate the degree of impairment they have actually suffered. In the vast majority of patients, problem solving is spared. This latter contention is strongly supported by studies using the Wisconsin Card Sorting Test (WCST), a putative measure of hypothesis formation, set shifting, and nonverbal problem solving; the majority of these studies have found HIV-infected subjects to be unimpaired (on this test Stern et al., 1989; Claypoole et al., 1988). In our own laboratory, we compared the performance of patients with AIDS and uninfected controls on the WCST and found that the two groups performed virtually identically.

Motor Functions

With advanced disease, HIV-1-infected patients become increasingly slow. This slowing takes two basic forms: (1) slowing of motor movements and (2) slowing of cognition. Motor slowing is measured by tasks such as the Finger Tapping Test, a measure requiring patients to tap a key rapidly on a teletype-like machine, using the index finger. Some studies have found that patients with AIDS tend to perform worse (more slowly) on this task than do uninfected controls (Saykin et al., 1988), while others have not found this difference (Claypoole et al., 1990; Franzblau et al., 1991; Ollo, Johnson, & Grafman 1991). Although it is caused in part by central slowing, upper-extremity motor slowing may also be caused by myelopathy and myopathy, peripheral neuropathy, or simply the effects of physical illness. It is important to note that neuropathies and myopathies can occur as direct effects of HIV infection or as side effects of pharmacological treatment (Brew, 1993).

Slowing of cognition, especially when speed of thought is linked to action (psychomotor slowing), is considered the cardinal sign of HIV-associated dementia (Hinkin et al., 1995), with the majority of studies to date having found differences between HIV-infected patients and noninfected controls on measures of psychomotor speed (Miller et al., 1990; Poutiainen et al., 1988; van Gorp et al., 1989). Clinical measures, such as the Digit Symbol subtest of the WAIS-R and the Trail Making Test, are particularly well suited for detecting psychomotor slowing. Slowed cognition, or "bradyphrenia," can also be sensitively detected via computerized measures of speeded information processing (Miller & Wilkie, 1994), which are discussed next.

Mr. Smith's Neuropsychological Performance Pattern

To return to Mr. Smith's case, inspection of his performance on neuropsychological testing revealed that his pattern of neuropsychological strengths and deficits was fairly typical of HIV-1 infection. He encountered the greatest difficulty on measures of memory. A comparison of his ability to recognize information with his free recall suggested that his memory problem was based more in retrieval than in encoding or storage. After a 20-minute delay, Mr. Smith was only able to recall 6 of the 16 words on the California Verbal Learning Test, but was able to accurately recognized 14 of the 16 words when he was presented with multiple-choice options. As can be seen in Table 1.1, other notable findings from his neuropsychological examination in-cluded the presence of marked psychomotor slowing. Tasks such as the Digit Symbol subtest of the WAIS-R and Part B of the Trail Making test posed considerable difficulty for him. Comparing those scores with his average performance on the Finger Tapping Test, a measure of pure motor speed, suggested that his slowing was more cognitive than motoric in nature. His difficulty on the ACT test, on which he scored at the 4th percentile, reflected his problems in dividing attention between two simultaneous activities. Equally important was considera-tion of the neuropsychological tasks on which Mr. Smith performed well. No evidence of language or visual–spatial impairment was ob-served. Had major deficits been seen in these domains, this would have suggested that an additional disease process, such as a CNS opportun-istic infection, was present.

COMPUTERIZED ASSESSMENT IN HIV-1 INFECTION

As mentioned above, both motor slowing and psychomotor slowing are considered hallmarks of HIV-related cognitive impairment; both are also quite amenable to computer assessment. In fact, in the early stages of HIV-1 infection, conventional neuropsychological measures may lack the necessary sensitivity to detect the often subtle cognitive changes that occur in a subset of patients (Miller & Wilkie, 1994). Computerized assessment measures may be more sensitive than are conventional neuropsychological tasks in demonstrating cognitive impairment (Miller & Wilkie, 1994), especially during the earlier stages of HIV infection.

The majority of studies using computerized assessment tools have measured reaction time and early-stage information-processing efficiency. Many of these instruments, which were developed according to the tenets of cognitive and experimental psychology, have shown promise in identifying deficits in a sizeable minority of HIV-infected patients (A. Martin et al., 1992; E. M. Martin, Sorensen, Edelstein, & Robertson, 1992b; Miller, Satz, van Gorp, Visscher, & Dudley, 1989; Law et al., 1993). Clearly, the sometimes subtle decrements in reaction time or information-processing speed do not always correlate with functional impairment, but it may be that these deficits are indicative of the onset of brain disease or an impending dementing process (Miller & Wilkie, 1994). Obviously, the ability to identify at-risk individuals as early in the disease process as possible could be of tremendous value.

As defined in most studies, "reaction time" is a composite measure of motor speed and the time required for such mental events as perception, stimulus processing, and decision making (Miller & Wilkie, 1994). "Simple reaction time" (SRT) is the time it takes an individual to respond to a single stimulus, such as the appearance of a visual cue or of an auditory tone. SRT, as it is generally conceptualized, does not involve higher cognitive processing (i.e., decision making) and is thought to measure mainly stimulus registration and motor speed. "Choice reaction time" (CRT) is the time it takes an individual to respond to one of at least two distinct stimuli that may occur, with each stimuli associated with a different response (e.g., "Push the button if you see a blue stimulus; don't push it if you see a red stimulus"). CRT, as the name implies, involves higher cognitive processing (i.e., making a decision about the status of a given stimulus) and can vary considerably in difficulty or in the information-processing demands required. The difference between SRT and CRT for any individual represents the speed of information processing for a particular choice decision and has been referred to as "decision-making time" (Miller & Wilkie, 1994). A limitation of much of the computerized reaction time research is that investigators have used different computerized measures of SRT and CRT, which make comparisons across groups more difficult.

Most reaction time studies have concluded that CRT is more likely than SRT to be impaired in HIV-1 infection. Perdices and Cooper (1989) found that asymptomatic patients performed similarly to seronegative controls on measures of both SRT and CRT, whereas symptomatic patients were significantly slower on measures of CRT but not SRT compared with controls. Although some investigators have found no differences between asymptomatic subjects and HIV-seronegative controls on either SRT or CRT tasks (Martin, Robertson, Edelstein, Jagust, & Sorensen, 1992a; Miller, Satz, & Visscher, 1991; Perdices & Cooper, 1989), others have found both asymptomatic and symptomatic subjects to be significantly slower than control subjects on measures of CRT (E. M. Martin et al., 1992b). It appears that SRT is less affected in HIV infection, or that if it is, this occurs in the later, symptomatic stages of the disease (A. Martin et al., 1992).

A study conducted by Alex Martin's group (1992) studied reaction time in both asymptomatic and symptomatic HIV-seropositive subjects, as well as HIV-seronegative psychiatric patients with adjustment disorders and HIV-seronegative controls with no medical or psychiatric illness. They found that both seropositive groups were slower on SRT and CRT measures than were both seronegative groups. Also, at a 6-month followup, on average, both seropositive groups were significantly slower than they were previously. Interestingly, there was a significant correlation between slowing of reaction time over time and cerebrospinal fluid levels of an endogenous neurotoxin, quinolinic acid.

Although some debate exists, a consensus is beginning to emerge that most symptomatic HIV-seropositive patients show signs of slowing on computerized measures of reaction time, relative to seronegative controls. This slowing may be more pronounced on measures of CRT (Perdices & Cooper, 1989), but it has also been observed on measures of SRT as well (Miller et al., 1990; A. Martin et al., 1992). With regards to asymptomatic patients, there is some evidence that they may show slowing on measures of CRT when compared with seronegative controls (E. M. Martin et al., 1992b; but also see Miller et al., 1991); however, they show roughly comparable performance on measures of SRT.

DEPRESSION AND HIV INFECTION

Considering the chronic and life-threatening nature of HIV, it is probably not surprising that HIV-infected individuals show high rates of depressed mood. The prevalence of depressed mood has been reported at nearly 80% in some studies (Boccellari, Dilley, & Shore, 1988; Perry & Tross, 1984), while the prevalence of a clinical syndrome of major depression in HIV-infected individuals has been reported at between 10% and 15% (Boccellari et al., 1988; Dilley, Ochitill, Perl, & Volberding, 1985). These elevated rates of depression are seen regardless of whether self-report measures (Cleary et al., 1993; Kelly et al., 1993) or interactive diagnostic interviews (Atkinson et al., 1988; Bornstein et al., 1993b) are used to ascertain depressive symptomatology. Clearly, these rates exceed those found in the general population.

As suggested above, depressive symptomatology in HIV-infected individuals may be a reaction to the life-altering, chronic, and ultimately terminal nature of the illness. Studies have found higher rates of depression and psychiatric disturbance immediately after patients learn that they have tested HIV-positive (Bix et al., 1995; Cleary, Singer, & Rogers, 1988; Ostrow et al., 1989). Also, immediately prior to HIV testing and while awaiting testing results, patients may show prominent symptoms of mood disturbance. Psychiatric support and, if necessary, crisis intervention may be most required at these times. Although psychiatric distress generally tends to lessen over time (Fell et al., 1993), some studies have suggested that depression may reemerge at transitional points of the disease (Grant & Atkinson, 1990). These transitions are often identified by physical symptoms (e.g., advent of AIDS-defining illness), with research suggesting that patients with the most HIV-related medical complications are more likely to be anxious and depressed (Gorman et al., 1991; Fell et al., 1993). Such issues as social stigmatization and marginalization are also important to consider as potential contributors to feelings of isolation and depression.

Certainly depression may be directly related to the involvement of subcortical brain structures (Cummings, 1993). Increased rates of depression have been reported in several neurological disorders that differentially affect subcortical structures (e.g., Parkinson's disease, Huntington's disease), suggesting that the presence of depression in some HIV-infected patients may relate, at least in part, to actual CNS changes. There is considerable overlap between the symptomatology characteristic of unipolar major depression and the presentation of various subcortical dementias; in fact, researchers have suggested that major depression is causally related to subcortical pathology (King & Caine, 1990; Cummings, 1993). Accordingly, depression and cognitive decline are perhaps best conceptualized as dual-pronged manifestations of an underlying disease process.

Issues Involved in Assessing Depression

Several issues concerning the measurement of depression in patients with HIV or AIDS warrant consideration. A primary complication in assessing depression in HIV-infected patients is the often considerable overlap between symptoms of depression and physical illness. Such signs and symptoms as fatigue, diminished sleep and appetite, weight loss, and somatic complaints may be diagnostically ambiguous. When somatic symptoms occur independently of affective distress, they may not be indicative of the vegetative signs of a mood syndrome, but instead simply signs of physical illness (Drebing, van Gorp, Hinkin, et al., 1994). Research with medical populations (Volk, Pace, & Parchman, 1993) in general, and HIV patients specifically (Drebing et al., 1994; Harker et al., 1995), has shown that the inclusion of somatic items in the measurement of depression often leads to increased rates of false positives. Clinicians and researchers working with HIV-infected patients should therefore use caution when interpreting measures containing somatic items, such as the BDI (Beck & Steer, 1987), the Hamilton Rating Scale for Depression Scale (Hamilton, 1960), and the MMPI-2. It is perhaps more prudent to emphasize cognitive and affective symptoms and signs of depression, especially with patients in the later, symptomatic stages of HIV disease. One such measure that minimizes the influence of physical symptoms in the assessment of depression is the Geriatric Depression Scale, a test originally designed for the elderly, which omits questions assessing neurovegetative symptomatology.

It is well established that severe depression can lead to cognitive impairment, especially in the elderly (Cassens, Wolfe, & Zola, 1990; La Rue, 1992). This phenomenon, which has been termed "pseudodementia," is more properly termed the "dementia syndrome of depression." Given the high prevalence of depression in HIV-1 infected individuals, it is reasonable to wonder whether depression is leading to potentially reversible dementias in this population. Studies that have addressed this question have almost uniformly concluded that, *on a group level,* depressed HIV-1 infected patients do not perform significantly poorer on more poorly on neuropsychological testing than do HIV-1 patients without depression (Atkinson et al., 1988; Bix et al., 1995; Grant et al., 1993; Hinkin et al., 1992; Pace, Rosenberger, Nasrallah & Bornstein, 1993). This is not meant to suggest that, *on an individual basis,* depression cannot result in a significant decrement in cognition.

Subjective Complaints of Cognitive Decline

Among the common manifestations of depression are hypersensitivity to and exaggeration of difficulties real or imagined. From a clinical perspective, we have observed that many HIV-infected patients will complain of cognitive deficits that cannot be detected on a thorough neuropsychological evaluation. Conversely, we have also encountered a subgroup of patients who, despite incontrovertible signs of severe neuropsychological impairment, will nevertheless deny that they have suffered any cognitive decline. The relationship between patients' complaints of self-perceived cognitive decline and performance on neuropsychological testing has also been empirically studied (Hinkin et al., 1996; Mapou et al., 1993; Poutiainen & Elovaara, 1996; van Gorp et al., 1991). This issue is of considerable importance to practicing clinicians, in that many treatment decisions (e.g., altering medication regimens) are based in large part on patients' self-report. Several studies have found that medically asymptomatic subjects' complaints of functional decline are indeed associated with poorer performance on objective neuropsychological testing (Mapou et al., 1993; Poutiainen & Elovaara, 1996). In contrast, several other studies have found that subjects who complain of cognitive decline do *not* perform worse on neuropsychological testing (Hinkin et al., in press; van Gorp et al., 1991; Wilkins et al., 1991). Rather, in a study of 223 HIV-infected asymptomatic subjects, we (van Gorp et al., 1991) found that subjects who complained of cognitive impairment tended instead to be more depressed. Since patient complaint of cognitive decline is often at variance with objective neuropsychological findings and instead tends to be related to level of depression, clinicians should obtain correlative data (e.g., interviews with significant others) prior to making diagnostic and treatment decisions.

HIV-RELATED COGNITIVE DECLINE COMPARED WITH THE NORMAL AGING PROCESS

Clinicians not formally trained in neuropsychology may experience some understandable difficulty incorporating the information detailed in this chapter in their own work with HIV-infected patients. A helpful heuristic for better understanding the neuropsychological effects of HIV infection is to view the cognitive sequelae of HIV/AIDS as similar to the neuropsychological changes associated with the normal aging process. In both instances, individuals may become both motorically and cognitively slower; similarly, both the elderly and patients with AIDS may become forgetful and have difficulty engaging in several tasks at once. Because both groups may face a foreshortened life span, similar psychodynamic issues may also arise. Noting the overlapping symptomatology between the normal elderly and younger patients with AIDS, we (Hinkin et al., 1990) compared the neuropsychological performance of three groups of individuals: (1) uninfected younger males with a mean age of 36; (2) older uninfected males with a mean age of 70; and (3) a group of younger men (mean age = 36) diagnosed with AIDS. As can be seen in Figure 1.2, the younger subjects with AIDS performed virtually identically to the elderly, uninfected group. Those tasks that were problematic for the older subjects (e.g., Part B of the Trail Making Test) also proved difficult for the younger subjects with AIDS, whereas those tasks which were normal in the elderly cohort were also within normal limits for the AIDS subjects. These data suggest that clinicians seeking to gain insight into the cognitive changes caused by HIV-1 infection can utilize the normal aging process as a useful heuristic model.

WHEN SHOULD A PATIENT BE REFERRED FOR EVALUATION?

One critical question that practicing clinicians must address is "When should I refer my patient for a neuropsychological evaluation?" Although no hard and fast answer can be provided, several guiding principles exist. Should a patient's family and/or friends complain of changes in the patient's thinking or behavior, this is almost always cause

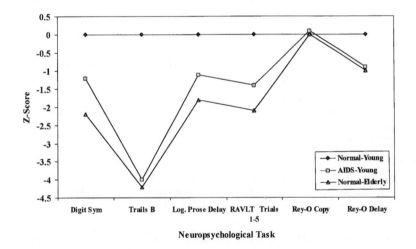

FIGURE 1.2. Pattern of neuropsychological performance for three groups: AIDS patients, normal elderly, and normal young. Digit Sym, Wechsler Adult Intelligence Scale–Revised, Digit Symbol subtest; Log Prose, Wechsler Memory Scale, Logical Prose subtest; RAVLT, Rey Auditory Verbal Learning Test; Rey-O, Rey–Osterrieth Complex Figure. From Hinkin et al. (1990). Copyright 1990 by *Canadian Journal on Aging*. Reprinted by permission.

for further workup and referral. In contrast, as discussed above, the validity of patients' self-complaint is often debatable. A conservative and prudent course is to take a patient's self-report at face value and refer for testing. Another clear reason for referral for neuropsychological testing is evidence that the patient's ability to perform at work or to discharge higher-level activities of daily living (e.g., balancing a checkbook) is beginning to suffer. Neuropsychological evaluation can also be helpful in establishing legal competence such as the ability to enter into contracts or execute a will, as well as in providing medical evidence to support a disability claim.

Resources permitting, neuropsychological testing concurrent with important disease milestones such as patient's CD4 count dropping below $200/mm^3$, viral load climbing above 20,000–30,000 copies/mm^3, onset of AIDS, or the institution of antiretroviral therapies—has also been proven to be a useful adjunct.

NEUROPSYCHOLOGICAL BATTERIES FOR THE ASSESSMENT OF DEMENTIA DUE TO HIV DISEASE

There has been considerable debate regarding what measures are most appropriate for investigating HIV-related cognitive dysfunction. Practical considerations such as patient tolerance, test administration costs, and fatigue effects must be balanced against the goal of thoroughly assessing all relevant cognitive domains. Some studies have used brief screening batteries lasting less than 1 hour (e.g., McArthur et al., 1989; Miller et al., 1990), while others have used assessment batteries requiring up to 7–9 hours of testing (Saykin et al., 1988; Heaton et al., 1995). Not surprisingly, the likelihood of identifying a problem appears to be related to the length of the battery administered. Brief screening batteries, developed out of necessity for large-scale longitudinal research, run the risk of increased false negatives or the failure to detect actual deficits. On the other hand, patients' inability to tolerate day-long testing frequently precludes using more lengthy assessment batteries.

Assigned with the task of constructing an ideal assessment battery for evaluating HIV-infected individuals, a National Institute of Mental Health (NIMH) working group chaired by the late Nelson Butters proposed the following 10 areas of examination: (1) premorbid intelligence, (2) attention, (3) speed of processing, (4) memory, (5) abstraction, (6) language, (7) visual perception, (8) constructional abilities, (9) motor abilities, and (10) psychiatric symptoms (Butters et al., 1990). The battery recommended by this group takes between 7 and 9 hours to administer, with additional time required for scoring, interpretation, and report preparation. A shortened version of the original NIMH battery, requiring between 1 and 2 hours of patient contact, has also been suggested. Table 1.6 lists the neuropsychological tests recommended by Butters et al. (1990) for the assessment of HIV-infected persons.

The Multicenter AIDS Cohort Study (MACS), assigned the task of testing large number of subjects longitudinally, used a multistage approach to develop a brief screening neuropsychological assessment battery (see Selnes & Miller, 1994, for details). Initially, they determined which measures from among 24 originally given to HIV-infected (asymptomatic and symptomatic) patients and seronegative controls best discriminated the performance of patients with AIDS from control subjects. Next, they identified major domains of cognitive functioning

TABLE 1.6. Neuropsychological Tests Recommended by the NIMH Working Group

Intelligence
    Wechsler Adult Intelligence Scale–Revised (WAIS-R)
    National Adult Reading Test–Revised
Simple and divided attention and sustained concentration
    WAIS-R Digit Span
    Paced Auditory Serial Addition Task
    Trail Making test (Parts A and B)
Language
    Boston Naming Test
    Verbal fluency tests
Visual–spatial function
    WAIS-R Block Design
Verbal memory
    California Verbal Learning Test
Nonverbal memory
    Wechsler Memory Scale–Revised, Visual Reproductions I and II
Motor speed
    Finger Tapping Test
    Grooved Pegboard Test
Psychomotor speed and speed of information processing
    Trail Making Test
    WAIS-R Digit Symbol
    Sternberg Search Task
    Simple and choice reaction time
Executive and frontal systems functions
    Category Test
Mood, affect, and personality
    Beck Depression Inventory or Hamilton Rating Scale for Depression
    State–Trait Anxiety Inventory
    Diagnostic Interview Schedule

Note. Adapted from Butters et al. (1990, p. 966). Copyright 1990 by Swets & Zeitlinger. Adapted by permission.

by performing factor analyses on the 24 original measures. They then eliminated any redundancy by selecting the one measure from each cognitive domain that showed the greatest power to discriminate AIDS patients from seronegative controls. The resulting assessment battery is both brief, taking approximately 45 minutes to administer, and sensitive to the earliest cognitive symptoms of HIV infection. Table 1.7 contains the MACS neuropsychological screening battery.

SUMMARY

To summarize, some degree of cognitive decline will occur in the majority of HIV-1-infected patients. This decline can range from very subtle psychomotor slowing and forgetfulness to profound dementia. Although the types of cognitive problems seen in HIV-infected individuals vary, the most common deficits are forgetfulness, psychomotor slowing, and trouble dividing attention between competing activities. Depression, apathy, anxiety, and irritability are also common. Should practicing clinicians suspect the presence of neuropsychological decline, they should screen for incipient cognitive decline, if they are appropriately trained to do so. Positive findings on screening should then trigger referral for a more comprehensive neuropsychological evaluation.

TABLE 1.7. MACS Neuropsychological Screening Battery

1. Trail Making Test, Parts A and B
2. Grooved Pegboard Test (dominant and nondominant hands)
3. Symbol Digit Modalities
   Raw score
   Paired recall
4. Rey Auditory Verbal Learning Test
   Trials 1–5
   Interference
   Recall after interference
   Delayed recall
   Delayed recognition
5. Rey–Osterrieth Complex Figure Test
   Copy
   Immediate recall
   Delayed recall
6. Stroop Task
7. California Computerized Assessment Package
   Simple reaction time
   Choice reaction time
   Serial pattern matching (sequential reaction time)

Note. Adapted from Selnes and Miller (1994). Copyright 1994 by Oxford University Press. Adapted by permission.

REFERENCES

American Academy of Neurology (AAN). (1991). Nomenclature and research case definitions for neurological manifestations of human immunodeficiency virus—type 1 (HIV-1) infection: Report of a working group of the American Academy of Neurology AIDS Task Force. *Neurology, 41*(6), 778–785.

American Psychiatric Association. (1994). *Diagnostic and statistical manual of mental disorders* (4th ed.). Washington, DC: Author.

Atkinson, J. H., Grant, I., Kennedy, C. J., et al. (1988). Prevalence of psychiatric disorders among men infected with human immunodeficiency virus. *Archives of General Psychiatry, 45,* 859–864.

Baddeley, A. D., Della Sala, S., Papagno, C., & Spinnler, H. (1997). Dual-task performance in dysexecutive and nondysexecutive patients with a frontal lesion. *Neuropsychology, 11,* 187–194.

Bartok, J. A., Martin, E. A., Pitrak, D. L., Novak, R. M., Pursell, K. J., Mullane, K. M., & Harrow, M. (1997). Working memory deficit in HIV-seropositive drug users. *Journal of the International Neuropsychological Society, 3,* 451–456.

Beck, A. T., & Steer, R. A. (1987). *Beck Depression Inventory: Manual.* San Antonio, TX: Psychological Corporation.

Benton, A. L., & Hamsher, K. (1989). *Multilingual Aphasia Examination.* Iowa City: AJA Associates.

Bix, B. C., Glosser, G., Holmes, W., Ballas, C., Meritz, M., Hutelmyer, C., & Turner, J. (1995). Relationship between psychiatric disease and neuropsychological impairment in HIV seropositive individuals. *Journal of the International Neuropsychological Society, 1,* 581–588.

Blessed, G., Tomlinson, B. E., & Roth, R. (1968). The association between quantitative measures of dementia and of senile change in the cerebral grey matter of elderly subjects. *British Journal of Psychiatry, 114,* 797–811.

Boccellari, A., Dilley, J. W., Chambers, D. B., Yingling, C. D., Tauber, M. A., Moss, A. R., & Osmond, D. H. (1993). Immune function and neuropsychological performance in HIV-1 infected homosexual men. *Journal of Acquired Immune Deficiency Syndromes, 6,* 592–601.

Boccellari, A., Dilley, J. W., & Shore, M. D. (1988). Neuropsychiatric aspects of AIDS dementia complex: A report on a clinical series. *Neurotoxicology, 9,* 381–390.

Bornstein, R. A. (1994). Methodological and conceptual issues in the study of cognitive change in HIV infection. In I. Grant & A. Martin (Eds.), *Neuropsychology of HIV infection* (pp. 3–19). New York: Oxford University Press.

Bornstein, R. A., Nasrallah, H. A., Para, M. F., Fass, R. J., et al. (1991). Rate of CD4 decline and neuropsychological performance in HIV infection. *Archives of Neurology, 48,* 704–707.

Bornstein, R. A., Nasrallah, H. A., Para, M. F., Whitacre, C. C., et al. (1992). Neuropsychological performance in asymptomatic HIV infection. *Journal of Neuropsychiatry and Clinical Neurosciences, 4,* 386–394.

Bornstein, R. A., Nasrallah, H. A., Para, M. F., Whitacre, C. C., Rosenberger, P.,

& Fass, R. J. (1993a). Neuropsychological performance in symptomatic and asymptomatic HIV infection. *AIDS, 7,* 519–524.

Bornstein, R. A., Pace, P., Rosenberger, P., Nasrallah, H. A., Whitacre, C. C., & Fass, R. J. (1993b). Depression and neuropsychological performance in asymptomatic HIV infection. *American Journal of Psychiatry, 150,* 922–927.

Brew, B. J. (1993). HIV-1 related neurological disease. *Journal of Acquired Immune Deficiency Syndromes, 6*(Suppl. 1), S10–S15.

Butters, N., Grant, I., Haxby, J., Judd, L. L., Martin, A., McClelland, J., Pequegnat, W., Schacter, D., & Stover, E. (1990). Assessment of AIDS related cognitive changes: Recommendations of the NIMH Workshop on Neuropsychological Assessment Approaches. *Journal of Clinical and Experimental Neuropsychology, 12,* 963–978.

Cassens, G., Wolfe, L., & Zola, M. (1990). The neuropsychology of depressions. *Journal of Neuropsychiatry, 2,* 202–213.

Centers for Disease Control (CDC). (1987). Revision of the CDC surveillance case definition for acquired immunodeficiency syndrome. *Morbidity and Mortality Weekly Report, 36*(Suppl.), 1S–16S.

Centers for Disease Control and Prevention. (1992). Centers for Disease Control 1993 revised classification system for HIV infection and expanded surveillance case definition for AIDS among adolescents and adults. *Morbidity and Mortality Weekly Report, 41,* 1–10.

Centers for Disease Control and Prevention. (1997). Update: Trends in AIDS incidence—United States, 1996. *Morbidity and Mortality Weekly Report, 46*(37), 861–867.

Claypoole, K., Townes, B., Collier, A., et al. (1990). *Neuropsychological aspects of early HIV infection.* Paper presented at the Eighteenth Annual Conference of the International Neuropsychological Society, Orlando, FL.

Cleary, P. D., Singer, E., & Rogers, T. F. (1988). Sociodemographic and behavioral characteristics of HIV antibody-positive blood donors. *American Journal of Public Health, 78,* 953–957.

Cleary, P. D., Van Devanter, N., Rogers, T., Singer, E., Shipton-Levy, R., Steilen, M., Stuart, A., Avorn, J., & Pindyck, J. (1993). Depressive symptoms in blood donors notified of HIV infection. *American Journal of Public Health, 83,* 534–539.

Collier, A. C., Gayle, T. C., & Bahls, F. H. (1987). Clinical manifestations and approach to management of HIV infection and AIDS. *AIDS: A Guide for the Primary Physician, 13,* 27–33.

Cummings, J. L. (1993). The neuroanatomy of depression. *Journal of Clinical Psychiatry, 54*(Suppl.), S14–S20.

Dilley, J. W., Ochitill, H. N., Perl, M., & Volberding, P. (1985). Findings in psychiatric consultation with patients with acquired immune deficiency syndrome. *American Journal of Psychiatry, 142,* 82–86.

Drebing, C. E., van Gorp, W. G., Hinkin, C. H., Miller, E. N., Satz, P., Kim, D. S., Holston, S., & D'Elia, L. F. (1994). Confounding factors in the measurement of depression of HIV. *Journal of Personality Assessment, 62,* 68–83.

Dunbar, N., Perdices, M., Grunseit, A., & Cooper, D. A. (1992). Changes in neuropsychological performance of AIDS-related complex patients who progress to AIDS. *AIDS, 6,* 691–700.

Elovaara, I., Poutiainen, E., Raininko, R., Valanne, L., Vira, A., Valle, S.-L., Lahdevirta, J., & Iivanainen, M. (1990). Mild brain atrophy in early HIV infection: The lack of association with cognitive deficits and HIV-specific intrathecal immune response. *Journal of the Neurological Sciences, 99,* 121–136.

Fell, M., Newman, S., Herns, M., Durrance, P., et al. (1993). Mood and psychiatric disturbance in HIV and AIDS: Changes over time. *British Journal of Psychiatry, 162,* 604–610.

Folstein, M. F., Folstein, S. E., & McHugh, P. R. (1975). Mini-Mental State. *Journal of Psychiatric Research, 12,* 189–198.

Franzblau, A., Letz, R., Hershman, D., Mason, P., Wallace, J. I., & Bekesi, J. G. (1991). Quantative neurologic and neurobehavioral testing of persons infected with human immunodeficiency virus type 1. *Archives of Neurology, 48,* 263–268.

Gabrieli, J. D., Singh, J., Stebbins, G. T., & Goetz, C. G. (1996). Reduced working memory span in Parkinson's disease: Evidence for the role of a frontal-striatal system in working and strategic memory. *Neuropsychology, 10,* 322–332.

Goldman-Rakic, P. S., & Friedman, H. R. (1991). The circuitry of working memory revealed by anatomy and metabolic imaging. In H. S. Levin, H. M. Eisenberg, & A. L. Benton (Eds.), *Frontal lobe function and dysfunction* (pp. 72–91). New York: Oxford University Press.

Gorman, J. M., Kertzner, R., Cooper, T., et al. (1991). Glucocorticoid level and neuropsychiatric symptoms in homosexual men with HIV infection. *American Journal of Psychiatry, 148,* 41–45.

Grant, I., & Atkinson, J. H. (1990). The evolution of neurobehavioral complications of HIV infection. *Psychological Medicine, 20,* 747–754.

Grant, I., & Atkinson, J. H. (1995). Psychiatric aspects of acquired immune deficiency syndrome. In H. I. Kaplan & B. J. Sadock (Eds.), *Comprehensive textbook of psychiatry* (Vol. 6, pp. 1644–1668). Baltimore: Williams & Wilkins.

Grant, I., Atkinson, J. H., Hesselink, J. R., Kennedy, C. J., Richman, D. D., Spector, S. A., & McCutchan, J. A. (1987). Evidence for early central nervous system involvement in the acquired immunodeficiency syndrome (AIDS) and other human immunodeficiency virus (HIV) infections. *Annals of Internal Medicine, 107,* 828–836.

Grant, I., & Martin, A. (1994). Neurocognitive disorders associated with HIV-1 infection. In I. Grant & A. Martin (Eds.), *Neuropsychology of HIV infection* (pp. 3–19). New York: Oxford University Press.

Grant, I., Olshen, R. A., Atkinson, J. H., Heaton, R. K., Nelson, J., McCutchan, J. A., & Weintrich, J. D. (1993). Depressed mood does not explain neuropsychological deficits in HIV-infected persons. *Neuropsychology, 7,* 53–61.

Green, T. A., Karon, J. M., & Nwanyanwu, D. C. (1992). Changes in AIDS incidence trends in the United States. *Journal of Acquired Immune Deficiency Syndromes, 5,* 547–555.

Hall, M., Whaley, R., Robertson, K., & Hamby, S. (1996). The correlation between neuropsychological and neuroanatomic changes over time in asymptomatic and symptomatic HIV-1 infected individuals. *Neurology, 46,* 1697–1702.

Hamilton, M. (1960). A rating scale for depression. *Journal of Neurology, Neurosurgery and Psychiatry, 23,* 56–62.

Harker, J. O., Satz, P., Jones, F. D., Verma, R. C., Gan, M. P., Poer, H. L., Gould, B. D., & Chervinsky, A. B. (1995). Measurement of depression and neuropsychological impairment in HIV-1 infection. *Neuropsychology, 9,* 110–117.

Heaton, R. K., Grant, I., Butters, N., White, D. A., Kirson, D., Atkinson, J. H., McCutchan, J. A., Taylor, M. J., et al. (1995). The HNRC 500: Neuropsychology of HIV infection at different disease stages. *Journal of the International Neuropsychological Society, 1,* 231–251.

Hinkin, C. H., Cummings, J. L., van Gorp, W. G., Satz, P., Mitrushina, M., & Freeman, D. (1990). Frontal/subcortical features of normal aging: An empirical analysis. *Canadian Journal on Aging, 9,* 104–119.

Hinkin, C. H., van Gorp, W. G., Mandelkern, M. A., Gee, M., Satz, P., Holston, S., Marcotte, T. D., Evans, G., Paz, D. H., Ropchan, J. R., Quinones, N., Khonsary, A., & Blahd, W. H. (1995a). Cerebral metabolic change in patients with AIDS: Report of a six-month follow-up using positron-emission tomography. *Journal of Neuropsychiatry and Clinical Neurosciences, 7,* 180–187.

Hinkin, C. H., van Gorp, W. G., & Satz, P. (1995b). Neuropsychological and neuropsychiatric aspects of HIV infection in adults. In H. I. Kaplan & B. J. Sadock (Eds.), *Comprehensive textbook of psychiatry* (Vol. 6). Baltimore: Williams & Wilkins.

Hinkin, C. H., van Gorp, W. G., Satz, P., Marcotte, T., Durvasula, R. S., Wood, S., Campbell, L., & Baluda, M. (1996). Actual versus self-reported cognitive dysfunction in HIV-1 infection: Memory–metamemory dissociations. *Journal of Clinical and Experimental Neuropsychology, 18,* 431–443.

Hinkin, C. H., van Gorp, W. G., Satz, P., Weisman, J. D., Thommes, J., & Buckingham, S. (1992). Depressed mood and its relationship to neuropsychological test performance in HIV-1 seropositive individuals. *Journal of Clinical and Experimental Neuropsychology, 14,* 289–297.

Janssen, R., Saykin, J., Cannon, L., Campbell, J., Pinsky, P. F., Hessol, N. A., O'Malley, P. M., Lifson, A. R., Doll, L. S., & Rutherford, G. W. (1989). Neurological and neuropsychological manifestations of human immunodeficiency virus (HIV-1) infection: Association with AIDS-related complex but not asymptomatic HIV-1 infection. *Annals of Neurology, 26,* 592–600.

Kalichman, S. C., & Sikkema, K. J. (1994). Psychological sequelae of HIV infection and AIDS: Review of empirical findings. *Clinical Psychology Review, 14,* 611–632.

Kelly, J. A., Murphy, D. A., Bahr, G. R, Koop, J., Morgan, M., Kalichman, S. C., Stevenson, L. Y., Brasfield, T. L., Bernstein, B., & St. Lawrence, J. (1993). Factors associated with severity of depression and high-risk sexual behavior among persons diagnosed with human immunodeficiency virus (HIV) infection. *Health Psychology, 12,* 215–219.

Kelly, M. D., Grant, I., Heaton, R. K., Marcotte, T. D., et al. (1997). Neuropsychological findings in HIV infection and AIDS. In I. Grant & K. Adams (Eds.), *Neuropsychological assessment of neuropsychiatric disorders* (2nd ed., pp. 403–422). New York: Oxford University Press.

King, D. A., & Caine, E. D. (1990). Depression. In J. L. Cummings (Ed.), *Subcortical dementia* (pp. 218–230). New York: Oxford University Press.

Krikorian, R., Wrobel, A. J., Meinecke, C., Liang, W. M., & Kay, J. (1990). Cognitive deficits associated with human immunodeficiency virus encephalopathy. *Journal of Neuropsychiatry and Clinical Neurosciences, 2,* 256–260.

La Rue, A. (1992). *Aging and neuropsychological disorders.* New York: Plenum Press.

Law, W. A., Martin, A., Mapou, R. L., Roller, T. L., Salazar, A. M., Temoshok, L. R., & Rundell, J. R. (1994). Working memory in individuals with HIV infection. *Journal of Clinical and Experimental Neuropsychology, 16,* 173–182.

Lunn, S., Skydsjerg, M., Schulsinger, H., Parnas, J., Pedersen, C., & Mathiesen, L. (1991). A preliminary report on the neuropsychologic sequelae of human immunodeficiency virus. *Archives of General Psychiatry, 48,* 139–142.

Maj, M., Satz, P., Janssen, R., Zaudig, M., Starace, F., D'Elia, L., Sughondbabirom, B., Mussa, M., Naber, D., Ndetei, D., Schulte, G., & Sartorius, N. (1994). WHO Neuropsychiatric AIDS Study, Cross-Sectional Phase II: Neuropsychological and neurological findings. *Archives of General Psychiatry, 51,* 51–61.

Mapou, R. L., & Law, W. A. (1994). Neurobehavioral aspects of HIV disease and AIDS: An update. *Professional Psychology: Research and Practice, 25,* 132–140.

Mapou, R. L., Law, W. A., Martin, A., Kampen, D., Salazar, A. M., & Rundell, J. R. (1993). Neuropsychological performance, mood, and complaints of cognitive and motor difficulties in individuals infected with the human immunodeficiency virus. *Journal of Neuropsychiatry and Clinical Neurosciences, 5,* 86–93.

Martin, A., Heyes, M. P., Salazar, A. M., Kampen, D. L., Williams, J., Law, W. A., Coats, M. E., & Markey, S. P. (1992). Progressive slowing of reaction time and increasing cerebrospinal fluid concentrations of quinolinic acid in HIV-infected individuals. *Journal of Neuropsychiatry and Clinical Neurosciences, 4,* 270–279.

Martin, E. M., Pitrak, D. L., Robertson, L. C., Novak, R. M., et al. (1995). Global–local analysis in HIV-1 infection. *Neuropsychology, 9,* 102–109.

Martin, E. M., Robertson, L. C., Edelstein, H., Jagust, W., Sorensen, D. J., et al. (1992a). Performance of patients with early HIV-1 infection on the Stroop task. *Journal of Clinical and Experimental Neuropsychology, 14,* 857–868.

Martin, E. M., Sorensen, D. J., Edelstein, H. E., & Robertson, L. C. (1992b). Decision-making speed in HIV-1 infection: A preliminary report. *AIDS, 6,* 109–113.

Mauri, M., Sinforiani, E., Muratori, S., et al. (1993). Three-year neuropsychological follow-up in a selected group of HIV-infected homosexual/bisexual men. *AIDS, 7,* 241–245.

McAllister, R. H., Herns, M. V., Harrison, M. J. G., et al. (1992). Neurological and neuropsychological performance in HIV seropositive men without symptoms. *Journal of Neurology, Neurosurgery and Psychiatry, 55,* 143–148.

McArthur, J. C., Cohen, B. A., Selnes, O. A., Kumar, A. J., et al. (1989). Low prevalence of neurological and neuropsychological abnormalities in otherwise healthy HIV-1 infected individuals: Results from the Multicenter AIDS Cohort Study. *Annals of Neurology, 26,* 601–611.

McArthur, J. C., Hoover, D. R., Bacellar, H., Miller, E. N., Cohen, B. A., Becker, J. T., Graham, N. M., McArthur, J. H., Selnes, O. A., Jacobsen, L. P., et al.

(1993). Dementia in AIDS patients: Incidence and risk factors, Multicenter AIDS Cohort Study. *Neurology, 43,* 2245–2252.

McArthur, J. C., Selnes, O. A., Glass, J. D., Hoover, D. R., & Bacellar, H. (1994). HIV dementia: Incidence and risk factors. In R. W. Price & S. Perry III (Eds.), *Research publications of the Association for Research in Nervous and Mental Disease: Vol. 72. HIV, AIDS and the brain* (pp. 251–272). New York: Raven Press.

McKegney, F. P., O'Dowd, M. A., Feiner, C., et al. (1990). A prospective comparison of neuropsychologic function in HIV-seropositive and seronegative methadone-maintained patients. *AIDS, 4,* 565–569.

Miller, E. N., Satz, P., van Gorp, W. G., Visscher, B., & Dudley, J. (1989). Computerized screening for HIV-related cognitive decline in gay men: Cross-sectional analyses and one-year follow-up. *Abstract of the International Conference on AIDS, 5,* 465.

Miller, E. N., Satz, P., & Visscher, B. (1991). Computerized and conventional neuropsychological assessment of HIV-1 infected homosexual men. *Neurology, 41,* 1608–1616.

Miller, E. N., Selnes, O. A., McArthur, J. C., Satz, P., Becker, J. T., Cohen, B. A., Sheridan, K., Machado, A. M., van Gorp, W. G., & Visscher, B. (1990). Neuropsychological performance in HIV-1-infected homosexual men: The Multicenter AIDS Cohort Study (MACS). *Neurology, 40,* 197–203.

Miller, E. N., & Wilkie, F. L. (1994). Computerized testing to assess cognition in HIV-positive individuals. In R. W. Price & S. Perry III (Eds.), *Research publications of the Association for Research in Nervous and Mental Disease: Vol. 72. HIV, AIDS and the brain* (pp. 161–175). New York: Raven Press.

Navia, B., Cho, E. S., Petito, C., & Price, R. (1986a). The AIDS dementia complex: II. Neuropathology. *Annals of Neurology, 19,* 525–535.

Navia, B. A., Jordan, B. D., & Price, R. W. (1986b). The AIDS dementia complex: I. Clinical features. *Annals of Neurology, 19,* 517–524.

Ollo, C., Johnson, R., & Grafman, J. (1991). Signs of cognitive change in HIV disease: An event-related brain potential study. *Neurology, 41,* 209–215.

Ostrow, D. G., Monjan, A., Joseph, J., Van Raden, M., Fox, R., Kingsley, L., Dudley, J., & Phair, J. (1989). HIV-related symptoms and psychological functioning in a cohort of homosexual men. *American Journal of Psychiatry, 146,* 737–742.

Pace, P. L., Rosenberger, P., Nasrallah, H. A., & Bornstein, R. A. (1993). Depression and neuropsychological performance in symptomatic HIV infection. *Journal of Clinical and Experimental Neuropsychology, 15,* 95.

Perdices, M. A., & Cooper, D. A. (1989). Simple and choice reaction time in patients with human immunodeficiency virus infection. *Annals of Neurology, 25,* 460–467.

Perry, S. W., & Tross, S. (1984). Psychiatric problems of AIDS inpatients at a New York hospital: Preliminary report. *Public Health Reports, 99,* 20–25.

Poutiainen, E., & Elovaara, I. (1996). Subjective complaints of cognitive symptoms are related to psychometric findings of memory deficits in patients with HIV-1 infection. *Journal of the International Neuropsychological Society, 2,* 219–225.

Poutiainen, E., Iivanainen, M., Elovaara, I., Valle, S., & Lahdevirta, J. (1988).

Cognitive changes as early signs of HIV infection. *Acta Neurologica Scandinavica, 78,* 49–52.

Price, R. W., & Brew, B. J. (1988). The AIDS dementia complex. *Journal of Infectious Diseases, 158,* 1079–1083.

Raininko, R., Elovaara, I., Vira, A., Valanne, L., Haltia, M., & Valle, S. L. (1992). Radiological study of the brain at various stages of human immunodeficiency virus infection: Early development of brain atrophy. *Neuroradiology, 34,* 190–196.

Resnick, L., de Marzio-Veronese, F., Schupbach, J., Tourtellotte, W., Ho, D., Muller, F., Shapshak, P., Vogt, M., Groopman, J., Markham, P., & Gallo, R. (1985). Intra-blood–brain-barrier synthesis of HTLV-III specific IgG in patients with neurological symptoms associated with AIDS or ARC. *New England Journal of Medicine, 313,* 1498–1504.

Rottenberg, D. A., Moeller, J. R., Strother, S. C., et al. (1987). The metabolic pathology of the AIDS dementia complex. *Annals of Neurology, 22,* 700–706.

Rubinow, D., Berettini, C., Brouwers, P., & Lane, H. (1988). Neuropsychiatric consequences of AIDS. *Annals of Neurology, 23*(Suppl.), S24–S26.

Sahakian, B. J., Elliot, R., Low, N., Mehta, M., Clark, R. T., & Pozniak, A. L. (1995). Neuropsychological deficits in tests of executive function in asymptomatic and symptomatic HIV-1 seropositive men. *Psychological Medicine, 25,* 1233–1246.

Saykin, A., Janssen, R., Sprehn, G., et al. (1988). Neuropsychological dysfunction in HIV-infection: Characterization in a lymphadenopathy cohort. *International Journal of Clinical Neuropsychology, 10,* 81–95.

Schwamm, L. H., Van Dyke, C., Kiernan, R. J., et al. (1987). The Neurobehavioral Cognitive Status Examination. *Annals of Internal Medicine, 107,* 486–491.

Selnes, O. A., Galai, N., Bacellar, H., Miller, E. N., Becker, J. T., Wesch, J., van Gorp, W. G., & McArthur, J. C. (1995). Cognitive performance after progression to AIDS: A longitudinal study from the Multicenter AIDS Cohort Study. *Neurology, 45,* 267–275.

Selnes, O. A., & Miller, E. N. (1994). Development of a screening battery for HIV-related cognitive impairment: The MACS experience. In I. Grant & A. Martin (Eds.), *Neuropsychology of HIV infection* (pp. 176–187). New York: Oxford University Press.

Sorenson, D. J., Martin, E. M., & Robertson, L. C. (1994). Visual attention in HIV-1 infection. *Neuropsychology, 8,* 424–432.

Stern, Y., Liu, X., Marder, K., Todak, G., Sano, M., Ehrhardt, A., & Gorman, J. (1995). Neuropsychological changes in a prospectively followed cohort of homosexual and bisexual men with and without HIV infection. *Neurology, 45,* 467–472.

Stern, Y., Marder, K., Bell, K., Chen, J., Dooneief, G., Goldstein, S., Mindry, D., Richards, M., Sano, M., Williams, J., Gorman, J., Ehrhardt, A., & Mayeux, R. (1991). Multidisciplinary baseline assessment of homosexual men with and without human immunodeficiency virus infection: III. Neurologic and neuropsychological findings. *Archives of General Psychiatry, 48,* 131–138.

Stern, Y., Sano, M., Williams, J., & Gorman, J. (1989). Neuropsychological consequences of HIV infection. *Journal of Clinical and Experimental Neuropsychology, 11,* 78.

Stout, J. C., Salmon, D. P., Butters, N., Taylor, M., Peavy, G., Heindel, W. C., Delis, D. C., Ryand, L., Atkinson, J. H., Chandler, J. L., Grant, I., & the HNRC Group. (1995). Decline in working memory associated with HIV infection. *Psychological Medicine, 25,* 1221–1232.

Tross, S., Price, R., Navia, B., et al. (1988). Neuropsychological characterization of the AIDS dementia complex: A preliminary report. *AIDS, 2,* 81–88.

van Gorp, W. G., Hinkin, C. H., Satz, P., Miller, E. N., Weisman, J., Holston, S., Drebing, C., Marcotte, T. D., & Dixon, W. (1993). Subtypes of HIV-related neuropsychological functioning: A cluster analysis approach. *Neuropsychology, 7,* 62–72.

van Gorp, W. G., Mandelkern, M. A., Gee, M., et al. (1992). Cerebral metabolic dysfunction in AIDS: Findings in a sample with and without dementia. *Journal of Neuropsychiatry and Clinical Neurosciences, 4,* 280–287.

van Gorp, W. G., Miller, E. N., Satz, P., & Visscher, B. (1989). Neuropsychological performance in HIV-1 immunocompromised patients: A preliminary report. *Journal of Clinical and Experimental Neuropsychology, 11,* 763–773.

van Gorp, W. G., Satz, P., Hinkin, C. H., Selnes, O. A., Miller, E. N., McArthur, J. C., Cohen, B., Paz, D., & the Multicenter AIDS Cohort Study (MACS). (1991). Metacognition in HIV-1 seropositive asymptomatic individuals: Self-ratings versus objective neuropsychological performance. *Journal of Clinical and Experimental Neuropsychology, 13,* 812–819.

Ventura, S. J., Peters, K. D., Martin, J. A., & Maurer, J. D. (1997). Births and deaths: United States, 1996. *Monthly Vital Statistics Report, 45*(12) (Suppl.).

Volk, R. J., Pace, T. M., & Parchman, M. L. (1993). Screening for depression in primary care patients: Dimensionality of the short form of the Beck Depression Inventory. *Psychological Assessment, 5,* 173–181.

Wechsler, D. (1981). *Wechsler Adult Intelligence Scale–Revised.* New York: Psychological Corporation.

White, D. A., Heaton, R. K., Monsch, A. U., & the HNRC Group. (1995). Neuropsychological studies of asymptomatic human immunodeficiency virus-type-1 infected individuals. *Journal of the International Neuropsychological Society, 1,* 304–315.

Wilkie, F. L., Eisdorfer, C., Morgan, R., Loewenstein, D. A., & Szapocznik, J. (1990). Cognition in early human immunodeficiency virus infection. *Archives of Neurology, 47,* 433–440.

Wilkins, J. W., Robertson, K. R., Snyder, C. R., et al. (1991). Implications of self-reported cognitive and motor dysfunction in HIV-positive patients. *American Journal of Psychiatry, 148,* 641–643.

2

Neurobiological Basis of Behavioral Changes in HIV-1 Encephalopathy

CARLA BACK
BRUCE MILLER
JEFFREY CUMMINGS

INTRODUCTION

Human immunodeficiency virus (HIV) infection is frequently complicated by a syndrome of central nervous system (CNS) dysfunction
known as "HIV-1 related encephalopathy" (also called "acquired immunodeficiency syndrome [AIDS] dementia complex" and, more recently,
"HIV-1-associated cognitive/motor complex"). HIV-1 or HIV encephalopathy (as we call it in this chapter) is often characterized by motor
symptoms and signs, neuropsychological impairment, and neuropsychiatric abnormalities. The diverse manifestations of HIV encephalopathy are produced by a retroviral infection of the brain.
Oligodondrocytes are more often affected than other CNS cellular
elements. The behavioral changes of HIV encephalopathy are a product
of white matter dysfunction early in the illness and of cortical changes
in the late stages of the disease. HIV encephalopathy is thought to be
a model neuropsychiatric illness, in which behavior is linked to dysfunc-

tion of specific brain regions. HIV encephalopathy is typically characterized as a subcortical dementia involving deep gray matter structures.

In this chapter, we review two of the most commonly observed classes of neurobehavioral disorders in HIV-1 encephalopathy: neuropsychological impairment and neuropsychiatric alterations. We then relate these behavioral changes to the neurobiology of HIV.

NEUROPSYCHOLOGICAL DEFICITS IN HIV-1

Prevalence

The reported frequency of neuropsychological changes in HIV/AIDS patients has varied considerably and is influenced by the study venue, the stage of HIV infection of the study population, and the criteria used for diagnosing cognitive impairment (Maj, 1990). In addition, recent research suggests that extraneous factors—such as substance use/misuse (Claypoole et al., 1993; Del Pesce et al., 1993; Egan, Crawford, Brettel, & Goodwin, 1990; Wilkins et al., 1990), level of education (Satz et al., 1993; Wilkins et al., 1990), depression (Wilkins et al., 1990), history of head injury (Claypoole et al., 1993; Wilkins et al., 1990), developmental disability (Wilkins et al., 1990), and age (Satz et al., 1993; Sinforiani et al., 1991)—may affect the frequency of cognitive deficits in HIV-1 encephalopathy.

Reported rates of neuropsychological dysfunction in HIV-1-infected individuals in most studies range from 25% to 66%. Navia, Jordan, and Price (1986a) reported that 66% (46 out of 70) of AIDS patients exhibited progressive dementia when assessed by bedside mental status testing, according to the criteria for dementia in the third edition of the *Diagnostic and Statistical Manual of Mental Disorders* (DSM-III). Saykin et al. (1988) found that 50% (9 out of 18) of seropositive gay men with lymphadenopathy syndrome evidenced cerebral dysfunction, as determined by specific cutoff scores on neuropsychological testing. Tross et al. (1988) examined the neuropsychological performance of AIDS patients at different stages of the disease; they reported that 32% of early AIDS patients and 71% of AIDS patients referred for neurological evaluation exhibited cognitive deficits as measured by abnormal scores on two or more neuropsychological tests. Grant et al. (1992) reported that 50% of nondemented patients with HIV-1-associated mild neurocognitive disorder (e.g., disturbance in two or more cognitive functions, which does not cause major disruption in daily functioning) were rated as impaired on the Halstead–Reitan Neuropsychological Test Battery (Halstead, 1947; Reitan & Wolfson,

1985). In a very small sample of hemophiliacs with AIDS (n = 4), Turnbull, Saling, Kaplan-Solms, Cohn, and Schoub (1991) reported a 25% frequency of neuropsychological impairment.

In contrast to the studies above, several investigators have reported lower prevalence rates of cognitive impairment in HIV-1 infection. Perriens et al. (1992) reported a 12.5% prevalence of HIV-1-associated cognitive/motor complex in Kinshasa, Zaire, based on bedside mental status screening. The Multicenter AIDS Cohort Study (MACS) reported only a 5% frequency of probable HIV encephalopathy in 289 cases of homosexual or bisexual men with AIDS (Bacellar et al., 1994; McArthur et al., 1993). Similarly, Maj et al. (1994) obtained prevalence rates of dementia from five different geographic locations (Germany, Brazil, Zaire, Kenya, and Thailand) and found frequencies ranging from 5.4% to 6.9% (when *International Classification of Diseases,* 10th revision [ICD-10] criteria were used) and from 4.4% to 6.5% (when DSM-III-R criteria were used) in all sites except Thailand, where no case of dementia was diagnosed.

There is a general consensus that neuropsychological impairment of varying degrees is common in the later stages of HIV-1 infection (Heaton et al., 1995; Bornstein, Nasrallah, Para, Whitacre, & Fass, 1993a). A number of studies have suggested that mild changes in cognitive performance may also be seen in a subgroup of patients at the asymptomatic stage prior to immunosuppression (White, Heaton, & Monsch, 1995; Maj et al., 1994; Bornstein et al., 1993b; Wilkie et al., 1992; Sinforoni et al., 1991; Stern et al., 1991; Grant et al., 1987). Thus, the cognitive changes in HIV-1 infection present a spectrum of cognitive disabilities, ranging from subtle early manifestations to severe dementia (Stern, 1994; van Gorp, Satz, Hinkin, Evans, & Miller, 1989c).

Pattern of Neuropsychological Changes

Following is a brief review of the findings from neuropsychological studies on HIV-1-infected individuals according to specific cognitive domains. (The reader is referred to Chapter 1 of this volume for a more extensive discussion of the cognitive deficits found in patients with HIV.)

Intelligence/Gross Cognitive Functioning

Research examining basic cognitive abilities in HIV-infected individuals—as measured by such tests as the Mini-Mental State Exam (Folstein, Folstein, & McHugh, 1975), the National Adult Reading Test—Revised (Nelson, 1982), and Raven's Progressive Matrices (Raven, 1938)—suggests that these abilities are generally preserved (Marsh & McCall, 1994; Maruff et al., 1994; Sinforiani et al., 1991; Gibbs, Andrews, Szmukler, Mulhall, & Bowden, 1990; Perdices & Cooper, 1990; van Gorp, Miller, Satz, & Visscher, 1989a). Several studies using the Wechsler Adult Intelligence Scale–Revised (WAIS-R; Wechsler, 1981) have documented poorer performance in AIDS patients than in seronegative controls (Bornstein et al., 1993b; van Gorp et al., 1989a; Rubinow, Berrettini, Brouwers, & Lane, 1988; Joffe et al., 1986). However, the AIDS patients still scored within the average to high-average range of intellectual functioning.

Attention and Information-Processing Speed

Immediate attention appears to be intact in HIV-1 encephalopathy, but selective deficits may be present in sustained and divided attention. Numerous studies have found that HIV-1-infected individuals do not differ significantly from controls on the WAIS-R Digit Span subtest (Maruff et al., 1994; Bornstein et al., 1993b; E. N. Miller et al., 1990; Sinforiani et al., 1991; van Gorp et al., 1989a; Tross et al., 1988; Grant et al., 1987; Rottenberg et al., 1987), although Stern et al. (1991) did report significant differences between HIV-1-infected patients and seronegative controls on this task. Deficits in divided attention, as measured by the Paced Auditory Serial Addition Task (Gronwall, 1977), have been observed in HIV-positive symptomatic individuals (Marsh & McCall, 1994; Bornstein et al., 1993b) and AIDS patients (Grant et al., 1987). Similarly, Perdices and Cooper (1990) documented impaired performance on the backward portion of the WAIS-R Digit Span subtest, a mental control test, in AIDS and AIDS-related complex patients.

Information-processing speed generally appears to be impaired in AIDS patients, particularly on tasks requiring psychomotor speed, visual–spatial tracking, and cognitive flexibility. Most reports note slowing on the Trail Making Test A (Army Individual Test Battery, 1944), a timed task requiring the subject to connect numbers rapidly and sequentially (Sackter et al., 1996; Maj et al., 1994; Marsh & McCall, 1994; Maruff et al., 1994; Perdices & Cooper, 1990; van Gorp et al., 1989a; Saykin et al., 1988; Rottenberg et al., 1987); however, Bornstein et al. (1993b) and Joffe et al. (1986) did not find this effect. Impaired performance on a more complex version of this test requiring cognitive flexibility (Trail Making Test B) has consistently been documented across numerous studies (Marsh & McCall, 1994; Maruff et al., 1994; Bornstein et al., 1993b; E. N. Miller et al., 1990; Perdices & Cooper, 1990; van Gorp et al., 1989a; Rubinow et al., 1988; Saykin et al., 1988; Tross et al., 1988; Rottenberg et al., 1987; Joffe et al., 1986). Perdices and Cooper (1990) and Saykin et al. (1988) reported that HIV-1 symptomatic patients performed significantly more poorly than controls on another test of sustained attention, visual scanning, and psychomotor speed, the Stroop task (Color Naming and Interference sections; Stroop, 1935).

Language

Studies examining language functioning in AIDS patients generally suggest that naming, vocabulary range, and word retrieval are preserved, although some inconsistent findings have been reported. Numerous reports document no significant difference between HIV-1-infected individuals and controls on the Vocabulary subtest of the WAIS-R (van Gorp et al., 1989a; Saykin et al., 1988; Tross et al., 1988; Grant et al., 1987; Rottenberg et al., 1987). Two studies found impaired performance on the WAIS-R Vocabulary subtest (Rubinow et al., 1988; Joffe et al., 1986), but these results may be attributable to failure to control for level of education and/or premorbid intellectual levels. Maruff et al. (1994), Wilkie et al. (1992), van Gorp et al. (1989a), and Tross et al. (1988) observed normal scores in AIDS patients on the Boston Naming Test (Kaplan, Goodglass, & Weintraub, 1978). In contrast, Saykin et al. (1988) found significantly lower performance in lymphadenopathy patients than in controls on the Boston Naming Test, although the HIV patients still scored within the average range. Results on tests of verbal fluency (e.g., tests requiring subjects to generate words beginning with a specific letter or words belonging to a particular category: see Spreen & Benton, 1969) have been variable. The majority of empirical studies suggest that this area of language is intact (Maruff et al., 1994; Bornstein et al., 1993b; Wilkie et al., 1992; Sinforiani et al., 1991; Krikorian, Wrobel, Meinecke, Liang, & Kay, 1990; E. N. Miller et al., 1990; Perdices & Cooper, 1990; van Gorp et al., 1989a; Tross et al., 1988; Rottenberg et al., 1987). However, a few studies have found poorer performance in HIV patients (Maj et al., 1994; Marsh & McCall, 1994; Stern et al., 1991; Saykin et al., 1988; Spreen & Benton, 1969).

Visual–Spatial–Constructional Skills

Most visual–spatial–constructional abilities appear to be intact in HIV-1 encephalopathy (e.g., paper-and-pencil copying/drawing, nonverbal intelligence) (Marsh & McCall, 1994; Maruff et al., 1994; Sinforiani et al., 1991; Krikorian et al., 1990; Perdices & Cooper, 1990; van Gorp et al., 1989a; Joffe et al., 1986). In contrast, variable performance has been noted on the Block Design subtest of the WAIS-R (a measure of puzzle solving), with some reports documenting significant differences between AIDS patients and controls (Maj et al., 1994; van Gorp et al., 1989a; Tross et al., 1988) and others finding no significant group differences (Wilkie et al., 1992; Perdices & Cooper, 1990; Saykin et al., 1988).

Learning and Memory

Research on HIV-1 encephalopathy and memory provides inconsistent findings as to impairment in both verbal and nonverbal memory functioning. Several investigators (Wilkie et al., 1992; Sinforiani et al., 1991; Perdices & Cooper, 1990; Saykin et al., 1988) have reported significant differences between HIV-1-infected individuals and controls on the Logical Memory subtests of the Wechsler Memory Scale (Wechsler, 1987), which are tests of paragraph learning; others have not found significant group differences on this task (van Gorp et al., 1989a; Tross et al., 1988; Grant et al., 1987). Results of list-learning tasks, such as the Rey Auditory Verbal Learning Test (Rey, 1941, 1964), the California Verbal Learning Test (Delis, Kramer, Kaplan, & Ober, 1983), and the World Health Organization Auditory Verbal Learning Test (Maj et al., 1993), have also been variable. Some reports have documented impaired list-learning performance in HIV-1-infected individuals (Maj et al., 1994; Gibbs et al., 1990; E. N. Miller et al., 1990), and others have noted no change (Perdices & Cooper, 1990; van Gorp et al., 1989a; Saykin et al., 1988). Studies of nonverbal memory have also reported inconsistent and contradictory results. Deficits in memory for simple line drawings, as assessed via the Visual Reproductions subtests of the Wechsler Memory Scale, have been observed in some studies (Marsh & McCall, 1994; Wilkie et al., 1992; Perdices & Cooper, 1990; van Gorp et al., 1989a) but not others (Saykin et al., 1988; Tross et al., 1988; Grant et al., 1987). Delayed recall on the Rey–Osterrieth Complex Figure Test (Rey, 1941, 1964) has been reported to be impaired in AIDS patients (van Gorp et al., 1989a), although two subsequent studies have failed to support this finding (McManis et al., 1993; Perdices & Cooper, 1990). In summary, deficits in verbal and nonverbal memory may occur in some HIV-1-infected individuals, but are not present in all. This variability reflects the heterogenous severity of CNS involvement in AIDS patients.

Frontal Lobe/Executive Abilities

"Executive functions" are cognitive processes that allow an individual to respond and adapt appropriately to his or her environment. From a neuropsychological standpoint, executive/frontal lobe functions include categorization, set shifting, abstract reasoning, concept formation, and response inhibition. Variable findings have been reported on executive/frontal lobe functioning in HIV-1-infected individuals. Mixed results have been observed on card-sorting tasks requiring categorization and mental flexibility. Maruff et al. (1994), Bornstein et al. (1993b), and Krikorian et al. (1990) documented significant differences between HIV-1-seropositive symptomatic patients and controls on the Wisconsin Card Sorting Test (Heaton, 1983), but Joffe et al. (1986) did not.

Investigation of abstract reasoning tasks has also produced inconsistent results, with some studies finding deficits (Perdices & Cooper, 1990; van Gorp et al., 1989a; Grant et al., 1987; Joffe et al., 1986), and others reporting intact performance (Gibbs et al., 1990; Sinforiani et al., 1990; Rubinow et al., 1988; Tross et al., 1988). As previously mentioned in regard to information-processing speed, several investigators have observed impaired response inhibition abilities in HIV infected individuals as measured by the Interference section of the Stroop task (Martin et al., 1992; Saykin et al., 1988).

Motor Functioning

Numerous investigators have demonstrated impairment in motor dexterity as measured by the Purdue Grooved Pegboard in HIV-1-seropositive patients, while inconsistent findings have been observed on the Finger Tapping Test. Most studies have documented bilateral slowing on the Purdue Grooved Pegboard (Tiffin, 1968), which measures fine motor coordination and speed (Maj et al., 1994; Bornstein et al., 1993b; E. N. Miller et al., 1990; Tross et al., 1988; Rottenberg et al., 1987); however, Stern et al. (1991) found no significant differences between HIV seropositive individuals and seronegative controls on the Purdue Grooved Pegboard. Rottenberg et al. (1987) observed impaired performance bilaterally in AIDS dementia complex patients on the Finger Tapping Test (Reitan & Wolfson, 1985). In contrast, Tross et al. (1988) reported no significant deterioration on this test in HIV patients.

Summary of Neuropsychological Changes

In summary (see also Table 2.1), the most common deficits in HIV-1 infection include psychomotor slowing and impaired fine motor control. Declines in verbal fluency and complex attentional abilities (sustained and divided attention) are also frequent. Impairment in verbal and nonverbal memory, frontal lobe/executive skills, and visual–spa-

TABLE 2.1. Neuropsychological Deficits in HIV-1 Encephalopathy

Most common

  Cognitive slowing
  Impaired fine motor control
  Decreased verbal fluency
  Attentional difficulties (sustained and divided attention)

Less frequent

  Memory deficits (verbal and nonverbal)
  Impaired executive/frontal lobe skills
  Visual–spatial–constructional declines

---

tial–constructional abilities may also occur. In contrast, overall intelligence appears to be relatively preserved. There is substantial variability in the severity of cognitive changes observed among patients.

Subcortical Dementia

A subset of HIV-1-infected individuals exhibit a dementia consisting of moderate to severe deficits on neuropsychological testing in the areas of complex attention, memory (primarily retrieval of information), and executive functions, as well as cognitive and motor slowing.

This pattern of neuropsychological declines is consistent with a subcortical dementia (Maruff et al., 1994; Perdices & Cooper, 1990; Krikorian et al., 1990; Saykin et al., 1988; Sidtis, Amitai, Ornitz, & Price, 1988; Tross et al., 1988). Early in the clinical course of this dementia, HIV-1-infected individuals exhibit impaired concentration and a memory disturbance characterized by forgetfulness. Slowing in cognition and difficulty maintaining a train of thought are common. Memory deficits become more noticeable with progression of the disease, and impairment in abstraction, mental flexibility, verbal fluency, and categorization (executive skills) may occur. As the disease approaches the preterminal stage, patients manifest more severe psychomotor retardation as well as confusion. In the terminal stage, many are in an awake state, but are mute and immobile. Mood and personality changes (e.g., depression and apathy) are common in the subcortical dementia of AIDS, and delusions and hallucinations can also occur. Associated neurological features include gait disturbance, dysarthria, tremor, lower-limb hyperflexia, headaches, and seizures (Navia et al., 1986a). The neurocognitive deficits in subcortical dementia are typically assessed with standard neuropsychological measures, such as those mentioned in the previous discussion on the specific cognitive domains (e.g., Parts A and B of the Trail Making Test, the Wechsler Memory

Scale, the Rey Auditory Verbal Learning Test, the Wisconsin Card Sorting Test, the WAIS-R, and the Purdue Grooved Pegboard).

HIV affects subcortical structures to a greater extent than cortical structures. The virus invades oligodendrocytes and may produce toxins that exert local effects. Dysfunction of the subcortical white matter produces the clinical syndrome of subcortical dementia observed in patients with HIV encephalopathy (Wilkinson et al., 1996) discussed below.

NEUROPSYCHIATRIC ALTERATIONS IN HIV ENCEPHALOPATHY

Most of the literature concerning HIV-1-associated neurobehavioral disorders has focused on neuropsychological dysfunction and dementia. Limited research exists on the frequency of other types of neuropsychiatric disorders, such as apathy, delirium, depression, psychosis, and anxiety. In addition, the symptoms and signs of the neuropsychiatric disorders in HIV-1 encephalopathy are often associated with, or coexist with, those of preexisting psychiatric disorders, such as depression (Maj, 1990). Below we briefly review the most frequently reported neuropsychiatric disorders in AIDS patients; Table 2.2 summarizes these disorders and their reported prevalence rates. Neuropsychiatric disorders are discussed in greater detail in Chapter 4 of this volume.

TABLE 2.2. Neuropsychiatric Disorders in HIV-1 Encephalopathy and Reported Prevalence Rates

Neuropsychiatric disorder	Prevalence in HIV-1 encephalopathy
Apathy	
Early stages	32–36%
Later stages	50%
Delirium	Unknown
Major depression	
Current	5–8%
Lifetime rate	13–38%
Psychosis	
Early stages	0.1%
Later stages	15%
Generalized anxiety	
Current	5–20%
Lifetime rate	5–40%
Mania	Unknown

Apathy

Apathy and social withdrawal are common in early stages of HIV-1 infection, with prevalence rates ranging from 32% to 36%. As the disease progresses, apathy develops in nearly half of AIDS patients (Perriens et al., 1992; Navia et al., 1986a).

Delirium

Delirium, or "acute confusional state," may present either with hyperactive and agitated features or with hypoactive and withdrawn symptoms (Atkinson & Grant, 1994). The prevalence of delirium in HIV-1 encephalopathy is unknown, but it is thought to be common even in ambulatory AIDS patients (Atkinson & Grant, 1994). Prior substance use and prior brain damage are risk factors for the development of delirium (Ochitill & Dilley, 1988). Differentiating delirium from dementia, and then determining the etiology of the delirium, are of utmost importance, as delirium may be reversible with appropriate treatment.

Depression

The prevalence of current major depression in HIV-1-infected individuals has been estimated to range from 5% to 8% and is approximately two times greater than the expected rates for the community (Atkinson & Grant, 1994; Rabkin, Ferrando, Jacobsberg, & Fishman, 1997). Lifetime prevalence rates of major depression range from 13% to 38%, with most studies documenting that about one-third of AIDS patients have had a major depressive episode (Williams, Rabkin, Remien, Gorman, & Ehrhardt, 1991; Atkinson et al., 1988). Depression is not markedly elevated in patients with HIV encephalopathy compared to seronegative gay men. Depressive symptoms may be difficult to differentiate from dementia (psychomotor slowing, attention and memory impairment) and HIV-1-associated neurovegetative changes (fatigue, sleep disturbance, weight loss, loss of sexual interest) (Maj, 1990). Thus, the neuropsychiatrist should obtain a detailed psychiatric history, as well as neuropsychological testing, to aid in the differential diagnosis (Atkinson & Grant, 1994).

Psychosis

Hallucinations (auditory, visual, or tactile), delusions (grandiose or persecutory), and thought disorder (loosening of associations or disorganization) may appear in HIV-1 encephalopathy. Psychotic symptoms have been reported in 0.1% of AIDS patients in the early stages (Navia et al., 1986a), but are more frequent in later stages of the illness, with prevalence rates of up to 15% (Atkinson & Grant, 1994; Navia et al., 1986a).

Mania

Mania has also been reported in HIV-1 encephalopathy. Manic syndromes may be secondary to neuromedical disease (e.g., cryptococcal meningitis) or pharmacological agents such as zidovudine, steroids, or ganciclovir (Johannessen & Wilson, 1988; O'Dowd & McKegney, 1988; Schmidt & Miller, 1988). They have also infrequently been associated specifically with HIV-1 infection (Lyketsos et al., 1993; Kieburtz, Zettelmaier, Ketonen, Tuite, & Caine, 1991; Schmidt & Miller, 1988). The incidence of manic conditions in HIV-1 encephalopathy is unknown, but is thought to be low (Atkinson & Grant, 1994).

Anxiety

Anxiety episodes lasting from one to several months are relatively common in HIV-1-infected individuals. Lifetime rates have been reported to exceed 40% (Atkinson et al., 1988), whereas the 6-month prevalence rates of generalized anxiety (defined according to DSM-III criteria) range from 11% to 20% (Perriens et al., 1992; Williams et al., 1991). However, lifetime and current rates of generalized anxiety drop to about 5% when more stringent criteria requiring a minimum duration of symptoms for 6 months are used (DSM-III-R) (Williams et al., 1991). Other anxiety disorders (e.g., obsessive–compulsive disorder or panic disorder) do not appear to be any more prevalent in AIDS patients than in the general population (Williams et al., 1991; Atkinson et al., 1988).

NEUROBIOLOGICAL BASIS
OF COGNITIVE DISTURBANCES
AND NEUROPSYCHIATRIC ALTERATIONS

Despite more than a decade of intensive research, the neurobiological mechanisms that underlie the dementia and behavioral syndromes associated with HIV are still poorly understood. Currently, there are many areas of controversy regarding the etiology, pathogenesis, and anatomical regions associated with HIV-1 encephalopathy. Although most investigators believe that HIV itself is the major cause for encephalopathy in HIV-infected patients (Navia, Petito, & Gold, 1986b), other viruses—such as cytomegalovirus (Vinters, Kwok, & Ho, 1989), papovavirus (J. R. Miller, Barrett, & Britton, 1982), herpes simplex virus (Hall et al., 1991), and varicella virus—cause, or contribute to, the dementia in many HIV-infected patients.

Hypotheses regarding the cellular mechanisms leading to the pathogenesis of HIV-1 encephalopathy also vary. Most agree that the macrophage is the cell with the highest concentration of HIV. Similarly, the macrophage is thought to be the cell where HIV replicates. However, some argue that the encephalopathy is secondary to an immune-mediated cascade that kills neurons and other cells within the brain (Pulliam, Herndier, Tang, & McGrath, 1991), whereas others contend that a toxic effect of virus on neurons is the cause for the syndrome (Brenneman, Westbrook, & Fitzgerald, 1988).

The specific anatomical site critical for HIV-1 encephalopathy is poorly understood. The basal ganglia, thalamus, subcortical white matter, frontal lobes, and diffuse cortical regions are all involved. The pattern of neuropsychological deficits is most consistent with dysfunction of frontal–subcortical circuits, primarily through effects on the subcortical white matter that connects the member structures of the circuit. Likewise, the types of neuropsychiatric disturbances observed in patients with HIV encephalopathy are also most consistent with dysfunction of subcortical brain structures and white matter.

There are disappointingly few data regarding the relative contribution of systemic illness and medications to the cognitive syndromes associated with AIDS, despite the facts that many of these patients show severe end-stage pulmonary, renal, and sometimes hepatic disorders, and that nearly all patients take multiple medications with CNS actions.

Secondary Infections and Tumors

Before HIV-1 encephalopathy can be diagnosed, it is essential that the focal infections, tumors, and meningitic lesions that invade the brain with HIV/AIDS be excluded as causes for the encephalopathy. Because AIDS leads to severe immunosuppression, infections and tumors develop that are not seen in healthy individuals. Similarly, the brain's ability to suppress the growth of infections and tumors is diminished, so that fulminant spread of these lesions is common. In addition, patients with meningitis do not always generate fever or develop a stiff neck, and the main manifestation of meningitis in the setting of HIV/AIDS can be dementia or cognitive slowing.

The four most common focal lesions seen in patients with AIDS are toxoplasmosis, lymphoma, progressive multifocal leukoencephalopathy, and cryptococcoma (Chang, Cornford, Chiang, Ernst, & Miller, 1995a; Chang et al., 1995b). Toxoplasmosis causes multifocal abscesses with a predilection for the thalamus, basal ganglia, and frontal lobes. Although seizures and focal motor or sensory deficits often differentiate toxoplasmosis patients from those with uncomplicated HIV-1 encephalopathy, slower presentations with lethargy and cognitive impairment are common. Lymphomas often spread around the ventricular system, so that focal motor or sensory symptoms can be absent, while lethargy or global dementia are the main presenting symptoms. Progressive multifocal leukoencephalopathy infects multiple areas of white matter, and progressive focal findings typically dominate the clinical picture. However, if white matter lesions are sufficiently diffuse, dementia can predominate, and the clinical and imaging picture overlaps with the white matter lesions of HIV encephalopathy. Finally, there are various possible causes of meningitis in HIV patients, and all need to be excluded with cerebrospinal fluid examinations. Reported infections include syphilis, listeria, nocardia, tuberculosis, cryptococcosis, candida, herpes, and bacterial infections.

HIV-1 Encephalopathy

The Role of HIV

Wiley and Achim (1995) have summarized many of the important neurobiological issues related to HIV-1 encephalopathy. Shaw, Harper, and Hahn (1985) demonstrated in AIDS patients with moderate and severe dementia that the concentration of HIV was higher in the brain than in the spleen. Others have shown that HIV can be cultured from the brain and cerebrospinal fluid of patients with HIV-1 encephalopathy, and antibodies against the HIV are found within the cerebrospinal fluid early in the course of HIV (Glass, Wesselingh, Selnes, & McArthur, 1993). Shaw et al. (1985) were the first to suggest that HIV might enter the CNS and cause progressive neurological deterioration. Subsequently, Navia et al. (1986b) noted the presence of a characteristic neuropathology in 16 of 34 patients with HIV-1 encephalopathy. These individuals had multinucleated cells within microglial nodules, which most severely affected the frontal and temporal lobes. Many showed white matter changes that varied from pallor to severe degeneration.

Glass et al. (1993) reported that about one-half of a sample of patients with HIV-1 encephalopathy showed microglial nodules and multinucleated cells. This finding of a specific neuropathology in approximately 50% of HIV-1 encephalopathy patients confirmed the original observations made by Navia et al. (1986b). Wiley and Achim (1995) found that in patients without opportunistic infection, HIV antigen generally correlated with the severity of encephalopathy. In contrast, Brew, Rosenblum, Cronin, and Price (1995) found that the infection with HIV-1 encephalopathy was localized primarily to the macrophages present in subcortical gray and white matter. They found that pathology in HIV-1 encephalopathy was greater than would have been expected from the severity of brain infection, suggesting that a mechanism other than viral load accounted for the dementia syndrome. Together, these studies suggest that HIV plays an important role in the pathogenesis of HIV-1 encephalopathy.

Clinical–Pathological Correlations

One presentation of HIV-1 encephalopathy is a relentlessly progressive dementia associated with worsening brain atrophy and progressively enlarging white matter lesions (Navia et al., 1986b). Global atrophy is present in nearly every patient with HIV-1 encephalopathy, whereas low-density white matter lesions demonstrated by computerized tomography (CT) are found in approximately one-third of patients. The white matter changes are typically present within the periventricular region and the centrum semiovale. Magnetic resonance imaging (MRI) is better for detecting these white matter lesions (Grafe, Press, Berthoty, Hesselink, & Wiley, 1990).

Studies of elderly patients with white matter hyperintensities suggest that these lesions are clinically silent until a threshold of volume is reached (Boone et al., 1992). This threshold typically occurs when the white matter lesions are confluent and surround the frontal and occipital horns. When this occurs, patients show subtle mental slowing, lethargy, and deficits on frontal systems tasks, with relative sparing of language. As the lesions become more confluent, more severe dementia supervenes (Liu et al., 1992). Similiar lesions are common in the setting of HIV-1 encephalopathy; however, as noted previously, about two-thirds of these patients do not show extensive white matter hyperintensities. Unfortunately, few studies have correlated the cognitive or psychiatric patterns found in HIV patients with atrophy patterns or white matter hyperintensities.

The anatomical localization of the pathology tends to correlate with the results of functional neuroimaging studies using positron emission tomography (PET). Initially, there is increased uptake of glucose in the basal ganglia, where HIV-infected macrophages are greatest in number. Eventually there is global hypometabolism, which correlates with progression of the infection. When patients with HIV-1 encephalopathy are treated with zidovudine, one can see both clinical improvement and improvement in metabolic patterns with PET (Sidtis et al., 1993).

Although most patients with HIV-1 encephalopathy have subcortical dementia, a clinical syndrome exhibited by some patients varies from this pattern. Ortego et al. (1994) evaluated 10 patients with HIV-1 encephalopathy and found that only 3 showed a classical subcortical dementia. The others demonstrated amnestic syndromes, frontal dementias, and a right parietal syndrome. Another manifestation of HIV-1 encephalopathy is a confusional state with hallucinations and paranoid delusions. In one such patient, severe global brain hypoperfusion was observed with single-photon emission computed tomography (SPECT) (Ortego et al., 1994). In general, there have been few systematic attempts to correlate the anatomical and neurochemical basis for the neuropsychiatric syndromes that are so commonly found in HIV-1 encephalopathy patients. Often these syndromes are multifactorial, with the combination of anatomical and neurochemical deficits interacting with the medications and systemic illnesses that occur in late-stage AIDS.

Impact of Subcortical Neuropathology on Cognition and Emotional States

As previously noted, HIV encephalopathy has typically been characterized as a subcortical dementia. The subcortical structures of the brain include the striatum, the globus pallidus/substantia nigra, and the thalamus. A series of parallel circuits has been found to link these subcortical structures to regions of the frontal lobes (Mega & Cummings, 1994; Cummings, 1993). Frontal–subcortical circuits mediate many aspects of human behavior, such as executive functions, personality, and mood, and may be implicated in HIV-related subcortical dementia. Neurobehavioral disorders of frontal–subcortical circuits include impaired executive functions, disinhibition, depression, mania, lability, and apathy. Similar behavioral changes are seen with damage to the prefrontal cortex.

The dorsolateral prefrontal–subcortical circuit mediates executive function. The neuropsychiatric disorders of depression and anxiety are also associated with dysfunction of this circuit. Irritability, mania, lability, and disinhibition have been related to the lateral orbitofrontal–subcortical circuit. Lastly, the anterior cingulate–subcortical circuit mediates motivation, and apathy is the neuropsychiatric disorder commonly observed with damage to the structures of this circuit. Differential involvement of this circuitry may contribute to the variability of symptoms observed in patients with HIV encephalopathy.

Cytomegalovirus Infection

Cytomegalovirus is a DNA virus that rarely causes symptomatic infections in individuals who are not immunosuppressed. However, in the setting of HIV/AIDS, cytomegalovirus commonly causes an opportunistic infection. In patients with advanced immunosuppression, cytomegalovirus can cause life-threatening hepatitis, enterocolitis, pneumonitis, and retinitis (Holland et al., 1994). Cytomegalovirus encephalopathy is still poorly characterized. Apathy, disorientation, and withdrawal associated with delirium are common. In Holland et al.'s (1994) study, cranial nerve findings were more typical of cytomegalovirus than of HIV, while motor abnormalities were more common in HIV. Seizures are uncommon with both. Cytomegalovirus encephalopathy is rapidly progressive; symptoms at presentation have been noted for less than 1 month. In contrast, HIV encephalopathy is less acute, with symptoms typically present for more than 4 months when the patient seeks medical attention. Encephalopathy is more likely to occur when patients demonstrate cytomegalovirus in other organ systems outside of the brain. In one study of cytomegalovirus encephalopathy (Holland et al., 1994), 92% of the patients showed infection of the adrenal glands, 58% had retinitis, and 42% had pneumonitis. The adrenal infection caused hyponatremia in 58% of patients.

Cytomegalovirus has a predilection for endothelial cells, so that periventricular infection and vasculitis are both common at autopsy. With the periventriculitis, there is often enhancement around the ventricles on CT or MRI. Holland et al. (1994) described a case with severe ventriculitis leading to hydrocephalus associated with amnesia. Although periventricular infections are common with cytomegalovirus, toxoplasmosis can also cause periventricular infection (Falangola & Petito, 1993).

SUMMARY

HIV-1-related encephalopathy has been extensively studied for the past decade, and there is substantial documentation of the neurological, neuropsychological, neuropsychiatric, neuroimaging, and neuropathological bases for this condition. However, further research is needed to better define the diversity of clinical syndromes found with

AIDS beyond the typical subcortical dementia pattern. The biological basis for HIV-1 encephalopathy also requires further investigation. In particular, the mechanisms associated with the dementia are still poorly understood; both direct injury by the virus itself and indirect injury by viral particles have been hypothesized. The location and type of neuronal injury found with HIV-1 encephalopathy is not well defined, and the relationship between this dementia and cytomegalovirus requires further study.

REFERENCES

Army Individual Test Battery. (1944). *Manual of directions and scoring.* Washington, DC: U.S. War Department, General's Office.

Atkinson, J. H., & Grant, I. (1994). Natural history of neuropsychiatric manifestations of HIV disease. *Psychiatric Clinics of North America, 17*(1), 17–33.

Atkinson, J. H., Grant, I., Kennedy, C. J., Richman, D. D., Spector, S. A., & McCutchan, J. A. (1988). Prevalence of psychiatric disorders among men infected with human immunodeficiency virus. *Archives of General Psychiatry, 45,* 859–864.

Bacellar, H., Munoz, A., Miller, E. N., Cohen, B. A., Besley, D., Selnes, O. A., Becker, J. T., & McArthur, J. C. (1994). Temporal trends in the incidence of HIV-1 related neurologic diseases: Multicenter AIDS Cohort Study, 1985–1992. *Neurology, 44,* 1892–1900.

Boone, K. B., Miller, B. L., Lesser, I. M., Mehringer, C. M., Hill, E., & Berman, N. (1992). Cognitive deficits with white-matter lesions in healthy elderly. *Archives of Neurology, 49,* 549–554.

Bornstein, R. A., Nasrallah, H. A., Para, M. F., Whitacre, C. C., & Fass, R. J. (1993a). Change in neuropsychological performance in asymptomatic HIV infection: 1-year follow-up. *AIDS, 7,* 1607–1611.

Bornstein, R. A., Nasrallah, H. A., Para, M. F., Whitacre, C., Rosenberger, P., & Fass, R. J. (1993b). Neuropsychological performance in symptomatic and asymptomatic HIV infection. *AIDS, 7,* 519–524.

Brenneman, D. E., Westbrook, G. L., & Fitzgerald, S. F. (1988). Neuronal cell killing by the envelope protein of HIV and its prevention by vasoactive intestinal peptide. *Nature, 335,* 639–642.

Brew, B. J., Rosenblum, M., Cronin, K., & Price, R. W. (1995). AIDS-dementia complex and HIV-1 brain infection: Clinical–virological correlations. *Annals of Neurology, 38,* 563–570.

Chang, L., Cornford, M. E., Chiang, F. L., Ernst, T., & Miller, B. L. (1995a). Radiologic–pathologic correlation: Cerebral toxoplasmosis and lymphoma in AIDS. *American Journal of Neuroradiation, 16,* 1653–1664.

Chang, L., Miller, B. L., McBride, D. Q., Chiang, F., Oropilla, G., & Buchthal, S. (1995b). Differentiation in AIDS between brain toxoplasmosis, lymphoma, and PML with 1H magnetic resonance spectroscopy. *Radiology, 197*(2), 525–532.

Claypoole, K. H., Collier, A. C., Marra, C., Cohen, W., Martin, D., Coombs, R. W., Goldstein, D., Sanches, P., & Handsfield, H. H. (1993). Cognitive risk factors and neuropsychological performance in HIV infection. *International Journal of Neuroscience, 70,* 13–27.

Cummings, J. L. (1993). Frontal–subcortical circuits and human behavior. *Archives of Neurology, 50,* 873–880.

Delis, D. C., Kramer, J. H., Kaplan, E., & Ober, B. A. (1983). *California Verbal Learning Test, research edition.* San Antonio, TX: Psychological Corporation.

Del Pesce, M., Franciolini, B., Censori, B., Bartolini, M., Ancarani, R., Petrelli, E., & Provinciali, L. (1993). Cognitive behavior in asymptomatic (CDC stage II and III) HIV-seropositive intravenous drug users (IVDUs). *Italian Journal of Neurological Sciences, 14*(9), 619–625.

Egan, V. G., Crawford, J. R., Brettel, R. P., & Goodwin, G. M. (1990). The Edinburgh cohort of HIV-positive drug users: Current intellectual function is impaired, but not due to early AIDS dementia complex. *AIDS, 4,* 651–656.

Falangola, M. F., & Petito, C. K. (1993). Choroid plexus infection in cerebral toxoplasmosis in AIDS patients. *Neurology, 43,* 2035–2040.

Folstein, M. F., Folstein, S. E., & McHugh, P. R. (1975). Mini Mental State: A practical method for grading the cognitive state of patients for the clinician. *Journal of Psychiatric Research, 12,* 189–198.

Gibbs, A., Andrews, D. G., Szmukler, G., Mulhall, B., & Bowden, S. C. (1990). Early HIV-related neuropsychological impairment: Relationship to stage of viral infection. *Journal of Clinical and Experimental Neuropsychology, 12*(5), 766–780.

Glass, J. D., Wesselingh, S. L., Selnes, O. A., & McArthur, J. C. (1993). Clinical-neuropathologic correlation in HIV-asssociated dementia. *Neurology, 43,* 2230–2237.

Grafe, M. R., Press, G. A., Berthoty, D. P., Hesselink, J. R., & Wiley, C. J. (1990). Abnormalities of the brain in AIDS patients: Correlation of postmortem MR findings with neuropathology. *American Journal of Neuroradiology, 11,* 905–911.

Grant, I., Atkinson, J. G., Hesselink, J. R., Kennedy, C. J., Richman, D. D., Spector, S. A., & McCutchan, J. A. (1987). Evidence for early central nervous system involvement in the acquired immunodeficiency syndrome and other HIV infections. *Annals of Internal Medicine, 107,* 828–836.

Grant, I., Heaton, R. K., Atkinson, J. H., Wiley, C. A., Kirson, D., Velin, R., Chandler, J., & McCutchan, J. A. (1992). HIV-1 associated neurocognitive disorder. *Clinical Neuropharmacology, 15*(Suppl. 1, Pt A), 364A–365A.

Gronwall, D. (1977). Paced Auditory Serial Addition Task: A measure of recovery from concussion. *Perceptual and Motor Skills, 44,* 367–373.

Hall, W. W., Farmer, P. M., Takahashi, Tanaka, S., Fututa, Y., & Nagashima, K. (1991). Pathological features of virus infections of the central nervous system (CNS) in the acquired immunodeficiency syndrome. *Japanese Society of Pathology, 41,* 172–181.

Halstead, W. D. (1947). *Brain and Intelligence.* Chicago: University of Chicago Press.

Heaton, R. K. (1983). *Wisconsin Card Sorting Test manual.* Odessa, FL: Psychological Assessment Resources.

Heaton, R. K., Grant, I., Butters, N., White, D. A., Kirson, D., Atkinson, J. H., McCutchan, J. A., Taylor, M. J., Kelly, M. D., Ellis, R. J., Wolfson, T., Velin, R., Marcotte, T. D., Hesselink, J. R., Jernigan, T. L., Chandler, J., Wallace, M., & Abrahamson, I. (1995). The HNRC 500: Neuropsychology of HIV infection at different disease stages. *Journal of the International Neuropsychological Society, 1,* 231–251.

Holland, N. R., Power, C., Mathews, V. P., Glass, J. D., Foreman, M., & McArthur, J. C. (1994). Cytomegalovirus encephalitis in acquired immunodeficiency syndrome (AIDS). *Neurology, 44,* 507–514.

Joffe, R. T., Rubinow, D. R., Squillace, K., Lane, C. H., Cuncan, C. C., & Fauci, A. S. (1986). Neuropsychiatric aspects of AIDS. *Psychopharmacology Bulletin,* 22(3), 684–688.

Johannessen, D. J., & Wilson, L. G. (1988). Mania with cryptococcal meningitis in two AIDS patients. *Journal of Clinical Psychiatry, 49,* 200–201.

Kaplan, E. F., Goodglass, H., & Weintraub, S. (1978). *The Boston Naming Test* (2nd ed.). Philadelphia: Lea & Febiger.

Kieburtz, K., Zettelmaier, A. E., Ketonen, L., Tuite, M., & Caine, E. D. (1991). Manic syndromes in AIDS. *American Journal of Psychiatry, 148*(8), 1068–1070.

Krikorian, R., Wrobel, A. J., Meinecke, C., Liang, W. M., & Kay, J. (1990). Cognitive deficits associated with human immunodeficiency virus encephalopathy. *Journal of Neuropsychiatry and Clinical Neurosciences, 2,* 256–260.

Liu, C. K., Miller, B. L., Cummings, J. L., Goldberg, M., Mehringer, C. M., Howng, S. L., & Benson, D. F. (1992). A quantitative MRI study of vascular dementia. *Neurology, 42,* 138–143.

Lyketsos, C. G., Hanson, A. L., Fishman, M., Rosenblatt, A., McHugh, P. R., & Treisman, G. J. (1993). Manic syndromes early and late in the course of HIV. *American Journal of Psychiatry, 150*(2), 326–327.

Maj, M. (1990). Organic mental disorders in HIV-1 infection. *AIDS, 4*(9), 831–840.

Maj, M., D'Elia, L., Satz, P., Janssen, R., Zaudig, M., Uchiyama, C., Starace, F., Galderisi, S., & Chervinsky, A. (1993). Evaluation of three new neuropsychological tests designed to minimize cultural bias in the assessment of HIV-1 seropositive persons: A WHO study. *Archives of Clinical Neuropsychology, 8,* 123–135.

Maj, M., Satz, P., Janssen, R., Zaudig, M., Starace, F., D'Dlia, L., Sughondhabirom, B., Mussa, M., Naber, D., Ndetei, D., Schulte, G., & Sartorius, N. (1994). WHO Neuropsychiatric AIDS Study, Cross-Sectional Phase II. *Archives of General Psychiatry, 51,* 51–61.

Marsh, N. V. & McCall, D. W. (1994). Early neuropsychological change in HIV infection. *Neuropsychology, 8*(1), 44–48.

Martin, E. M., Robertson, L. C., Edelstein, H. E., Jagust, W. J., Sorensen, D. J., San Giovanni, D., & Chirurgi, V. A. (1992). Performance of patients with early HIV-1 infection on the Stroop task. *Journal of Clinical and Experimental Neuropsychology, 14*(5), 857–868.

Maruff, P., Currie, J., Malone, V., McArthur-Jackson, C., Mulhall, B., & Benson, E. (1994). Neuropsychological characterization of the AIDS dementia complex and rationalization of a test battery. *Archives of Neurology, 51,* 689–695.

McArthur, J. C., Hoover, D. R., Bacellar, H., Miller, E. N., Cohen, B. A., Becker, J. T., Graham, N. M. H., McArthur, J. H., Selnes, O. A., Jacobson, L. P., Visscher, B. R., Concha, M., & Saah, A. (1993). Dementia in AIDS patients: Incidence and risk factors. *Neurology, 43,* 2245–2252.

McManis, S. E., Brown, G. R., Zachary, R., & Rundell, J. R. (1993). A screening test for subtle cognitive impairment early in the course of HIV infection. *Psychosomatics, 34*(5), 424–431.

Mega, M. S., & Cummings, J. L. (1994). Frontal–subcortical circuits and neuropsychiatric disorders. *Journal of Neuropsychiatry, 6*(4), 358–370.

Miller, E. N., Selnes, O. A., McArthur, J. C., Satz, P., Becker, J. T., Cohen, B. A., Sheridan, K., Machado, A. M., van Gorp, W. G., & Visscher, B. (1990). Neuropsychological performance in HIV-infected homosexual men: The Multicenter AIDS Cohort Study (MACS). *Neurology, 40,* 197–203.

Miller, J. R., Barrett, R. E., & Britton, C. B. (1982). Progressive multifocal leukoencephalopathy in a male homosexual with T-cell immune deficiency. *New England Journal of Medicine, 307,* 1436–1438.

Navia, B. A., Jordan, B. D., & Price, R. W. (1986a). The AIDS dementia complex: I. Clinical features. *Annals of Neurology, 19*(6), 517–524.

Navia, B. A., Petito, C. K., & Gold, J. W. (1986b). Cerebral toxoplasmosis complicating the acquired immune deficiency syndrome: Clinical and neuropathological findings in 27 patients. *Annals of Neurology, 19,* 224–238.

Nelson, H. E. (1982). National Adult Reading Test (NART): Test manual. Windsor, United Kingdom: NFER Nelson.

Ochitill, H. N., & Dilley, J. W. (1988). Neuropsychiatric aspects of acquired immunodeficiency syndrome. In M. L. Rosenblum, R. M. Levy, & D. E. Bredesen (Eds.), *AIDS and the nervous system* (pp. 315–325). New York: Raven Press.

O'Dowd, M. A., & McKegney, F. P. (1988). Manic syndrome associated with zidovudine. *Journal of the American Medical Association, 260,* 3587.

Ortego, J. N., Chang, L., Miller, B., Oropilla, G., Meyer, H., Satz, P., & Mena, I. (1994). Neurobehavioral and neuroimaging correlations in HIV-1-associated dementia complex. *Neurology, 44*(Suppl. 2), A248.

Perdices, M., & Cooper, D. A. (1990). Neuropsychological investigation of patients with AIDS and ARC. *Journal of Acquired Immune Deficiency Syndromes, 3*(6), 555–564.

Perriens, J. H., Mussa, M., Luabeya, M. S., Kayembe, K., Kapita, B., Brown, C., Piot, P., & Janssen, R. (1992). Neurological complications of HIV-1 seropositive internal medicine inpatients in Kinshasa, Zaire. *Journal of Acquired Immune Deficiency Syndromes, 5*(4), 333–340.

Pulliam, L., Herndier, B. G., Tang, N. M., & McGrath, M. (1991). Human immunodeficiency virus-infected macrophages produce soluable factors that cause histological and neurochemical alterations in cultured human brains. *Journal of Clinical Investigation, 81,* 503–512.

Rabkin, J. G., Ferrando, S. J., Jacobsberg, L. B., & Fishman, B. (1997). Prevalence of axis I disorders in an AIDS cohort: A cross sectional, controlled study. *Comprehensive Psychiatry, 38*(3), 146–154.

Raven, J. C. (1938). *Progressive Matrices: A perceptual test of intelligence (Individual Form)*. London: H. K. Lewis.

Reitan, R. M., & Wolfson, D. (1985). *The Halstead–Reitan Neuropsychological Test Battery: Theory and interpretation*. Tucson, AZ: Neuropsychology Press.

Rey, A. (1941). L'examen psychologique dans les cas d'encéphalopathie traumatique. *Archives de Psychologie, 28,* 286–340.

Rey, A. (1964). *L'examen clinique en psychologie*. Paris: Presses Universitaires de France.

Rottenberg, D. A., Moeller, J R., Strother, S. C., Sidtis, J. J., Navia, B. A., Dhawan, V., Ginos, J. Z., & Price, R. W. (1987). The metabolic pathology of the AIDS dementia complex. *Annals of Neurology, 22,* 700–706.

Rubinow, D. R., Berrettini, C. H., Brouwers, P., & Lane, H. C. (1988). Neuropsychiatric consequences of AIDS. *Annals of Neurology, 23*(Suppl.), S24–S26.

Sackter, N. C., Bacellar, H., Hoover, D. R., Nance-Sproson, T. E., Selnes, O. A., Miller, E. N., Dan Pan, G. J., Kleenberger, C., Brown, A., & Sash, A. (1996). Psychomotor slowing in HIV infection: A predictor of dementia, AIDS and death. *Journal of Neurobiology, 2*(6), 404–410.

Satz, P., Morgenstern, H., Miller, E. N., Selnes, O. A., McArthur, J. C., Cohern, B. A., Wesch, J., Becker, J. T., Jacobson, L., D'Elia, L. F., van Gorp, W., & Visscher, B. (1993). Low education as a possible risk factor for cognitive abnormalities in HIV-1: Findings from the Multicenter AIDS Cohort Study (MACS). *Journal of Acquired Immune Deficiency Syndromes, 6*(5), 503–511.

Saykin, A. J., Janssen, R. S., Sprehn, G. C., Kaplan, J. E., Spira, T. J., & Weller, P. (1988). Neuropsychological dysfunction in HIV-infection: Characterization in a lymphadenopathy cohort. *International Journal of Clinical Neuropsychology, 10*(2), 81–95.

Schmidt, U., & Miller, D. (1988). Two cases of hypomania in AIDS. *British Journal of Psychiatry, 152,* 839–842.

Seilhean, P., Duyckaerts, C., Vazeux, R., Bolgert, F., Brunet, P., Katlama, C., Gentilini, M., & Hauw, J. J. (1993). HIV-1 associated cognitive/motor complex: Absence of neuronal loss in the cerebral neocortex. *Neurology, 43*(8), 1492–1499.

Shaw, G. M., Harper, M. E., & Hahn, B. H. (1985). HTLV-III infection in brains of children and adults with AIDS encephalopathy. *Science, 227,* 177–182.

Sidtis, J. J., Amitai, H., Ornitz, D., & Price, R. W. (1988). Neuropsychological and neurological characterization of the AIDS dementia complex. *Journal of Clinical and Experimental Neuropsychology, 10*(1), 76. (Abstract)

Sidtis, J. J., Gatsonis, C., Price, R. W., Singer, E. J., Collier, A. C., Richman, D. D., Hirsch, M. S., Schaerf, F. W., Fisch, M. A., Kieburtz, K., Simpson, D., Kock, M. A., Feinberg, J., Dafni, U., & the AIDS Clinical Trials Group. (1993). Zidovudine treatment of the AIDS dementia complex: Results of a placebo-controlled trial. *Annals of Neurology, 33,* 342–349.

Sinforiani, E., Mauri, M., Bono, G., Murator, S., Alessi, E., & Minoli, L. (1991). Cognitive abnormalities and disease progression in a selected population of asymptomatic HIV positive subjects. *AIDS, 5,* 117–1120.

Spreen, O., & Benton, A. (1969). *Neurosensory Center Comprehensive Examination for Aphasia (NCCEA).* Victoria, British Columbia: University of Victoria, Neuropsychological Laboratory.

Stern, Y. (1994). Neuropsychological evaluation of the HIV patient. *Psychiatric Clinics of North America, 17*(1), 125–134.

Stern, Y., Marder, K., Bell, K., Chen, J., Doonief, G., Golstein, S., Mindry, D., Richards, M., Sano, M., Williams, J., Gorman, J., Ehrhardt, A., & Mayeux, R. (1991). Multi-disciplinary baseline assessment of homosexual men with and without human immunodeficiency virus infection: III. Neurologic and neuropsychological findings. *Archives of General Psychiatry, 48,* 131–138.

Stroop, J. R. (1935). Studies of interference in serial verbal reaction. *Journal of Experimental Psychology, 18,* 643–662.

Tiffin, J. (1968). *Purdue Grooved Pegboard: Examiner manual.* Chicago: Science Research Associates.

Tross, S., Price, R. W., Navia, B., Thaler, H. T., Gold, J., Hirsch, D.A., & Sidtis, J. J. (1988). Neuropsychological characterization of the AIDS dementia complex: A preliminary report. *AIDS, 2,* 81–88.

Turnbull, O., Saling, M. M., Kaplan-Solms, K., Cohn, R., & Schoub, B. (1991). Neuropsychological deficit in haemophiliacs with human immunodeficiency virus. *Journal of Neurology, Neurosurgery and Psychiatry, 54,* 175–177.

van Gorp, W. G., Miller, E. N., Satz, P., & Visscher, B. (1989a). Neuropsychological performance in HIV-1 immunocompromised patients: A preliminary report. *Journal of Clinical and Experimental Neuropsychology, 11*(5), 763–773.

van Gorp, W. G., Satz, P., Hinkin, C., Evans, G., & Miller, E. N. (1989b). The neuropsychological aspects of HIV-1 spectrum disease. *Psychiatric Medicine, 7*(2), 59–78.

Vinters, H. V., Kwok, M. K., & Ho, H. W. (1989). Cytomegalovirus in the nervous system of patients with the acquired immune deficiency syndrome. *Brain, 112,* 245–268.

Wechsler, D. (1981). *Wechsler Adult Intelligence Scale– Revised.* New York: Psychological Corporation.

Wechsler, D. (1987). *Wechsler Memory Scale–Revised.* New York: Psychological Corporation.

White, D. A., Heaton, R. K., & Monsch, A. U. (1995). Neuropsychological studies of asymptomatic human immunodeficiency virus-type-1 infected individuals. *Journal of the International Neuropsychological Society, 1,* 304–315.

Wiley, C. A., & Achim, C. L. (1995). Human immunodeficiency virus encephalitis and dementia. *Annals of Neurology, 38,* 559–560.

Wilkie, F. L., Morgan, R., Fletcher, M. A., Blaney, N., Baum, M., Komaroff, E., Szapocznik, J., & Eisdorfer, C. (1992). Cognition and immune function in HIV-1 infection. *AIDS, 6,* 977–981.

Wilkins, J. W., Robertson, K. R., Van der Horst, C., Robertson, W. T., Fryer, J. G., & Hall, C. D. (1990). The importance of confounding changes in patients infected with human immunodeficiency virus. *Journal of Acquired Immune Deficiency Syndromes, 3*(10), 938–942.

Wilkinson, I. D., Chinn, R. T., Jall-Craggs, M. A., Kendall, B. E., Paley, M. N., Plummer, D. L., Miller, R. F., & Harrison, M. J. (1996). Sub-cortical white-grey matter contrast on MRI as a quantitative marker of diffuse HIV-rekated parenchymal abnormality. *Clinical Radiology, 51*(7), 475–479.

Williams, J. G., Rabkin, J. B., Remien, R. H., Gorman, J. M., & Ehrhardt, A. A. (1991). Multidisciplinary baseline assessment of homosexual men with and without human immunodeficiency virus infection: II. Standardized clinical assessment of current and lifetime psychopathology. *Archives of General Psychiatry, 48*(2), 124–130.

3

Differential Diagnosis of HIV-1 Neurological Disease

ELYSE J. SINGER

INTRODUCTION

Mental health professionals who work with HIV-1-infected clients encounter neuropsychiatric problems that cut across disciplinary boundaries. An approach to such problems incorporates the neurological and medical aspects of HIV, as well as the psychiatric, psychological, and social approaches traditionally employed in mental health settings.

Why should busy therapists learn about the effects of HIV on the central nervous system (CNS)? All too often, HIV-related neuropsychiatric problems are deemed to be untreatable (see the case report below). This attitude is dangerously out of date. However, an early diagnosis is essential for people with HIV/AIDS to benefit from modern therapy.

Mental health professionals are often the first persons consulted by HIV-infected clients for such problems as pain, sleep disorders, altered level of consciousness, and cognitive dysfunction. These clients may lack the knowledge and resources to obtain treatment for such symptoms and depend upon their therapists for guidance in seeking care. Therapists on the "front line" of HIV/AIDS care may be asked to evaluate patients for possible organic causes of their behavioral abnormalities and to make referrals to other professionals.

This chapter outlines an approach to the differential diagnosis of HIV-1 neurological disease for the nonphysician mental health professional. Case reports illustrate many of the points made. First, important aspects of the natural medical and neurological history of HIV/AIDS are reviewed briefly. Next, the basic diagnostic approach is outlined; questions about the factors discussed here can be incorporated into a therapist's existing psychological and social evaluation. The following section includes brief descriptions of common HIV-related CNS diseases that may present with behavioral changes, together with descriptions of diagnostic procedures and treatments. However, the HIV-1 field is evolving so rapidly that treatment information may be out of date within a few months. Thus, information on current treatment regimens should be confirmed by consultation with an appropriate professional.

CASE REPORT

Mr. W, a 47-year-old man with AIDS, was brought to an HIV clinic by a friend in June 1997. The friend stated that Mr. W had tested HIV-seropositive in 1986, but had not sought treatment because he had no symptoms. In 1990, Mr. W began to abuse cocaine and alcohol. From 1990 to 1992, Mr. W gradually became rude, inappropriate, loud, disruptive, intrusive, and disheveled. In June 1992, Mr. W stopped working. Shortly thereafter, he began to make frequent, repetitive telephone calls at all hours to his friends; he would apparently forget these calls as soon as they were finished. Mr. W was also banned from his community center because he fought with other patrons.

His behavior was attributed to drug and alcohol abuse.

In December 1992, Mr. W was taken to a psychiatric hospital because of bizarre behavior and inability to care for himself. His family was informed that Mr. W had "schizophrenia" and "AIDS encephalopathy," that there was no treatment available, and that Mr. W would die within 6 months. Mr. W was then treated with antipsychotic medication to control his outbursts and discharged to a hospice. For the next 5 years he was shuffled in and out of several hospices and chronic care facilities. During that time he gradually became incontinent and lost the ability to walk, but he received no HIV-specific treatment of any kind.

In 1997, an old friend visited Mr. W, who was residing in a locked nursing home. The friend insisted that Mr. W receive medical care from an HIV specialist, and escorted him to the clinic.

On examination, Mr. W was thin and "wasted." He had fungal infections of his mouth, skin, and nails, but no other HIV-related infections or tumors. Despite his medical condition, Mr. W was alert, unconcerned, and cheerful, with a euphoric demeanor. Formal testing was difficult, because Mr. W was easily distracted and would interrupt the testing to make crude comments. He was oriented to name but not to date or place. His speech was sparse, mildly dysarthric, loud, and punctuated by inappropriate remarks. Mr. W could not remember his Social Security number, his friend's last name, or any of three words after 3 minutes. He was unable to perform all but the simplest calculations. He could read simple words slowly, correctly name most of the objects that he was shown, and distinguish right from left. His handwriting was illegible, and he was unable to copy simple figures. Mr. W could not walk without assistance. His legs were weak and spastic, with hyperactive deep tendon reflexes. He had prominent frontal release signs (snout, jaw jerk, palmomental, and grasp). Mr. W also had repetitive lip-smacking movements.

Mr. W was severely immunodeficient, with a CD4 cell count of 41 cells/mm^3 (normal 500–1,200), and an HIV viral load of 200,000 copies/ml (normal is nondetectable). A brain magnetic resonance imaging scan (MRI) showed severe atrophy. Tests of blood and cerebrospinal fluid (CSF) revealed no pathogens other than HIV.

Mr. W was diagnosed with severe HIV-1-associated dementia complex. This diagnosis was based on the presence of progressive cognitive impairment (dementia), central motor dysfunction (weakness, spasticity, incoordination), and behavioral changes (uninhibited and inappropriate behavior), as well as on the absence of any other probable organic cause for his symptoms. Mr. W's frontal systems appeared to have been preferentially affected, resulting in his distractible, impulsive, and uninhibited behavior.

Mr. W's new physicians concluded that his behavioral problems had been the initial manifestation of HIV-1-associated dementia complex, exacerbated by drug and alcohol abuse. However, he had continued to deteriorate despite 5 years of enforced sobriety. Schizophrenia was unlikely because the patient exhibited no evidence of a thought disorder, had had an excellent level of functioning well into adult life, and had no family history of mental illness. Mr. W also had tardive dyskinesia from antipsychotic medications.

After several weeks of highly active antiretroviral therapy (HAART), Mr. W gained weight and was able to participate in physical therapy. He began to walk with a cane, to recognize family members, and to engage in short conversations. However, he continued to require constant supervision and never regained the ability to live independently.

NATURAL HISTORY

HIV-1 enters the brain early during the initial or "primary" HIV infection (the process that precedes seroconversion). The evidence for "early penetration" includes a case in which an HIV-negative patient was accidentally transfused with HIV-infected white blood cells (WBCs) (Davis et al., 1992). The patient died of unrelated causes 2 weeks later. An autopsy revealed abundant HIV within his brain. Autopsies of asymptomatic, neurologically normal HIV-infected persons who died in accidents also demonstrated HIV in their brains. Up to 90% of asymptomatic, neurologically normal HIV+ adults have abnormalities in their CSF (the clear fluid that surrounds the brain and spinal cord), such as elevated CSF WBC count, total protein, and antibody synthesis (Marshall, Brey, & Cahill, 1988; Singer et al., 1994b, 1994c). These laboratory abnormalities are markers for HIV infection of the CNS, although they do not indicate clinical CNS disease. Studies using polymerase chain reaction (PCR, a technique that can detect very small amounts of viral nucleic acids) found evidence of HIV in the CSF of up to 90% of all HIV-infected persons (Schmid et al., 1994).

The mere presence of HIV in the CNS does not correlate with clinical neurological disease. Almost all HIV-infected persons have HIV in their CNS, but all HIV-infected persons do not develop neurological disease. There are a number of hypotheses to explain why some individuals are more likely to develop neurologic problems, such as infection by a strain of HIV that preferentially replicates in the brain; the presence of "activated" macrophages (scavenger WBCs that can enter the brain), which can secrete neurotoxic substances; higher levels of HIV within the CNS of neurologically abnormal persons; an accumulation of viral proteins that are toxic to CNS cells; or the accumulation of by-products of inflammation that are toxic to CNS cells and alter CNS metabolism (Lipton & Gendelman, 1995).

APPROACH TO HIV-1-ASSOCIATED
NEUROLOGICAL DISEASE

Mental health professionals are often asked to determine whether aberrant behavior is caused by HIV neurological disease, as opposed to an unrelated psychiatric disorder or substance use. Several HIV-related CNS disorders may present with changes in behavior. The most extensively studied changes have been those associated with cognitive dysfunction, but there are also reports of AIDS patients presenting with

the new onset of depressive, manic, or schizophrenic symptoms, attributed to HIV infection (Cummings, Cummings, Rapaport, Atkinson, &
Grant, 1987; Horwath, Kramer, Cournos, Empfield, & Gewirtz, 1989;
Lyketsos et al., 1993; Thomas & Szabadi, 1987). However, other authors
have critiqued the hypothesis that HIV infection plays a causal role in
new-onset mental illness (Vogel-Scibilia, Mulsant, & Keshavan, 1988).

Host Factors

Investigators have searched for demographic or constitutional host
characteristics or "risk factors" that could be used to identify individuals
at high risk for HIV neurological disease. Increased age has been
associated with HIV-1-associated dementia (Janssen, Nwanyanwu, Selik,
& Stehr-Green, 1992). A higher level of education, and an individual's
"cognitive reserve," appear to have a protective effect against neuropsychological impairment; however, education may be a surrogate for
other factors that have not been evaluated (Maj et al., 1994; Satz et al.,
1993; Stern, Silva, Chaisson, & Evans, 1996). Zidovudine (AZT) use may
provide some protection against the development of HIV-associated
dementia (Gray et al., 1994; Portegies et al., 1989). Injection drug use,
alcohol, head injury, gender, smoking, and nutritional status have also
been studied, and are less consistently associated with an increased risk
of HIV-associated dementia and other neurological diseases (Bornstein
et al., 1993; Chiesi et al., 1995; Conley et al., 1996; Egan, Crawford,
Brettle, & Goodwin, 1990; Herzlich & Schiano, 1993; Marder et al.,
1992; Selnes et al., 1992).

Other Risk Factors

The majority of individuals with HIV CNS disease have advanced HIV
systemic disease (McArthur et al., 1989; Miller, Satz, & Visscher, 1991),
and they are the most likely to have a brain infection or tumor
masquerading as a behavioral problem. A therapist can briefly assess a
client's risk for HIV CNS diseases by asking about specific HIV-related
medical illnesses and the results of key laboratory tests. This information can be elicited during the intake session or by means of a
preinterview checklist, and can be confirmed by the medical record.
Ascertainment of this specific information is preferable to asking
open-ended questions about the client's health, because such questions
tend to elicit highly subjective answers. Likewise, attempts to determine
the length of time that the client has been HIV-seropositive may also
elicit misleading information, because most people get tested for HIV

years after they actually become infected. Even if the date of infection is known, disease progression varies among individuals. The following areas should be included in the initial evaluation.

AIDS-Defining Illnesses

The therapist should ask the client about his or her previous HIV-1-associated diseases. The therapist may need to prompt the client by naming a few of the "AIDS-defining" diagnoses listed by the Centers for Disease Control (and Prevention) (CDC), or by giving the client a checklist of these before the interview (CDC, 1986, 1987, 1992). Most of these illnesses are opportunistic infections such as *Pneumocystis carinii* pneumonia, or malignancies such as lymphoma. AIDS-defining illnesses increase the risk for CNS disease. One study has correlated weight loss, low body mass, anemia, and low serum albumin (an index of poor nutritional status) with HIV-associated dementia (McArthur, Selnes, Glass, Hoover, & Bacellar, 1994).

Immune Status

The therapist should ask for the client's most recent CD4 cell count (absolute number and/or percentage of CD4 cells in the blood). The CD4 cell is a type of WBC or T cell that plays a major role in maintaining cell-mediated immunity, and it is a major target for destruction by HIV. A normal adult CD4 cell count typically ranges from 500 to 1,200 cells/mm^3, with a mean of about 900. A CD4 count below 200 cells/mm^3 (over two standard deviations below the mean) has been used as one definition of AIDS. More importantly, the risk of an AIDS-defining infection, tumor, or CNS disease increases greatly when the CD4 cell count dips below 200 cells/mm^3.

Clients who are treated with HAART may have their CD4 cell count increase dramatically after treatment. It is not known whether these new CD4 cells are as effective in preventing infections as the patient's original CD4 cells. Therefore, it may be useful to ask about the client's lowest CD4 cell count as well.

Viral Load

The therapist should also ask for the results of the client's most recent HIV "viral load" test. "Viral load" refers to the quantity of HIV-1 present in body tissues. The most commonly tested tissue is the plasma (clear liquid) portion of peripheral blood. Viral load is measured by the quantitative ribonucleic acid (RNA) PCR test or by the branched-chain deoxyribonucleic acid (bDNA) assay, and is expressed as the number of copies per milliliter.

Plasma viral load is a sensitive indicator of HIV-1 disease progression (Mellors et al., 1997). Patients with a "high" HIV viral load (usually defined as over 20,000 copies/ml) are at the greatest risk for progression to AIDS, whereas those with a "low" viral load (usually defined as under 5,000 copies/ml) are at less risk (Ferre et al., 1995; Hufert et al., 1991; Hughes et al., 1997; Mueller et al., 1996; Mullis & Faloona, 1987). The viral load also reflects the efficacy of antiretroviral therapy (O'Brien et al., 1997). A significant decrease (by at least one log) in the viral load is considered a favorable response to therapy (Hughes et al., 1997) , whereas a lesser decrease or an increase in the viral load may indicate that the drugs are ineffective or that the patient is not taking them properly.

Blood, or plasma, contains only a small fraction of total body HIV. Most HIV is located in lymph nodes or other tissues, and is not measured by testing the plasma (Mueller et al., 1996). In particular, HIV in the CNS may differ significantly from HIV in the blood in quantity and strain. It is not feasible to perform biopsies to measure the amount of HIV in the brain. Therefore, a number of tests—including the viral load in the CSF (which can be easily measured), neuroimaging tests, and neuropsychological tests—have been studied as substitutes for directly measuring the HIV activity in the CNS.

Several cross-sectional studies indicate that subjects with HIV-associated neurological disease have higher mean viral loads in blood and in CSF than do HIV-infected persons without neurological disease (Brew, Pemberton, Cunningham, & Law, 1997; Conrad et al., 1995; Ginocchio, Kaplan, & Wang, 1995; Pratt et al., 1996; Schmid et al., 1994; Sei et al., 1996). Although these differences have not always reached statistical significance, they support the relationship between higher levels of HIV replication and clinical neurological disease.

Differential Diagnosis

CNS diseases associated with HIV-1 infection have been categorized as primary HIV-1 neurological disease (disease due to HIV alone), or as secondary HIV-1 associated neurological disease (opportunistic infections and tumors associated with immunodeficiency). Prior to the AIDS epidemic, the latter were seen in immunodeficient individuals with leukemia, cancer, and organ transplants. In addition, adverse drug reactions, intoxication, delirium, sepsis (severe systemic infection), hypoxia (inadequate oxygen), inadequate nutrition, and premorbid neuropsychiatric diseases can all be mistaken for HIV CNS disease.

CASE REPORT

Mr. G, a 55-year-old HIV-infected attorney, was referred for evaluation of dementia associated with HIV. His major symptoms were short-term memory loss, insomnia, and fatigue. Mr. G's current CD4 cell count was 360, and his viral load was undetectable. There were no physical abnormalities consistent with systemic or neurological disease, and his brain MRI was normal. Mr. G was noted to be lethargic and emotionally labile. His daily medication was then reviewed. His usual regimen, prescribed by four different physicians, included three different benzodiazepines for insomnia and anxiety, four opiates for pain, an antihistamine for sinusitis, a tricyclic antidepressant, and two "muscle relaxers." Mr. G's memory problems improved after he was weaned from these medications.

Focal versus Nonfocal Presentation

There are many HIV-related neurological diseases, and only a few are covered here. Differential diagnosis requires that the therapist formulate a list of the most likely causes for a client's neuropsychiatric problem. This can require the memorization of a large amount of material, or the therapist may choose to obtain selected information about key clinical features of the client's case and to match them against the most common presentations of the most common HIV-related CNS diseases. (This approach may not be very helpful if the client has a rare disease or an atypical presentation of a common disease, but such persons usually require an extended evaluation from a specialist.)

Some CNS diseases, such as toxoplasmosis, are characterized by "focal" lesions, which selectively damage one or more areas of tissue while sparing other areas. In contrast, delirium, sepsis, and most toxic/metabolic problems or diffuse CNS infections are "nonfocal" (i.e., they affect diffuse areas of the brain).

Likewise, diseases such as HIV-associated cognitive/motor complex (HIV CMC) typically present with symmetrical (bilateral) deficits, which affect the right and left sides of the brain equally. In contrast, diseases such as progressive multifocal leukoencephalopathy (PML) tend to begin in an asymmetrical fashion, with one side or site affected more severely than its counterpart. Deficits in cortical function (such as aphasia, agnosia, and apraxia) are common features of PML. In contrast, HIV CMC typically presents with subcortical deficits (such as motor slowing or tremor).

The time course (acute, subacute, or chronic) of different CNS diseases varies with different pathogens. HIV CMC typically has a chronic course, in which deficits worsen over months or even years. In a few instances patients may decompensate rapidly over a period of days, but this decompensation is usually triggered by a systemic infection and may spontaneously improve when the infection clears (Navia, Jordan, & Price, 1986b). In contrast, the deficits of PML may progress over days, and the mean time from onset to death is 4 months.

CASE REPORT

Mr. J, a 42-year-old man with AIDS, was admitted to the hospital with a low-grade fever and altered mental status. His family stated that Mr. J had been restless and irritable for 2 days. On the day of admission he forgot to turn off a faucet, flooding his apartment. Mr. J was on disability because of fatigue and wasting, but had no known history of CNS symptoms. His admission MRI showed mild atrophy, and his CSF showed no pathogens other than HIV.

During the first 2 days of hospitalization, Mr. J developed more cognitive dysfunction, accompanied by leg weakness, stiffness, tremor, and mutism. A neurologist thought Mr. J had manifestations of HIV-associated dementia complex, but thought that this diagnosis was inconsistent with the rapid evolution of symptoms. On the third day, Mr. J developed shaking chills and a high fever, determined to be caused by a bacterial infection of his kidneys. After several days of antibiotic treatment, Mr. J's neurological problems improved. Subsequently, he confided that he had been forgetful for over 6 months. The neurologist concluded that Mr. J had probably met the criteria for mild HIV-associated dementia complex well before the onset of his acute illness, and that he had decompensated in the setting of a systemic infection.

Is This an Emergency?

There are few situations in which HIV serostatus directly affects the immediate management of a neurological or mental health emergency. Suicidality, coma, delirium, or seizures require an emergency evaluation in any patient. The immediate goal of emergency management is to protect the patient's life, and HIV does not alter that management.

COMMON HIV-RELATED CNS DISEASES

HIV Aseptic Meningitis

"Meningitis" refers to inflammation of the meninges (membranes that surround the brain and spinal cord). The most common cause of meningitis is an infection. Historically, the term "aseptic meningitis" described cases in which bacteria could not be detected in the CSF. This term also implied that there was no actual tissue damage to the brain (encephalitis) or the spinal cord (myelitis), and that the illness was expected to follow a relatively benign course.

HIV aseptic meningitis usually presents in an acute or subacute fashion, with nonfocal symptoms of severe headache, with or without a stiff neck and fever (Hollander & Stringari, 1987). Less commonly, aseptic meningitis may cause focal signs by damaging one or more of the cranial nerves, most commonly cranial nerve VII (in this case, it is known as Bell's palsy). Any meningitis may cause delirium or lethargy.

Unlike most of the CNS diseases to be discussed here, HIV-1 associated aseptic meningitis may occur early in the course of infection. For example, it may be a part of the primary infection syndrome, which is also characterized by fever, rash, swollen lymph nodes, sore throat, muscle pains, diarrhea, and other "flu-like" symptoms (Ho et al., 1985). The HIV antibody test may be negative during this period, although HIV may be detected by viral culture, PCR, or antigen testing.

The syndrome of HIV-1 aseptic meningitis resembles other types of viral meningitis. For this reason, all cases of aseptic meningitis should be tested for HIV. However, the initial symptoms of aseptic meningitis cannot be reliably distinguished from those of bacterial, fungal, or tubercular meningitis, which are potentially life-threatening. Meningitis is a medical emergency.

The diagnostic evaluation for meningitis begins with a neuroimaging scan, such as a computerized tomography (CT) or MRI scan, to identify any focal brain masses or brain edema (swelling) that might precipitate brain herniation (shift and compression of brain tissue associated with unequally distributed pressure within the brain, which is a cause of potential brain damage or death). In such situations, it may be unsafe to perform a lumbar puncture (spinal tap), a procedure used to sample CSF and measure CSF pressure. The CSF is analyzed for its WBC count, red blood cell count, total protein, and glucose. Depending on the suspected pathogen, the evaluation may include bacterial, fungal, and acid fast bacterial (AFB) cultures; serological tests for such diseases as syphilis and toxoplasmosis; or PCR tests for various viruses. Cytological tests can be performed to detect malignant cells in the CSF if cancer is suspected.

The typical CSF findings in HIV meningitis include an elevated (over 5 cells/mm^3) WBC count, which is usually composed of lymphocytes; an elevated CSF total protein (due to the elevated production of antibodies within the CNS, and the increased permeability of the blood–brain barrier to proteins from the blood); a normal or slightly low glucose; and an absence of other pathogens (Marshall et al., 1988; Singer et al., 1994c). There is no specific treatment for HIV-1 meningitis, although antiretroviral medications, pain medications, and steroids have been used empirically. Most persons have a single episode and recover completely with supportive care (bed rest, control of fever, intravenous hydration). In some patients HIV meningitis has been reported to recur and remit for several years.

CASE REPORT

> Mr. P was a 36-year-old bisexual male who presented to the emergency room with fever, nausea, and a severe headache 6 weeks after unprotected anal intercourse. On examination, Mr. P had swollen lymph nodes, a stiff neck, a sore throat, and a rash. His brain CT scan was normal. The CSF exam showed a WBC count of 25 cells/mm^3 (normal less than 5), elevated total protein of 59 (normal less than 45), and a normal glucose. Tests for syphilis, bacteria, fungi, and tuberculosis were all negative. An HIV antibody test was negative; however, a PCR test for HIV was positive. Mr. P was admitted to the hospital and treated for his pain, fever, and dehydration. After his discharge, he reported similar but less severe episodes of headache and stiff neck for the next 3 years.

HIV-1-Associated Cognitive/Motor Complex

HIV CMC is the most common HIV-related neurological problem found in most clinical and pathologic series. Previously, the syndrome was known by other names, including "subacute encephalitis," "HIV-related encephalopathy," and "AIDS dementia complex" (CDC, 1987; Navia, Cho, Petito, & Price, 1986a; Snider et al., 1983). The term "HIV CMC" was developed by the American Academy of Neurology (AAN) AIDS Task Force as part of a standardized nomenclature to define and study HIV-1-related neurological illnesses (AAN, 1991). The older terms did not provide research case definitions for the various diseases, and did not distinguish individuals with disabling cognitive impairment from individuals in whom the degree of cognitive impairment was minimal, and who did not meet the usual criteria for a dementia. Likewise, the older terms did not separate cases that predominantly involved the spinal cord (HIV-1-associated myelopathy) without significant cognitive impairment from those that primarily involved the brain. These distinctions are not merely semantic. The term "dementia" has frightening associations for many patients, as well as significant medicolegal repercussions. A "demented" person may be restricted from driving a car or from making independent decisions about such issues as medical care and finances. In addition, the older definitions were never validated, whereas the AAN nomenclature has been validated in a clinical study (Dana Consortium, 1996). A more complete discussion of these issues is found in Chapter 1 of this book.

HIV CMC is a syndrome characterized by cognitive, central motor, and behavioral changes; it typically presents in persons with advanced HIV-1 infection. In its more severe form (HIV-1-associated dementia complex), it is considered an AIDS-defining diagnosis (CDC, 1987). The diagnosis of HIV CMC remains a clinical diagnosis; it can be made when an HIV-infected person has sufficient characteristic clinical abnormalities, *and* the laboratory tests for other common causes of cognitive and motor dysfunction (such as thyroid disease, vitamin B_{12} deficiency, syphilis, CNS opportunistic infections, and CNS tumors) are negative or normal.

HIV CMC typically presents in a subacute or chronic fashion (over weeks to years). Occasionally, patients will decompensate rapidly during a systemic infection (Lopez et al., 1996). The deficits in HIV CMC patients usually involve both sides of the brain in a symmetrical fashion.

The most common cognitive deficits in HIV CMC are short-term memory loss, decreased concentration and attention span, problems with word finding, slowed thought processing, slowed psychomotor speed, and problems in executive function. In the late stages of disease, patients develop problems with visual–spatial function (Navia et al., 1986b). These deficits are localized to the subcortical and frontal systems of the brain. Severely impaired persons may develop mutism. The cognitive deficits may fluctuate in severity, especially in early disease. Because they can be subtle, the first symptoms of HIV CMC are often attributed to anxiety, depression, or the fatigue of systemic illness. In particular, a patient's psychomotor slowing may be misidentified as a symptom of depression.

The central motor deficits (sometimes called "upper motor neuron" lesions in the neurological literature) of HIV CMC are caused by lesions within the brain or spinal cord (Navia et al., 1986a, 1986b). In contrast, peripheral motor deficits ("lower motor neuron" lesions) are caused by damage to the peripheral nerves after they exit the spinal cord, or to the muscles. Both central and peripheral motor deficits are associated with weakness. However, central motor lesions are usually associated with increased motor tone (stiffness, rigidity, spasticity, or "cogwheeling" in the extremities). In contrast, peripheral nerve damage is associated with decreased motor tone (floppiness). Central motor lesions are associated with increased tendon reflexes or hyperreflexia (e.g., very brisk, rapid reflexes or spread of the muscle contraction to an adjacent muscle group) or with clonus (more than one muscle contraction after only one percussion of a muscle tendon). Clinically, these neurological deficits can result in painful spasms, inability to flex the legs, or a stiff, abnormal gait. Peripheral motor lesions (peripheral neuropathy) are characterized by decreased tendon reflexes or hyporeflexia (slow, weak, or absent reflexes) and by a floppy gait often associated with a foot drop.

The earliest motor abnormality in HIV CMC is typically a gradual slowing of movement and speed. This slowing may be so subtle at first that it can only be demonstrated by serial neuropsychological testing or timed motor tests. Another early problem is a breakdown in motor control or coordination. Patients may experience this as a lack of control of fine hand movement, exemplified by sloppy or illegible handwriting, difficulty with fastening buttons, or inability to thread a needle. Other common complaints include loss of balance, "drifting" to one side when walking, or falling. As the disease progresses, involuntary movements such as tremor or jerking may occur. The upper motor neuron deficits may cause a loss of ability to relax the muscle tone in the legs, leading to painful involuntary muscle spasms or contractures. Loss of voluntary motor control over bowel and bladder function may cause incontinence.

Behavioral disturbances are not required for a diagnosis of HIV CMC. However, changes in personality are frequently cited by patients and their families as the earliest and most disturbing aspects of this disease. Patients with advanced HIV CMC typically develop severe slowing of motor and thought processes. The loss of function in the muscles of facial expression gives the appearance of a "flat" affect. This in turn gives the impression of a depressive disorder, although feelings of guilt, worthlessness, sadness, or hopelessness are often absent. Slowing of thought processes can be interpreted as apathy, poor concentration, and loss of drive (Navia et al., 1986b). Patients with HIV CMC often appear to be withdrawn and quiet. If they frequently forget their medication, they may be labeled "noncompliant." Because many language skills (e.g., speech, reading, and comprehension) are relatively well preserved, patients with HIV CMC can often compensate for their deficits, and may elude attention until they become severely demented. A relatively small group of persons with HIV CMC present with "manic" symptoms. They are easily agitated and restless, have poor impulse control, and tend to be talkative but to have difficulty concentrating or focusing on a topic. Some of these patients become suspicious, paranoid, delusional, or even grandiose. Persons with HIV CMC who present with these "manic" symptoms draw attention to themselves quickly and are usually referred to a mental health professional. In particular, those patients with poor impulse control who are physically mobile are difficult to manage, because they may have aggressive, hypersexual, or belligerent behavior that can only be managed in a supervised environment. However, such patients are notoriously difficult to place and may require chemical restraints.

In summary, HIV-1-associated dementia complex resembles other "subcortical" dementias, such as those associated with Parkinson's disease and Huntington's chorea. In these illnesses, central motor dysfunction plays a prominent and early role. In contrast, the "cortical" dementias, typified by Alzheimer's disease, are associated with aphasia (disturbance in the comprehension or expression of language), agnosia (loss of ability to identify, comprehend the meaning of, or recognize the importance of various types of sensory stimulation, despite intact primary sensory modalities and otherwise normal cognitive function), apraxia (difficulty in performing a motor task in the absence of significant weakness or sensory loss), and other cortical functions.

Patients with dementia and other CNS disorders are at increased risk for delirium associated with adverse drug reactions, toxins, metabolic changes such as hypoxia (a lack of oxygen, such as occurs with pneumonia), or sepsis. HIV-associated neurological problems may be exacerbated by other infections, even if the brain is not directly involved (Lopez et al., 1996). Demented patients who become agitated or delirious are often given dopamine-blocking drugs to control their behavior. However, an increased incidence of drug-induced parkinsonism, other extrapyramidal movement disorders, and neuroleptic malignant syndrome has been reported in AIDS patients treated with dopamine-blocking drugs (Breitbart, Marotta, & Call, 1988; Hollander, Golden, Mendelson, & Cortland, 1985; Hriso, Kuhn, Masdeu, & Grundman, 1991).

Neuroimaging, blood, and CSF tests are part of the evaluation of HIV CMC, primarily in order to identify or exclude other treatable causes of CNS disease. Neuroimaging is important because of the need to identify structural brain lesions, such as brain tumors. Brain MRI is preferable to CT in AIDS patients. MRI involves no radiation; it is also more sensitive than CT in the detection of AIDS-related brain lesions. The MRI contrast material (gadolinium) has fewer adverse effects than does the iodine-containing CT contrast, which is associated with more frequent allergic reactions and with renal damage. However, patient movement may produce MRI artifacts that are impossible to interpret. The MRI magnet attracts magnetic metal devices such as pacemakers, so that patients with such devices cannot be scanned safely. A CT scan is preferable when the patient is restless, or if the scan must be performed very quickly. Despite the medical and scientific reasons for choosing a specific test, many institutions make this decision on a purely financial basis.

The CT or MRI scan in HIV CMC may be normal, or it may show atrophy of the cerebral hemispheres, enlarged ventricles (the large spaces within the brain that contain CSF), and/or patchy white matter disease. Scans that evaluate brain function (as opposed to structure) have also been used to study patients with HIV CMC. These include tests of cerebral blood flow (single-photon emission computed tomography, or SPECT), glucose metabolism (positron emission tomography, or PET), and "functional" MRI (Chang, 1995; Chang et al., 1995; Kuni et al., 1991; Menon et al., 1992; Post et al., 1988, 1992; Rottenberg et al., 1987). These scans may demonstrate physiological abnormalities (e.g., reduced cerebral blood flow) in persons with a "normal" routine brain CT or MRI.

Most patients with HIV-1 infection have abnormal CSF laboratory values (Marshall et al., 1988; Singer et al., 1994c) regardless of the presence or absence of neurological disease. The most common abnormalities include an elevated CSF WBC count, an elevated CSF total protein, elevated antibody synthesis, and elevations on tests (such as ß-2-microglobulin and neopterin) that are nonspecific measures of inflammation (Brew et al., 1989, 1990; Marshall et al., 1988; Singer et al., 1994b, 1994c). The quantitative p24 antigen test (which measures a protein made during viral replication) and the quantitative HIV PCR are often elevated in persons with HIV CMC, as well as in other HIV-related CNS infections (Fiala et al., 1993; Royal, Selnes, Concha, Nance-Sproson, & McArthur, 1994; Singer et al., 1994b). However, the most important reason for performing a CSF exam is to exclude other diseases, including syphilis, cryptococcal meningitis, toxoplasmosis, CNS lymphoma, and cytomegalovirus encephalitis. In the future, neuroimaging and CSF studies may be used to measure more disease-specific markers of HIV CMC, in order to follow disease progression and response to antiretroviral therapy.

Few controlled studies have been performed on antiretroviral therapy of HIV CMC, although there are several open or retrospective studies. Most of these studies have concentrated on zidovudine, and were conducted in the first 10 years of the AIDS epidemic. They did not adequately address the impact of factors now thought to be important in the pharmacological treatment of HIV CMC, such as the ability of the drug to penetrate the CNS, the development of resistance to antiretroviral drugs, and the impact of combination antiretroviral therapy.

Two double-blind, randomized, placebo-controlled studies found that zidovudine, given as a single antiretroviral therapy in oral doses of at least 1,000 mg per day, improved cognitive and motor function (as measured by neuropsychological test scores) both in unselected adults with AIDS or AIDS-related complex and in adults selected for HIV CMC (Schmitt et al., 1988; Sidtis et al., 1993). A retrospective study of AIDS dementia in The Netherlands suggested that the incidence of HIV CMC fell sharply after the introduction of zidovudine (1,000 mg per day) for the treatment of AIDS (Portegies et al., 1989, 1993). Several series reported clinical, neuropsychological, neuropathological, neuroepidemiological, neuroimaging, or neurovirological improvement in the CNS of zidovudine-treated patients (Brivio, Tornaghi, Musetti, Marchisio, & Principi, 1991; Brunetti et al., 1989; Chiesi et al., 1995; de Gans et al., 1988; DeCarli et al., 1989; Grafman et al., 1989; Gray et al., 1994; Maehlen et al., 1995; Portegies et al., 1989; Tozzi et al., 1993; Vago et al., 1993) although these effects were sometimes transient (Chiesi et al., 1995; Sidtis et al., 1993).

Open-label studies of the drug dideoxyinosine (didanosine; ddI) in HIV-infected children with progressive encephalopathy (the pediatric equivalent of HIV CMC) found that there was an improvement in neurological and neuropsychological function with treatment, and that this appeared to be dose-related (Butler et al., 1991). However, more serious adverse effects occurred at the higher doses.

A controlled study suggested that the effectiveness of zidovudine in the treatment of HIV CMC increased as a function of dose (2,000 mg orally per day appeared to be more effective than 1,000 mg per day), although the now-standard dose (600 mg per day) was not evaluated (Sidtis et al., 1993). However, this observation has been challenged. There is also some evidence that drugs that better CNS penetration (as indicated by a higher CSF-to-blood or brain-to-blood ratio) are more effective in the treatment of HIV CMC. For example, a study that compared HIV-infected adults treated with either zidovudine or ddI found that the risk of HIV CMC was higher in the ddI-treated subjects than in those who received zidovudine (Vella et al., 1994). Another study reported that subjects treated with zidovudine had lower levels of HIV in their CSF than did those treated with ddI (Sei et al., 1996). The antiretroviral drugs ddI, dideoxycytidine (ddC), saquinivir, and ritonavir appear to have relatively low penetration into the CNS, whereas stavudine (D4T), zidovudine (AZT), nevirapine (Viramune), and delavirdine (Rescriptor) have higher levels (Abbott Laboratories, 1994; Blaney, Daniel, Harker, Godwin, & Balis, 1995; Bristol-Myers Squibb, 1992; Burger et al., 1993, 1995; Devineni & Gallo, 1995; Havlir et al., 1995; Roche Laboratories, 1995, 1996). These studies do not take into account the relative potency of each drug or the effect of such drugs when given in combination.

The development of virus strains that are resistant to antiretroviral drugs may also contribute to neurological disease. In one study, children with antiretroviral-resistant HIV mutations in their CSF fared worse neurologically than children without such mutations (Sei et al., 1996).

Several new agents are under study as putative neuroprotective drugs, rather than as antiretroviral drugs, in HIV CMC. Theoretically, these drugs will protect neural cells from the toxicity of gp120 (glycoprotein), tat protein, nitric oxide, tumor necrosis factor, free radicals, and increased oxidative stress. These drugs include nimodepine (a calcium channel blocker), memantine (an *N*-methyl-D-aspartate antagonist), and OPC-14117, an antioxidant (Chen et al., 1992; Dana Consortium, 1997). No controlled study has demonstrated the efficacy of these drugs as yet.

Symptomatic treatment of HIV CMC is a valuable, but often overlooked, aspect of management. Behavioral strategies, such as structuring the environment, lessening distracting stimuli, and using reminders or prompts, are very helpful to maximize function and are described in more detail elsewhere (see Chapters 6, 7, and 9, this volume). Psychoactive drugs are used to maximize function and reduce the impact of cognitive and behavioral deficits. Stimulants such as amphetamines have been reported to improve motor speed and mood in HIV-infected persons (Fernández, Adams, & Levy, 1988a; Fernández, Levy, & Galizzi, 1988b; Holmes, Fernández, & Levy, 1989). Neuroleptic drugs have been used to reduce agitation, but a high incidence of adverse effects (e.g., extrapyramidal movement disorders and neuroleptic malignant syndrome) has been reported in AIDS patients (Breitbart et al., 1988; Kieburtz, Epstein, Gelbard, & Greenamyre, 1991; Manser & Warner, 1990). Antidepressants appear to be very effective in treating mood disorders in HIV-infected patients, but those drugs with anticholinergic, antihistaminic adverse effects may exacerbate memory disorders (Ayd, 1988; Rabkin & Harrison, 1990).

Other CNS Infections

Neurosyphilis

Syphilis is caused by a spirochete, *Treponema pallidum*. HIV and syphilis have many features in common: Both can be transmitted in a similar manner (through sex, through blood contact, or vertically from mother to child); both can have a long "latent" period, with few clinical symptoms despite abnormal laboratory tests; and in the United States, both are common in ethnic minority groups and in drug users.

Syphilis is not a true opportunistic infection. Most people infected with syphilis are immunologically intact and HIV-seronegative. However, some investigators contend that syphilis is accelerated by HIV infection; that HIV-infected persons may have negative serological tests for syphilis, despite positive clinical findings; and that standard therapy is less successful in eradicating syphilis in HIV-infected than in HIV-seronegative persons (Johns, Tierney, & Felsenstein, 1987; Malone et al., 1995; Musher, Hamill, & Baughn, 1990). These contentions are not uniformly accepted and require further study.

Syphilitic infection proceeds over a period of decades in the HIV-seronegative person. The primary (first) stage of syphilis is characterized by a painless sore or "chancre" on the mucous membranes or genitals (the entry site of the organism) and by swollen lymph nodes in the local area (regional lymphadenopathy). This disappears without treatment and is followed up to 2 years later by secondary syphilis, which is characterized by rash, swollen lymph nodes, fever, painless ulcers on the mucous membranes of the mouth or genitals, and other genital lesions. Many patients with secondary syphilis have abnormal CSF, indicating that the spirochete penetrates the CNS relatively early in the course of this disease. Most such patients have no clinical neurological symptoms, although a few develop a syphilitic meningitis characterized by headache, stiff neck, nausea, and occasionally cranial nerve deficits. Untreated secondary syphilis resolves in 1–3 months, and in many patients spirochetes can disappear from the CNS without treatment. During the next stage, latent syphilis, the serology remains positive although the clinical findings are minimal. The final stage is tertiary syphilis, in which syphilitic lesions cause clinical disease in various organs, including the heart, eyes, and CNS (neurosyphilis).

Neurosyphilis occurs in fewer than 10% of patients with untreated syphilis (Clark & Danbolt, 1955), and it can be asymptomatic (no clinical manifestations, but the CSF is abnormal) or symptomatic. Symptomatic neurosyphilis occurs many years after the initial infection and presents in a variable manner. The better-described syndromes include syphilitic meningitis; syphilitic stroke; syphilitic dementia (a common cause of admission to mental hospitals before the antibiotic era), also known as "general paresis," associated with seizures, mania, euphoria, and grandiose delusions; tabes dorsalis, which is characterized by ataxia (loss of balance), sensory loss and weakness in the legs, loss of reflexes, incontinence, and severe "lightning-like" pains; seizures; and "gummatous neurosyphilis." "Gummas" are areas of focal tissue degeneration that contain spirochetes and are surrounded by a wall of fibrous scarring. Rarely, gummas can cause a brain mass in HIV-infected persons.

Because of the common risk factors for both diseases, all HIV-infected persons should be tested for syphilis. However, *Treponema pallidum* is extraordinarily difficult to culture, so the diagnosis is made by examining a specimen from a lesion under a microscope, or by serological blood tests such as the Venereal Disease Research Laboratory (VDRL) test or the rapid plasma reagent (RPR) test. These screening tests must be confirmed by a microhemagglutination assay for *Treponema pallidum* (MH-ATP), or by the fluorescent treponemal antibody (FTA).

A lumbar puncture is recommended for all HIV-infected persons with syphilis, regardless of symptoms. By contrast, a lumbar puncture is recommended for HIV-negative persons with syphilis only if they have symptomatic syphilis, a high-titer RPR or VDRL test, or a history of treatment failure, or if treatment with antibiotics other than penicillin is planned (CDC, 1993).

The recommended treatment regimen for neurosyphilis is intravenous, high-dose aqueous penicillin G (12–24 million units per day for 14 days). Although a number of case reports suggest that relapse after therapy for neurosyphilis may be more common in HIV-infected than in HIV-negative patients, this has never been confirmed in a controlled study. However, it is recommended that HIV-infected persons who are treated for neurosyphilis should be followed up with monthly serum VDRL or RPR tests for 3 months and then every 3–6 months until these tests are nonreactive or have stabilized at a titer of 1:8. The CSF should be reexamined at 3 months posttreatment and then every 6 months thereafter until it is normal (CDC, 1993)

CASE REPORT

Mr. G was a 27-year-old, HIV-positive, homeless, male cocaine user. He was admitted to the Veterans Affairs hospital because of 2 weeks of right-sided headache, right-eye pain and redness, photophobia, and 2 days of decreased vision on the right, all of which were thought to be symptoms of a syphilitic eye infection. Mr. G had been diagnosed with syphilis 1 year prior at a clinic for sexually transmitted diseases. He was noncompliant with penicillin treatment of his syphilis and refused treatment for HIV infection. A CT scan of his brain was normal. A lumbar puncture showed CSF abnormalities consistent with syphilitic meningitis. Mr. G was admitted to the hospital for intravenous penicillin therapy, but left against medical advice after only 1 week of treatment.

Cryptococcal Meningitis

Cryptococcal meningitis is the infection of the meninges by *Cryptococcus neoformans*, a yeast (fungus) surrounded by a gelatinous capsule. *Cryptococcus* is a common CNS opportunistic infection in AIDS patients, affecting about 10% of adults. Most patients with cryptococcal meningitis are severely immunosuppressed.

Cryptococcus neoformans is transmitted by spores from pigeon droppings, dust, and soil. The spores are inhaled into the lungs, resulting in a self-limited respiratory infection. Most healthy people recover, although the organism persists for years. In immunocompromised hosts, however, *Cryptococcus* may reactivate and spread. It is uncommon for cryptococcal meningitis in AIDS to result from new infections.

Two-thirds of patients with disseminated *Cryptococcus* develop meningitis. About 10% of AIDS patients with cryptococcal meningitis also have abscesses within the brain tissue, called "cryptococcomas." Cryptococcomas are mass lesions that can compress adjacent brain tissue, causing swelling (edema) or impairing the free circulation of CSF.

The symptoms of cryptococcal meningitis develop over a few days to 3 weeks (acute–subacute). The early symptoms of cryptococcal meningitis are often nonspecific and nonfocal, such as fever, lethargy, persistent and increasingly severe headache, or seizures (Kovacs et al., 1985; Zuger, Louie, Holzman, Simberkoff, & Rahal, 1986). Some patients have a near-normal level of consciousness, while others become delirious. Meningismus (stiff neck caused by inflammation of the meninges) is not a constant feature. A subgroup of patients with cryptococcal meningitis present with focal symptoms, such as hemiparesis (weakness on one side of the body), hyperreflexia, or paralysis of one or more cranial nerves. In particular, cranial nerves II (optic) and VIII (cochlear and vestibular) may also be damaged, so that blindness and deafness can be permanent sequelae of this disease.

Cryptococcal meningitis is a medical emergency, and early diagnosis and treatment are the keys to reducing the sequelae of the disease. Complications include seizures, stroke (due to the thrombosis of cerebral blood vessels), coma, brain edema, increased intracranial pressure and/or brain herniation, or death, even if the infection is properly treated. Even treated patients may have serious long-term sequelae, such as hydrocephalus (an accumulation of CSF within the brain, resulting in large, fluid-filled ventricles and increased intracranial pressure); permanent damage to the cranial nerves, resulting in blindness; dysarthria (slurred speech); swallowing disorders; deafness; weakness in the extremities; or dementia.

The diagnosis is made by identifying the fungus in blood or CSF.

Tests for *Cryptococcus* include India ink slides, cryptococcal antigen tests, and fungal cultures. Elevated CSF pressure, elevated CSF WBC count, low to very low CSF glucose, and elevated CSF total protein are common but nondiagnostic findings. A few patients who had normal CSF have been reported.

The MRI and CT are usually normal. If cryptococcomas are present, they are usually seen in the basal ganglia. In fulminant disease, the cerebral ventricles may become inflamed (ventriculitis) and may enhance with contrast. Hydrocephalus may be present in advanced cases.

Treatment should be started immediately. The most commonly used first-line treatment is amphotericin B, an intravenously administered antibiotic. The usual dose in AIDS patients is 0.5–0.7 mg/kg/day (Kovacs et al., 1985; Zuger et al., 1986), but this may be modified if the patient has kidney disease. This drug can cause serious adverse reactions when administered, such as chills, fevers, vomiting, pain, phlebitis, and seizures. Kidney damage may occur, especially after cumulative treatment, but is usually reversible when the drug is stopped. Recently, a less toxic liposomal formulation of amphotericin B has been released. Another intravenous antifungal drug, 5-flucytosine, is sometimes given with amphotericin B at a dose of 100–150 mg/kg/day in divided doses, although its efficacy in AIDS patients is somewhat controversial (Kovacs et al., 1985; Zuger et al., 1986). These drugs are usually continued until the CSF is sterilized, generally 2–4 weeks. A new orally administered antifungal drug, fluconazole, has greatly improved the treatment of cryptococcal meningitis. Fluconazole has good CSF penetration and few serious adverse effects. It is not recommended for the acute treatment of treatment of fulminant cryptococcal meningitis, but is very effective for outpatient maintainance therapy (Sugar & Saunders, 1988). The usual doses are 200–400 mg per day.

CASE REPORT

Mr. U was a 47-year-old HIV-infected injection drug user with a history of "drug-seeking" behavior and poor compliance. He presented to the HIV clinic with 5 days of headache. Mr. U's exam was normal and he was afebrile, so he was sent home. He returned three times over the next 10 days with the same complaint. On his fourth clinic visit an outpatient CT scan of the brain, repeat CD4 count, and viral load test were ordered. Twenty days after symptom onset, Mr. U was brought to the emergency room because he was "hallucinating" and had a fever of 101.5F. In the emergency room, Mr. U had a seizure. A CT scan showed brain atrophy. His drug screen was positive for codeine only. His CD4 count was 75 cells/mm³, and his viral load was 42,000 copies/ml. Mr. U's CSF showed an elevated pressure of 320 (normal less than 220), elevated CSF WBC count, elevated CSF total protein, and very low CSF glucose. An India ink slide of his CSF showed budding yeast. A cryptococcal antigen titer was positive in CSF (1:1,024). Three days later, a CSF fungal culture confirmed the diagnosis of cryptococcal meningitis.

AIDS patients with cryptococcal meningitis must be treated for life, because relapse occurs in up to 58% of patients if treatment is discontinued. Therefore, compliance with continued treatment is very important.

Toxoplasmosis

Toxoplasmosis is caused by infection with the parasite *Toxoplasma gondii*. It is the most common cause of a CNS mass lesion in adults with AIDS, accounting for up to 70% of brain mass lesions in AIDS patients. Humans can acquire toxoplasmosis by eating *T. gondii* cysts in inadequately cooked infected food, by ingesting contaminated soil, by fecal–oral contamination, by contact with infected cat feces, or vertically (from mother to fetus). Toxoplasmosis is especially common in France, Haiti, Africa, and Florida (Dukes, Luft, & Durack, 1991).

The primary (initial) toxoplasmosis infection in a healthy person is characterized by swollen cervical lymph nodes or by a mononucleosis-type syndrome. Up to 40% of HIV-infected persons have prior exposure to *T. gondii*, as indicated by positive serological tests (Grant, Gold, Rosenblum, Biedzwiecki, & Armstrong, 1990; Luft & Remington, 1992). In immunosuppressed persons, such as AIDS patients and transplant recipients, *T. gondii* can reactivate and cause clinical disease (Grant et al., 1990). The mean CD4 counts of patients with AIDS and toxoplasmosis are usually below 100 cells/mm³ (Jones et al., 1996).

Few toxoplamosis infections in adult AIDS patients are acquired *de novo*. However, to avoid this possibility, AIDS patients who own cats should have someone else empty the litter box, or wear gloves and a mask when handling the litter. Immunosuppressed persons should wear gloves when gardening, and should avoid raw meat and other uncooked foods. Reactivation of toxoplasmosis may be prevented in patients who take drugs such as trimethoprim–sulfamethoxazole for *Pneumocystis* prophylaxis (Jones et al., 1996).

Toxoplasmosis causes an encephalitis (brain inflammation) characterized by multiple abscesses surrounded by areas of edema. Depending upon the stage of the illness and the location of the lesions, toxoplasmosis may present with nonfocal symptoms such as headache, fever, malaise, delirium, or lethargy, or with focal signs and symptoms that can be localized to specific abscesses (Dukes et al., 1991).

Most patients report that their symptoms began weeks before diagnosis (acute–subacute). The most common focal signs include unilateral weakness of the extremities (hemiparesis), unilateral numbness (hemisensory loss), unilateral visual loss (hemianopsia), aphasia, memory loss, and focal seizures. Stiff neck is relatively uncommon. As the disease progresses, the level of consciousness declines. Nausea, vomiting, and lethargy suggest increased intracranial pressure. This may occur if expanding lesions obstruct the outflow of CSF from the brain, bleed, or cause local or diffuse brain swelling. Such situations are likely to cause fatal brain herniation, which may be hastened if a lumbar puncture precipitously lowers the intracranial pressure. For this reason, persons with suspected mass lesions or increased intracranial pressure from any source should have an MRI or CT scan performed before they undergo a lumbar puncture, and the puncture should be deferred in situations that might result in herniation.

Most patients (97%) with toxoplasmosis have multiple brain lesions (Bishburg, Eng, Slim, Perez, & Johnson, 1989; Bonaventura et al., 1988; Porter & Sande, 1992). Cases with only a single lesion are more difficult to diagnose. The use of contrast material is very helpful in identifying these brain lesions. Most commonly toxoplasmosis abscesses have a "ring-enhancing" pattern (i.e., the contrast lights up the rim of the lesion), surrounded by edema. However, many other patterns of contrast enhancement have been reported. Unfortunately, no MRI or CT pattern definitively differentiates toxoplasmosis from brain lymphoma, so additional diagnostic tests (toxoplasmosis serology, a biopsy, or response to empirical antitoxoplasmosis therapy) are needed to confirm the diagnosis (Ciricillo & Rosenblum, 1990).

A lumbar puncture (CSF exam) should be performed only after an MRI or CT demonstrates that the patient is not at risk for herniation. The CSF findings are nonspecific, and there are instances reported of normal CSF profiles. False-negative CSF toxoplasmosis titers are common, so many physicians rely on serum titers. The major reason to obtain CSF in cases of suspected toxoplasmosis is that an alternative pathogen may be identified. Many AIDS patients have positive toxoplasmosis titers in blood, because exposure to the parasite is common in the general population, but there may be another cause for their brain mass. However, a negative blood toxoplasmosis serology indicates that toxoplasmosis is not likely.

Patients who have probable toxoplasmosis, based on characteristic lesions and positive toxoplasmosis serology, are usually treated for at least 2 weeks under close observation with oral pyrimethamine (50–100 mg per day), along with oral folinic (acid 5 mg per day) to prevent megaloblastic anemia, and oral sulfadiazine (1–1.5 g every 6 hours). Patients who are allergic to sulfonamides can be treated with oral clindamycin (450–600 mg every 6 hours) and pyrimethamine (Rolston & Hoy, 1987). If the CNS lesions respond within 1–2 weeks (disappearance of clinical symptoms and radiological improvement), an empirical diagnosis of toxoplasmosis can be made, and the patient is given secondary prophylaxis for life. If the patient does not respond or worsens, a stereotactic brain biopsy is indicated for definitive diagnosis and treatment.

CASE REPORT

Ms. R was a 40-year-old Afro-Caribbean woman with AIDS who presented with 7 days of increasing right-sided headache, nausea, "blurred" vision, low-grade fever, and loss of balance. On exam, she was slightly lethargic and had left-sided weakness and hyperreflexia. An emergency CT brain scan showed three contrast-enhancing mass lesions. The largest lesion was in the right cerebral hemisphere. The scan showed early signs of brain herniation. Serum toxoplasmosis tests were strongly positive, and tests for other pathogens were negative. Ms. R's physicians decided against a lumbar puncture. She was treated empirically for toxoplasmosis, with the plan to biopsy one of her brain lesions if she did not improve within 2 weeks.

A significant number of persons who recover from toxoplasmosis remain neurologically impaired, despite apparent resolution of their lesions. This impairment, which may take the form of a seizure disorders, weakness of the extremities, or forgetfulness, is probably due to tissue destruction by the abscess. Because of the high rate of relapse when therapy is discontinued in AIDS patients, treatment should be continued for life.

Progressive Multifocal Leukoencephalopathy

PML is a devastating CNS disease caused by a polyoma virus known as the John Cunningham virus (JCV; Astrom, Mancall, & Richardson, 1958). The JCV is ubiquitous in the general population. It is thought to be spread through respiratory infection, or from mother to fetus. By age 40, 90% of all adults worldwide have been infected, as indicated by antibodies to JCV (Brown, Tsai, & Gadjusek, 1975). JCV persists in a latent state in kidney cells, and is excreted in the urine of healthy, HIV-negative persons (Kitamura, Aso, Kunioshi, Hara, & Yogo, 1990). Thus, infection by JCV does not predict PML.

Before AIDS, PML was a very rare infection seen in immunosuppressed persons with cancer or lupus, or in those who were receiving immunosuppressive drugs for organ transplants (Weiner & Naravan, 1974). PML is much more frequent in AIDS patients (an estimated 3–7%) than in patients with other immunosuppressive diseases (Gillespie et al., 1991; Lang et al., 1989). This may occur because HIV tat protein increases the replication of JCV, which spreads to the CNS (Tada et al., 1990).

JCV infects and kills oligodendrocytes (CNS cells that make myelin, the fatty covering surrounding the nerve axons). Myelin speeds the transmission of electrical impulses in the nervous system, and JCV-induced demyelination slows or stops this conduction. Large areas of demyelination manifest themselves with focal neurological deficits, and radiologically as multiple lesions in the white matter of the brain.

The clinical symptoms of PML are highly individualized and are associated with the location of the single or multiple CNS lesions (Berger et al., 1987). The most common syndromes include cognitive deficits, unilateral weakness (hemiparesis), unilateral sensory loss (hemisensory loss), visual symptoms (e.g., loss of all or part of the visual field, double vision, or inability to interpret visual information), abnormalities in speech and language (e.g., slurred speech or dysarthria), incoordination, headache, or vertigo. Seizures also occur in about 10% of AIDS/PML patients (Berger, Gallo, & Concha, 1997). Most patients with PML do not have fever, stiff neck, or a headache. However, neurobehavioral abnormalities are common in PML, especially if the lesions affect the frontal or parietal areas. Examples include apraxia, aphasia, alexia (the acquired inability to read, despite normal visual function), and agnosia.

The laboratory evaluation for PML usually begins with a neuro-imaging scan. Brain MRI is more sensitive than CT to the white matter lesions of PML, which typically appear as multiple hyperintense (white) lesions on the T2-weighted portion of the MRI, and as hypodense (dark) on the T1 portion (Bishburg et al., 1989). The CT scan may be normal or may show lucent (dark) areas in the white matter. It is uncommon for PML lesions to be enhanced with contrast material, or to be surrounded by edema. PML lesions are actually space-occupying lesions (i.e., they take up space but do not compress the surrounding brain) rather than mass lesions, and do not increase the risk of brain herniation.

The new technique of magnetic resonance spectroscopy (MRS) is a promising noninvasive tool to diagnose PML and other CNS lesions in AIDS patients (Chang et al., 1997). An MRS study measures the quantity of certain brain metabolites (chemicals) within a small area (a voxel) of brain tissue. The voxel is selected from a lesion, which is first mapped on a routine MRI. Various brain infections, including PML, have characteristic chemical profiles on MRS.

No unique CSF WBC, protein, or glucose values distinguish PML. Until recently, the CSF exam was used to exclude other causes of white matter disease. A JCV PCR test has been developed, which can detect JCV in the CSF and blood (Weber et al., 1994); however, the usefulness of this test in clinical diagnosis has not yet been validated. Serology for JCV is not helpful, as most adults are positive. The diagnostic "gold standard" for PML remains a brain biopsy or autopsy that confirms the characteristic histological abnormalities and polyoma virus.

CASE REPORT

Mr. S is a 55-year-old HIV-positive bisexual male with a history of severe depression and a CD4 count of 169 cells/mm^3. He was brought in for psychiatric evaluation by his wife, who complained that for 4 days Mr. S had been behaving in an unusual manner: "He says that he can see the clock but that he can't tell the time." On exam, Mr. S was afebrile and systemically well, but he had a visual agnosia. MRI showed patchy lesions in the parietal and occipital white matter without enhancement or mass effect, as well as another very small white matter lesion in the right frontal lobe. A CSF exam was unremarkable except for an elevated total protein. A biopsy of the lesion was consistent with PML.

The prognosis for persons with AIDS and PML has been poor, with a mean lifespan estimated to be 4–5 months after the onset of symptoms (Berger et al., 1987; Fong, Toma, & the Canadian PML Study Group, 1995). Death usually results from neurological disease. However, a few PML patients survive for prolonged periods of time (Lortholary et al., 1994). Some PML patients, with or without AIDS, have stabilized spontaneously or after their underlying immune disorder was treated (Berger & Mucke, 1988; Mark & Atlas, 1989; Singer et al., 1994a). A few individuals have responded to high-dose antiretroviral therapy, such as zidovudine (Singer et al., 1994a). The antiretroviral drugs α-interferon and cytosine arabinoside have been reported to prolong life in some PML patients (Berger et al., 1992; Britton, Romagnoll, Sisti, & Powers, 1992; Portegies et al., 1991); however, a controlled study of patients with AIDS/PML did not find any survival advantage for this treatment (Hall & the AIDS Clinical Trials Group, 1997). Currently, several new antiretroviral drugs are under study for the treatment of AIDS/PML.

Primary CNS Lymphoma

Lymphoma is the second most common CNS mass lesion in adults with AIDS, affecting 5% of AIDS patients (Levine, 1991; So, Beckstead, & Davis, 1986). A brain lymphoma can be primary (i.e., it originates within the CNS) or metastatic (i.e., it originates outside the brain and spinal cord, and spreads to the CNS). AIDS-associated CNS lymphoma is most common in persons with severe immunodeficiency (mean CD4 count of about 50 cells/mm^3) and/or antecedent opportunistic infections or Kaposi's sarcoma (Straus, 1997).

Most cases of CNS lymphoma present in a subacute fashion, with symptoms preceding diagnosis by several weeks. Although nonfocal symptoms (e.g., headache, seizures, and lethargy) are common, most patients have one or more focal neurological deficits (e.g., aphasia, hemiparesis, or cranial nerve palsies) at the time of presentation (Baumgartner et al., 1990). Fever and stiff neck are not typical features of CNS lymphoma.

Primary CNS lymphoma usually appears on CT or MRI as one or more homogeneous, uniformly enhancing mass lesions, and less often with a ring-enhancing pattern surrounded by edema (Baumgartner et al., 1990; Ciricillo & Rosenblum, 1990). The majority of primary CNS lymphomas present with multiple lesions at the time of diagnosis; however, a single CNS lesion in an AIDS patient is much more likely to be lymphoma than toxoplasmosis. Still, there are no findings on MRI or CT that definitively distinguish lymphoma from toxoplasmosis (Dina, 1991).

Unless there is an associated lymphomatous meningitis, CSF cytology is usually not helpful. In the presence of a large mass lesion, a lumbar puncture may be dangerous. The major reason to perform a lumbar puncture at all would be to detect an infection that might mimic or accompany a lymphoma. Failure to respond to therapy for toxoplasmosis is not diagnostic of lymphoma, and empirical brain radiation is not recommended. The definitive diagnosis is made by a brain biopsy (Chappell, Guthrie, & Orenstein, 1992).

Lymphoma that metastasizes to the CNS from a systemic tumor can present as a mass lesion, as lymphomatous meningitis, or as an epidural mass in the spinal cord (Levine, 1991). Malignant cells are more likely to be found in the CSF if the meninges are involved.

Patients with primary CNS lymphoma may respond at least temporarily to radiation, steroids, and/or chemotherapy. The standard chemotherapy doses are usually reduced because of myelosuppression (Levine et al., 1991). Most patients with AIDS/lymphoma die from infection and not from tumor.

CASE REPORT

Mr. X, a previously pleasant and compliant 60-year-old man with AIDS, became belligerent and forgetful over a 1-month period. He was brought to the clinic after he lost his balance and fell, striking his head. On examination, Mr. X was afebrile and irritable. He denied headache. He had poor short-term memory, and his gait was wide based and unsteady. An emergency CT scan with contrast showed a large enhancing mass that compressed Mr. X's frontal lobes. A serum toxoplasmosis titer was negative. Brain biopsy revealed primary CNS lymphoma.

Cytomegalovirus Encephalitis

Cytomegalovirus (CMV) is related to the viruses that cause oral herpes (herpes simplex virus 1, or HSV-1), genital herpes (herpes simplex virus 2, or HSV-2), chickenpox (varicella zoster, or VZV), mononucleosis (Epstein–Barr virus, or EBV), roseola or exanthem subitem (human herpes virus 6, or HHV-6), and the recently identified Kaposi's sarcoma virus (human herpes virus 8, or HHV-8). However, CMV is probably the most common and serious opportunistic viral cause of CNS disease in AIDS.

Previous exposure to CMV is common in the general population, and occurs in up to 95% of persons with HIV infection (Collier et al., 1987). CMV can be spread through contact with blood or genital secretions, or from mother to child. Most primary infections with CMV are self-limited, nonspecific viral syndromes associated with fever and swollen lymph nodes. However, CMV can persist in a latent state within the body. Reactivation can occur when immunity declines in HIV and other situations (e.g., CMV is a common complication of organ transplants) and may also be stimulated by some HIV genes. Most patients with AIDS and active CMV disease have a CD4 count below 100 cells/mm^3, with an increased risk if the count drops below 50 (Gerard et al., 1997).

Clinical CMV disease (retinitis, pneumonia, esophagitis, colitis, adrenal infection, neurological disease, etc.) occurs in up to 30% of people with full-blown AIDS (Drew, 1992). Within the nervous system, CMV can cause multiple types of neurological disease, including encephalitis, myelitis, and peripheral neuropathy. Many persons thought to have HIV-associated dementia during life were found to have CMV encephalitis or a mixed HIV and CMV infection at autopsy (Arribas, Storch, Clifford, & Tselis, 1996; Fiala et al., 1993). Recently developed of tests such as CMV PCR have helped identify more cases of CMV encephalitis during life (Clifford, Buller, Mohammed, Robison, & Storch, 1993).

Up to 90% of AIDS patients with CMV encephalitis will have a history of CMV in another organ, especially the retina (Arribas et al., 1996). Most will be receiving some type of CMV therapy at the time they present with CNS disease (Arribas et al., 1996). Over half of patients with CMV encephalitis will have a nonfocal presentation (lethargy, confusion, coma, fever, seizures, headache, dementia) (Holland et al., 1994). A minority present with focal findings, such as cranial nerve palsies (especially the facial and ocular nerves), abnormal eye movements, and leg weakness. Myelitis and neuropathy can occur concurrently with encephalitis.

CMV encephalitis in AIDS may have been underdiagnosed, because a definitive diagnosis formerly required a brain biopsy. Antibody testing is not helpful, because most AIDS patients are positive for CMV. CMV in the blood (viremia) is common in advanced HIV infection, and is not necessarily associated with CMV end-organ disease (Zurlo et al., 1993). CSF CMV PCR is probably the best noninvasive test currently available to diagnose CMV encephalitis during life; the higher the levels of CMV DNA in CSF, the more likely the patient is to have serious CNS disease (Arribas et al., 1996; Clifford et al., 1993). MRI and CT occasionally demonstrate ventriculitis (enhancement of the cerebral ventricles) in cases of advanced CMV encephalitis (Grafe, Press, Berhoty, Hesselink, & Wiley, 1990).

CASE REPORT

Ms. F was a 42-year-old woman with AIDS and CMV retinitis, an infection of the eyes. She was treated with ganciclovir (an anti-CMV drug), and her condition was well controlled for 9 months. In her 10th month of treatment, Ms. F became irritable, argumentative, irrational, and disoriented over a 7-day period. She was taken to a psychiatric emergency room, where she was found to be delirious. Ms. F was then transferred to a medical ward. Results of her brain MRI and CSF exam confirmed that Ms. F had CMV encephalitis. Even though Ms. F was compliant with therapy, she nevertheless did not respond to a higher dose of ganciclovir. Her symptoms improved when she was treated with a different anti-CMV drug.

The first-line treatment for CMV encephalitis is intravenous ganciclovir (Novak et al., 1989). Because this drug must be given for life in persons with CNS disease, a catheter is usually implanted into the arm or chest. Neutropenia is a serious adverse effect of ganciclovir, and patients may require support with granulocyte colony-stimulating factor to continue the drug. An oral form of ganciclovir and drug-containing ocular implants are available but are not recommended for neurological disease. Treatment must be continued for life because of the possibility of relapse. If the patient cannot tolerate ganciclovir or is resistant to the drug, there are two alternatives, foscavir and cidofovir; however, very little has been published about their use in neurological disease (Blick, Garton, Hopkins, & La Gravinese, 1997; Cohen et al., 1993).

REFERENCES

Abbott Laboratories, Pharmaceutical Products Division, Research and Development. (1994, September). *Information for clinical investigators: ABT-538.* North Chicago, IL: Abbott Laboratories.

American Academy of Neurology (AAN). (1991). Nomenclature and research definitions for neurological manifestations of human immunodeficiency virus—type 1 (HIV-1) infection: Report of a working group of the American Academy of Neurology AIDS Task Force. *Neurology, 41*(6), 778–785.

Arribas, J., Storch, G., Clifford, D., & Tselis, A. (1996). Cytomegalovirus encephalitis. *Annals of Internal Medicine, 125,* 577–587.

Astrom, K., Mancall, E., & Richardson, E. J. (1958). Progressive multifocal leukoencephalopathy: Hitherto unrecognized complication of chronic lymphocytic leukemia and Hodgkin's disease. *Brain, 81,* 93–111.

Ayd, F. J. (1988). Psychopharmacotherapy for HIV-infected, AIDS-related complex (ARC), and AIDS patients. *International Drug Therapy Newsletter, 23,* 25–28.

Baumgartner, J., Rachlin, J., Beckstead, J., Meeker, T. C., Levy, R. M., Wara, W. M., & Rosenblum, M. L. (1990). Primary central nervous system lymphomas: Natural history and response to radiation therapy in 55 patients with acquired immunodeficiency syndrome. *Journal of Neurosurgery, 73,* 206–211.

Berger, J., Gallo, B., & Concha, M. (1997). Progressive multifocal leukoencephalopathy. In J. Berger & R. Levy (Ed.), *AIDS and the nervous system* (pp. 569–594). Philadelphia: Lippincott/Raven Press.

Berger, J., Kaszovitz, B., Post, M. J. D., et al. (1987). PML associated with human immunodeficiency virus infection. *Annals of Internal Medicine, 107,* 78–87.

Berger, J., & Mucke, L. (1988). Prolonged survival and partial recovery in AIDS-associated progressive multifocal leukoencephalopathy. *Neurology, 38,* 1060–1065.

Berger, J., Pall, L., McArthur, J., et al. (1992). A pilot study of recombinant alpha-2A interferon in the treatment of AIDS-related progressive multifocal leukoencephalopathy. *Neurology, 42*(Suppl. 3), 257. (Abstract)

Bishburg, E., Eng, R. H., Slim, J., Perez, G., & Johnson, E. (1989). Brain lesions in patients with acquired immunodeficiency syndrome. *Archives of Internal Medicine, 149*(4), 941–943.

Blaney, S., Daniel, M., Harker, A., Godwin, K., & Balis, F. (1995). Pharmacokinetics of lamivudine and BCH-189 in plasma and cerebrospinal fluid of nonhuman primates. *Antimicrobial Agents and Chemotherapy, 39,* 2779–2782.

Blick, G., Garton, T., Hopkins, U., & La Gravinese, L. (1997). Successful use of cidofovir in treating AIDS-related cytomegalovirus retinitis, encephalitis, and esophagitis. *Journal of AIDS, 15,* 84–85.

Bonaventura, I., Romero, F., Ortega, A., Navarro, C., Juste, C., & Codina-Puiggrós, A. (1988). Cerebral toxoplasmosis in the acquired immunodeficiency syndrome: Study of the clinical, radiological, and pathological findings in 10 cases. *Medicina Clínica, 91*(1), 1–6.

Bornstein, R. A., Fama, R., Rosenberger, P., Whitacre, C. C., Para, M. F., Nasrallah, H. A., & Fass, R. J. (1993). Drug and alcohol use and neuropsychological performance in asymptomatic HIV infection. *Journal of Neuropsychiatry and Clinical Neurosciences, 5*(3), 254–259.

Breitbart, W., Marotta, R. F., & Call, P. (1988). AIDS and neuroleptic malignant syndrome. *Lancet, ii*(8626–8627), 1488–1489.

Brew, B. J., Bhalla, R. B., Fleisher, M., Paul, M., Khan, A., Schwartz, M. K., & Price, R. W. (1989). Cerebrospinal fluid beta 2 microglobulin in patients infected with human immunodeficiency virus. *Neurology, 39*(6), 830–834.

Brew, B. J., Bhalla, R. B., Paul, M., Gallardo, H., McArthur, J. C., Schwartz, M. K., & Price, R. W. (1990). Cerebrospinal fluid neopterin in human immunodeficiency virus type 1 infection. *Annals of Neurology, 28,* 556–560.

Brew, B., Pemberton, L., Cunningham, P., & Law, M. (1997). Levels of human immunodeficiency virus type 1 RNA in cerebrospinal fluid correlate with AIDS dementia stage. *Journal of Infectious Diseases, 175,* 963–966.

Bristol-Myers Squibb, Pharmaceutical Research Institute. (1992). *Investigator brochure: Stavudine (2′, 3′-didehydro-3′-deoxythymidine, d4T).* Wallingford, CT: Bristol-Myers Squibb.

Britton, C., Romagnoll, M., Sisti, M., & Powers, J. (1992). Progressive multifocal leukoencephalopathy: Disease progression, stabilization, and response to intrathecal ARA-C in 26 patients. In *VIII International Conference on AIDS, Amsterdam, The Netherlands* (Abstract No. Th B3886).

Brivio, L., Tornaghi, R., Musetti, L., Marchisio, P., & Principi, N. (1991). Improvement of auditory brainstem responses after treatment with zidovudine in a child with AIDS. *Pediatric Neurology, 7*(1), 53–55.

Brown, P., Tsai, T., & Gadjusek, D. (1975). Seroepidemiology of human papovaviruses: Discovery of virgin populations and some unusual patterns of antibody prevalence among remote peoples of the world. *American Journal of Epidemiology, 102,* 331–340.

Brunetti, A., Berg, G., Di Chiro, G., Cohen, R. M., Yarchoan, R., Pizzo, P. A., Broder, S., Eddy, J., Fulham, M. J., Finn, R. D., et al. (1989). Reversal of brain metabolic abnormalities following treatment of AIDS dementia complex with 3'-azido-2',3'-dideoxythymidine (AZT, zidovudine): A PET-FDG study. *Journal of Nuclear Medicine, 30*(5), 581–590.

Burger, D., Kraayeveld, C. L., Meenhorst, P. L., Mulder, J. W., Hoetelmans, R., & Koks, C. (1995). Study on didanosine concentrations in cerebrospinal fluid: Implications for the treatment of AIDS dementia complex. *Pharmacy World and Science, 17,* 218–221.

Burger, D. M., Kraaijeveld, C., Meenhorst, P. L., Mulder, J. W., Koks, C. H., Bult, A., & Beijnen, J. (1993). Penetration of zidovudine into the cerebrospinal fluid of patients infected with HIV. *AIDS, 7,* 1581–1587.

Butler, K. M., Husson, R. N., Balis, F. M., Brouwers, P., Eddy, J., El-Amin, D., Gress, J., & Hawkins, M. (1991). Dideoxyinosine in children with symptomatic human immunodeficiency virus infection. *New England Journal of Medicine, 324,* 137–144.

Centers for Disease Control (CDC). (1986). Classification system for human T-lymphotropic virus type III/lymphadenopathy-associated virus infections. *Annals of Internal Medicine, 105,* 234–237.

Centers for Disease Control (CDC). (1987). Revision of the CDC surveillance case definition for acquired immunodeficiency syndrome. *Morbidity and Mortality Weekly Report, 36*(Suppl. 1), 1S–14S.

Centers for Disease Control and Prevention (CDC). (1992). 1993 revised classification system for HIV infection and expanded surveillance case definition for AIDS among adolescents and adults. *Morbidity and Mortality Weekly Report, 41*(RR-17), 1–19.

Centers for Disease Control and Prevention (CDC). (1993). 1993 sexually transmitted diseases treatment guidelines. *Morbidity and Mortality Weekly Report, 42*(RR-14), 1–102.

Chang, L. (1995). *In vivo* magnetic resonance spectroscopy in HIV and HIV-related brain diseases. *Reviews in the Neurosciences, 6,* 365–378.

Chang, L., Ernst, T., Tornatore, C., et al. (1997). Metabolite abnormalities in progressive multifocal leukoencephalopathy by proton magnetic resonance spectroscopy. *Neurology, 48,* 836–844.

Chang, L., Miller, B., McBride, D., Cornford, M., Oropilla, G., Buchthal, S., Chiang, F., Aronow, H., & Ernst, T. (1995). Brain lesions in patients with AIDS: H-1 MR spectroscopy. *Radiology, 197,* 525–531.

Chappell, E. T., Guthrie, B. L., & Orenstein, J. (1992). The role of stereotactic biopsy in the management of HIV-related focal brain lesions. *Neurosurgery, 30*(6), 825–829.

Chen, H. S. V., Pellegrini, J. W., Aggarwal, S. K., Lei, S. Z., Warach, S., Jensen, F. E., & Lipton, S. A. (1992). Open-channel block of *N*-methyl-D-aspartate (NMDA) responses by memantine: Therapeutic advantage against NMDA receptor-mediated neurotoxicity. *Journal of Neuroscience, 12,* 4427–4436.

Chiesi, A., Vella, S., Dally, L., Pedersen, C., Danners, S., Johnson, A., Schwanders, S., Croebel, F., Glauser, M., Antunes, F., et al. (1995). Epidemiology of AIDS dementia complex in Europe. *Journal of Acquired Immune Deficiency Syndromes and Human Retrovirology, 11,* 39–44.

Ciricillo, S. F., & Rosenblum, M. L. (1990). Use of CT and MRI to distinguish intracranial lesions and to define the need for biopsy in AIDS patients. *Journal of Neurosurgery, 73*(5), 720–724.

Clark, E., & Danbolt, N. (1955). The Oslo study of the natural history of untreated syphilis: An epidemiological investigation based on a restudy of the Boeck–Bruusgaard material—a review and appraisal. *Journal of Chronic Diseases, 2,* 311–344.

Clifford, D. B., Buller, R. S., Mohammed, S., Robison, L., & Storch, G. A. (1993). Use of polymerase chain reaction to demonstrate cytomegalovirus DNA in CSF of patients with human immunodeficiency virus infection. *Neurology, 43,* 75–79.

Cohen, B. A., McArthur, J. C., Grohman, S., Patterson, B., & Gloss, J. D. (1993). Neurologic prognosis of cytomegalovirus polyradiculomyelopathy in AIDS. *Neurology, 43,* 493–499.

Collier, A., Meyers, J., Corey, L., Murphy, V., Roberts, P., & Handsfield, H. (1987). Cytomegalovirus infection in homosexual men: Relationship to sexual practices, antibody to human immunodeficiency virus, and cell-mediated immunity. *American Journal of Medicine, 82,* 593–601.

Conley, L., Bush, T., Buchbinder, S., Penley, K., Judson, F., & Holmberg, S. (1996). The association between cigarette smoking and selected HIV-related medical conditions. *AIDS, 10,* 1121–1126.

Conrad, A., Schmid, P., Syndulko, K., Singer, E., Nagra, R., Russell, J., & Tourtellotte, W. (1995). Quantifying HIV-1 RNA using the polymerase chain reaction on cerebrospinal fluid and serum of seropositive individuals with and without neurologic abnormalities. *Journal of AIDS, 10,* 425–435.

Cummings, M. A., Cummings, K. L., Rapaport, M. H., Atkinson, J. H., & Grant, I. (1987). Acquired immunodeficiency syndrome presenting as schizophrenia. *Western Journal of Medicine, 146*(5), 615–618.

Dana Consortium on the Therapy of HIV Dementia and Related Cognitive Disorders. (1996). Clinical confirmation of the American Academy of Neurology algorithm for HIV-1-associated cognitive/motor disorder. *Neurology, 47,* 1247–1253.

Dana Consortium on the Therapy of HIV Dementia and Related Cognitive Disorders. (1997). Safety and tolerability of the antioxidant OPC-14117 in HIV-associated cognitive impairment. *Neurology, 49,* 142–146.

Davis, L. E., Hjelle, B. L., Miller, V. E., Palmer, D. L., Llewellyn, F. L., Merlin, T. L., Young, S. A., Mills, R. G., Wachsman, W., & Wiley, C. A. (1992). Early viral brain invasion in iatrogenic human immunodeficiency virus infection. *Neurology, 42,* 1736–1739.

DeCarli, C., Falloon, F. J., Eddy, J., Pizzo, P. A., Friedland, R. P., & Rapoport, S. I. (1989). Brain growth and cognitive improvement in children with human immunodeficiency virus-induced encephalopathy after 6 months of chronic infusion azidothymidine therapy. *Neurology, 39*(Suppl. 1), 186.

de Gans, J., Lange, J. M. A., Derix, M. M. A., De Wolf, F., Schattenkerk, J. K. M. E., Danner, S. A., De Visser, B.W.O., Cload, P., & Goudsmit, J. (1988). Decline of HIV antigen levels in cerebrospinal fluid during treatment with low-dose zidovudine. *AIDS, 2,* 37–40.

Devineni, D., & Gallo, J. M. (1995). Zalcitabine: Clinical pharmacokinetics and efficacy. *Clinical Pharmacokinetics, 28,* 351–360.

Dina, T. S. (1991). Primary central nervous system lymphoma versus toxoplasmosis in AIDS. *Radiology, 179*(3), 823–828.

Drew, W. (1992). Cytomegalovirus infection in patients with AIDS. *Clinical Infectious Diseases, 14,* 608–615.

Dukes, C., Luft, B., & Durack, D. (1991). Toxoplasmosis of the central nervous system. In W. Scheld, R. Whitley, & D. Durack (Eds.), *Infections of the central nervous system* (pp. 801–823). New York: Raven Press.

Egan, V. G., Crawford, J. R., Brettle, R. P., & Goodwin, G. M. (1990). The Edinburgh cohort of HIV-positive drug users: Current intellectual function is impaired, but not due to early AIDS dementia complex. *AIDS, 4,* 651–656.

Fernández, F., Adams, F., & Levy, J. K. (1988a). Cognitive impairment due to AIDS-related complex and its response to psychostimulants. *Psychosomatics, 29,* 38–46.

Fernández, F., Levy, J. K., & Galizzi, H. (1988b). Response of HIV-related depression to psychostimulants: Case reports. *Hospital and Community Psychiatry, 39,* 628–631.

Ferre, F., Moss, R., Daigle, A., Richieri, S., Jensen, F., & Carlo, D. (1995). Viral load in peripheral blood mononuclear cells as surrogate for clinical progression. *Journal of Acquired Immune Deficiency Syndromes and Human Retrovirology, 10*(Suppl. 2), S51–S56.

Fiala, M., Singer, E. J., Graves, M. C., Tourtellotte, W. W., Stewart, J. A., Schable, C. A., Rhodes, R. H., & Vinters, H. V. (1993). AIDS dementia complex complicated by cytomegalovirus encephalopathy. *Journal of Neurology, 240*(4), 223–231.

Fong, I., Toma, E., & the Canadian PML Study Group. (1995). The natural history of progressive multifocal leukoencephalopathy in patients with AIDS. *Clinical Infectious Diseases, 20,* 1305–1310.

Gerard, L., Leport, C., Flandre, P., Houhou, N., Salmon-Ceron, D., Pepin, J., Mandet, C., Brun-Vezinet, F., & Vilde, J. (1997). Cytomegalovirus (CMV) viremia and the CD4+ lymphocyte count as predictors of CMV disease in patients infected with human immunodeficiency virus. *Clinical Infectious Diseases, 24,* 836–840.

Gillespie, S., Chang, Y., Lemp, G., Arthur, R., Buchbinder, S., Steimle, A., Baumgartner, J., Rando, T., Neal, D., Rutherford, G., et al. (1991). Progressive multifocal leukoencephalopathy in persons infected with human immunodeficiency virus, San Francisco, 1981 to 1989. *Annals of Neurology, 30,* 597–604.

Ginocchio, C., Kaplan, M., & Wang, X. (1995). CSF HIV-1 RNA quantitation as a prognostic marker for the differential diagnosis of AIDs related encephalopathy. In *Third International Conference on Antiretrovirals, Washington, DC* (Abstract No. 57).

Grafe, M. R., Press, G. A., Berthoty, D. P., Hesselink, J. R., & Wiley, C. A. (1990). Abnormalities of the brain in AIDS patients: Correlation of postmortem MR findings with neuropathology. *American Journal of Neuroradiology, 11*(5), 905–911.

Grafman, J., Wichman, A., Dalakas, M., Yarchoan, R., Broder, S., & Sever, J. (1989). HIV dementia: Cognitive profiles and response to AZT. *Neurology, 39*(Suppl. 1), 225.

Grant, I., Gold, J., Rosenblum, M., Niedzwiecki, D., & Armstrong, D. (1990). *Toxoplasma gondii* serology in HIV-infected patients: The development of central nervous system toxoplasmosis in AIDS. *AIDS, 4,* 519–521.

Gray, F., Belec, L., Keohane, C., De Truchis, P., Clair, B., Durigon, M., Sobel, A., & Gherardi, R. (1994). Zidovudine therapy and HIV encephalitis: A 10-year neuropathological study. *AIDS, 8*(4), 489–493.

Hall, C., & the AIDS Clinical Trial Group. (1997). Manuscript in preparation.

Havlir, D., Cheeseman, S., McLaughlin, M., Murphy, R., Erice, A., Spector, S., Greenaugh, T., Sullivan, J., Hall, D., Myers, M., et al. (1995). High dose nevirapine: Safety, pharmacokinetics, and antiviral activity in patients with HIV. *Journal of Infectious Diseases, 171,* 537–545.

Herzlich, B. C., & Schiano, T. D. (1993). Reversal of apparent AIDS dementia complex following treatment with vitamin B12. *Journal of Internal Medicine, 233*(6), 495–497.

Ho, D. D., Sarngadharan, M. G., Resnick, L., Di Marzo-Veronese, F., Rota, T. R., & Hirsch, M. S. (1985). Primary human T-lymphotrophic virus type III infection. *Annals of Internal Medicine, 103,* 880–883.

Holland, N., Power, C., Mathews, V., Glass, J. D., Forman, H., McArthur, J. C. (1994). CMV encephalitis in acquired immunodeficiency syndrome. *Neurology, 44,* 507–514.

Hollander, H., Golden, J., Mendelson, T., & Cortland, D. (1985). Extrapyramidal symptoms in AIDS patients given low dose metoclopramide or chlorpromazine. *Lancet, ii,* 1186.

Hollander, H., & Stringari, S. (1987). Human immunodeficiency virus-associated meningitis: Clinical course and correlations. *American Journal of Medicine, 83,* 813–816.

Holmes, V. F., Fernández, F., & Levy, J. K. (1989). Psychostimulant response in AIDS-related complex patients. *Journal of Clinical Psychiatry, 50,* 5–8.

Horwath, E., Kramer, M., Cournos, F., Empfield, M., & Gewirtz, G. (1989). Clinical presentations of AIDS and HIV infection in state psychiatric facilities. *Hospital and Community Psychiatry, 40*(5), 502–506.

Hriso, E., Kuhn, T., Masdeu, J. C., & Grundman, M. (1991). Extrapyramidal symptoms due to dopamine-blocking agents in patients with AIDS encephalopathy. *American Journal of Psychiatry, 148,* 1558–1561.

Hufert, F. T., von Laer, D., Fenner, T. E., Schwander, S., Kern, P., & Schmitz, H. (1991). Progression of HIV-1 infection: Monitoring of HIV-1 DNA in peripheral blood mononuclear cells by PCR. *Archives of Virology, 120,* 233–240.

Hughes, M., Johnson, V., Hirsch, M., Bremer, J., Elbeik, T., Erice, A., Kurltzkes, D., Scott, W., Spector, S., Bosgoz, N., et al. (1997). Monitoring plasma HIV-1 RNA levels in addition to CD4+ lymphocyte count improves assessment of antiretroviral therapeutic response. *Annals of Internal Medicine, 126,* 929–938.

Janssen, R. S., Nwanyanwu, O. C., Selik, R. M., & Stehr-Green, J. K. (1992).

Epidemiology of human immunodeficiency virus encephalopathy in the United States. *Neurology, 42,* 1472–1476.

Johns, D. R., Tierney, M., & Felsenstein, D. (1987). Alteration in the natural history of neurosyphilis by concurrent infection with the human immunodeficiency virus. *New England Journal of Medicine, 316,* 1569–1572.

Jones, J., Hanson, D., Chu, S., Ciesielski, C., Kaplan, J., Ward, J., & Navin, T. (1996). Toxoplasmic encephalitis in HIV-infected persons: Risk factors and trends. *AIDS, 10,* 1393–1399.

Kieburtz, K. D., Epstein, L. G., Gelbard, H. A., & Greenamyre, J. T. (1991). Excitotoxicity and dopaminergic dysfunction in the acquired immunodeficiency syndrome dementia complex: Therapeutic implications. *Archives of Neurology, 48,* 1281–1284.

Kitamura, T., Aso, Y., Kunioshi, N., Hara, K., & Yogo, Y. (1990). High incidence of urinary JC Virus excretion in nonimmunocompromised older patients. *Journal of Infectious Diseases, 161,* 1128–1133.

Kovacs, J. A., Kovacs, A. A., Polis, M., et al. (1985). Cryptococcosis in the acquired immunodeficiency syndrome. *Annals of Internal Medicine, 103,* 533–538.

Kuni, C. C., Rhame, F. S., Meier, M. J., Foehse, M. C., Loewenson, R. B., Lee, B. C., Boudreau, R. J., & duCret, R. P. (1991). Quantitative I-123-IMP brain SPECT and neuropsychological testing in AIDS dementia. *Clinical Nuclear Medicine, 16*(3), 174–177.

Lang, W., Miklossy, J., Dervaz, J., Pizzolator, G. P., Probst, A., Schaffner, J., Gessaga, E., & Kleihues, P. (1989). Neuropathology of the acquired immunodeficiency syndrome (AIDS): Report of 135 consecutive autopsy cases from Switzerland. *Acta Neuropathologica, 77,* 379–390.

Levine, A. (1991). Epidemiology, clinical characteristics, and management of AIDs-related lymphoma. *Hematology/Oncology Clinics of North America, 5,* 331–342.

Levine, A., Wernz, J. C., Kaplan, L., Rodman, N., Cohen, P., Metroka, C., Bennett, J. M., Rarick, M. V., Walsh, C., Kahn, J., et al. (1991). Low-dose chemotherapy with central nervous system prophylaxis and zidovudine maintainance in AIDS-related lymphoma: A prospective multi-institutional trial. *Journal of the American Medical Association, 266,* 84–88.

Lipton, S. A., & Gendelman, H. E. (1995). Dementia associated with the acquired immunodeficiency syndrome. *New England Journal of Medicine, 332,* 934–940.

Lopez, O., Becker, J., Banks, G., Giconi, J., Sanchez, J., & Dorst, S. (1996). Development of subtle neurologic signs after systemic illness in HIV-infected individuals. *European Neurology, 36,* 71–75.

Lortholary, G., Pialous, B., Dupont, B., Trotot, P., et al. (1994). Prolonged survival of a patient with AIDS and progressive multifocal leukoencephalopathy. *Clinical Infectious Diseases, 18,* 826–827.

Luft, B., & Remington, J. (1992). Toxoplasmic encephalitis in AIDS. *Clinical Infectious Diseases, 15,* 211–222.

Lyketsos, C., Hanson, A., Fishman, M., Rosenblatt, A., Mc Hugh, R. R., & Trelsman, G. J. (1993). Manic syndrome early and and late in the course of HIV. *American Journal of Psychiatry, 150,* 326–327.

Maehlen, J., Dunlop, O., Liestol, K., Dobloug, J., Goplen, A., & Torvik, A. (1995). Changing incidence of HIV-induced brain lesions in Oslo, 1983–1994: Effects of zidovudine treatment. *AIDS, 9,* 1165–1169.

Maj, M., Satz, P., Janssen, R., Zaudig, M., Starace, F., D'Elia, L., Sughondhabirom, B., Mussa, M., Naber, D., Ndetei, D., et al. (1994). WHO Neuropsychiatric AIDS Study, Cross-Sectional Phase II: Neuropsychological and neurological findings. *Archives of General Psychiatry, 51,* 51–61.

Malone, J., Wallace, M., Hendrick, B., La Rocco, A., Tonon, E., Brodine, S., Bowler, W., Lavin, B., Hawkins, R., & Oldfield, E. (1995). Syphilis and neurosyphilis in a human immunodeficiency virus type-1 seropositive population: Evidence for frequent serologic relapse after therapy. *American Journal of Medicine, 99,* 55–63.

Manser, T., & Warner, J. (1990). Neuroleptic malignant syndrome associated with prochlorperazine. *Southern Medical Journal, 83,* 73–76.

Marder, K., Stern, Y., Malouf, R., Tang, M., Bell, K., Dooneief, G., El-Sadr, W., Goldstein, S., Gorman, J., Richards, M., Sano, M., Sorrell, S., Todak, G., Williams, J. B. W., Ehrhardt, A., & Mayeux, R. (1992). Neurologic and neuropsychological manifestations of human immunodeficiency virus infection in intravenous drug users without acquired immunodeficiency syndrome. *Archives of Neurology, 49,* 1169–1175.

Mark, A. S., & Atlas, S. W. (1989). Progressive multifocal leukoencephalopathy in patients with AIDS: appearance on MR images. *Radiology, 173*(2), 517–520.

Marshall, D. W., Brey, R. L., & Cahill, W. T. (1988). Cerebrospinal fluid (CSF) findings in asymptomatic (AS) individuals infected by human immunodeficiency virus (HIV). *Neurology, 38,* 167–168.

McArthur, J. C., Cohen, B. A., Selnes, O. A., Kumar, A. J., Cooper, K., McArthur, J. H., Soucy, G., Cornblath, D. R., Chmiel, J. S., Wang, M. C., Starkey, D. L., Ginzburg, H., Ostrow, D. G., Johnson, R. T., Phair, J. P., & Polk, B. F. (1989). Low prevalence of neurological and neuropsychological abnormalities in otherwise healthy HIV-1-infected individuals: Results from the Multicenter AIDS Cohort Study. *Annals of Neurology, 26*(5), 601–611.

McArthur, J. C., Hoover, D. R., Bacellar, H., Miller, E. N., Cohen, B. A., Becker, J. T., Graham, N. M. H., McArthur, J. H., Selnes, O. A., Jacobsen, L. P., Visscher, B. R., Concha, M., & Saah, A. (1993). Dementia in AIDS patients: Incidence and risk factors. *Neurology, 43,* 2245–2252.

McArthur, J. C., Selnes, O. A., Glass, J. D., Hoover, D. R., & Bacellar, H. (1994). HIV dementia: Incidence and risk factors. In R. W. Price & S. W. Perry (Ed.), *Research publications of the Association for Research in Nervous and Mental Disease: Vol. 72. HIV, AIDS and the brain* (pp. 251–271). New York: Raven Press.

Mellors, J., Munoz, A., Giorgi, J., Margolick, J., Tassoni, C., Gupta, P., Kingsley, L., Todd, J., Saah, A. J., Detels, R., et al. (1997). Plasma viral load and CD4+ lymphocytes as prognostic markers of HIV-1 infection. *Annals of Internal Medicine, 126,* 946–954.

Menon, D., Ainsworth, J., Cox, I., Coker, R., Sargentoni, J., Coutts, G., Baudouin, C., Kocsis, A., & Harris, J. (1992). Proton MR spectroscopy of the brain in

AIDS dementia complex. *Journal of Computer-Assisted Tomography, 16,* 538–542.

Miller, E., Satz, P., & Visscher, B. (1991). Computerized and conventional neuropsychological assessment of HIV-1-infected homosexual men. *Neurology, 41,* 1608–1616.

Mueller, B., Sei, S., Anderson, B., Luzuriaga, K., Farley, M., Venzon, D., Tudor-Williams, G., Schwartzentruber, D., Fox, C., Sullivan, J., et al. (1996). Comparison of virus burden in blood and sequential lymph node biopsy specimens from children infected with human immunodeficiency virus. *Journal of Pediatrics, 129,* 410–418.

Mullis, K. B., & Faloona, F. A. (1987). *Specific synthesis of DNA in* vitro *via a polymerase-catalyzed chain reaction. Methods in Enzymology, 155,* 335–350.

Musher, D., Hamill, R., & Baughn, R. (1990). Effect of human immunodeficiency virus (HIV) infection on the course of syphilis and on the response to treatment. *Annals of Internal Medicine, 113,* 872–881.

Navia, B. A., Cho, E.-S., Petito, C. K., & Price, R. W. (1986a). The AIDS dementia complex: II. Neuropathology. *Annals of Neurology, 19,* 525–535.

Navia, B. A., Jordan, B. D., & Price, R. W. (1986b). The AIDS dementia complex: I. Clinical features. *Annals of Neurology, 19,* 517–524.

Novak, I. S., Trujillo, J. R., Rivera, V. M., Conklin, R., Ussery, F., III, Stool, E. W., & Piot, D. F. (1989). Ganciclovir in the treatment of CMV infection in AIDS patients with neurologic complications. *Neurology, 39*(Suppl. 1), 379.

O'Brien, W., Hartigan, P., Daar, E., Simberkoff, M., Hamilton, J., & Veterans Affairs Cooperative Study Group on AIDS. (1997). Changes in plasma HIV RNA levels and CD4+ lymphocyte counts predict both response to antiretroviral therapy and therapuetic failure. *Annals of Internal Medicine, 126,* 939–945.

Portegies, P., Algra, P., Hollak, C., Prins, J. M., Reiss, P., Valk, J., & Lange, J. M. (1991). Response to cytarabine in progressive multifocal leucoencephalopathy in AIDS. *Lancet, 337,* 680–681.

Portegies, P., de Gans, J., Lange, J. M., Derix, M. M., Speelman, H., Bakker, M., Danner, S. A., & Goudsmit, J. (1989). Declining incidence of AIDS dementia complex after introduction of zidovudine treatment. *British Medical Journal, 299*(6703), 819–821.

Portegies, P., Enting, R. H., de Gans, J., Algra, P. R., Derix, M. M., Lange, J. M., & Goudsmit, J. (1993). Presentation and course of AIDS dementia complex: 10 years of follow-up in Amsterdam, The Netherlands. *AIDS, 7*(5), 669–675.

Porter, S., & Sande, M. (1992). Toxoplasmosis of the central nervous system in the acquired immunodeficiency syndrome. *New England Journal of Medicine, 327,* 1643–1648.

Post, M. J., Levin, B. E., Berger, J. R., Duncan, R., Quencer, R. M., & Calabro, G. (1992). Sequential cranial MR findings of asymptomatic and neurologically symptomatic HIV+ subjects. *American Journal of Neuroradiology, 13*(1), 359–370.

Post, M. J., Tate, L. G., Quencer, R. M., Hensley, G. T., Berger, J. R., Sheremata, W. A., & Maul, G. (1988). CT, MR, and pathology in HIV encephalitis and meningitis. *American Journal of Roentgenology, 151*(2), 373–380.

Pratt, R., Nichols, S., McKinney, N., Kwok, S., Danker, W., & Spector, S. (1996). Virologic markers of human immunodeficiency virus type 1 in cerebrospinal fluid of infected children. *Journal of Infectious Diseases, 174,* 288–293.

Rabkin, J., & Harrison, W. (1990). Effect of imiprimine on depression and immune status in a sample of men with HIV infection. *American Journal of Psychiatry, 147,* 782–784.

Roche Laboratories. (1995). *Investigational drug brochure Ro 31-8959.* Nutley, NJ: Hoffmann–La Roche.

Roche Laboratories. (1996). *Invirase*^{TM} *(saquinivir mesylate) package insert. Nutley, NJ: Hoffmann–La Roche.*

Rolston, K., & Hoy, J. (1987). Role of clindamycin in the treatment of central nervous system toxoplasmosis. *American Journal of Medicine, 83,* 551–554.

Rottenberg, D. A., Moeller, J. R., Strother, S. C., Sidtis, J. J., Navia, B. A., Dhawan, V., Ginos, J. Z., & Price, R. W. (1987). The metabolic pathology of the AIDS dementia complex. *Annals of Neurology, 22*(6), 700–706.

Royal, W. III, Selnes, O., Concha, M., Nance-Sproson, T., & McArthur, J. (1994). Cerebrospinal fluid human immunodeficiency virus type 1 (HIV-1) p24 antigen levels in HIV-1-related dementia. *Annals of Neurology, 36,* 32–39.

Satz, P., Morgenstern, H., Miller, E. N., Selnes, O. A., McArthur, J. C., Cohen, B. A., Wesch, J., Becker, J. T., Jacobson, L., D'Elia, L. F., et al. (1993). Low education as a possible risk factor for cognitive abnormalities in HIV-1: Findings from the Multicenter AIDS Cohort Study (MACS). *Journal of Acquired Immune Deficiency Syndromes, 6,* 503–511.

Schmid, P., Conrad, A., Syndulko, K., Singer, E., Handley, D., Li, X., Tao, G., Fahy-Chandon, B., & Tourtellotte, W. (1994). Quantifying HIV-1 proviral DNA using the polymerase chain reaction on cerebrospinal fluid and blood of seropositive individuals with and without neurologic abnormalities. *Journal of Acquired Immune Deficiency Syndrome, 7,* 777–788.

Schmitt, F. A., Bigley, J. W., McKinnis, R., Logue, P. E., Evans, R. W., & Drucker, J. L. (1988). Neuropsychological outcome of zidovudine (AZT) treatment of patients with AIDS and AIDS-related complex. *New England Journal of Medicine, 319*(24), 1573–1578.

Sei, S., Stewart, S., Farley, M., Mueller, B., Lane, J., Robb, M., Brouwers, P., & Pizzo, P. (1996). Evaluation of human immunodeficiency virus (HIV) type 1 RNA levels in cerebrospinal fluid and viral resistance to zidovudine in children with HIV encephalopathy. *Journal of Infectious Diseases, 174*(6), 1200–1206.

Selnes, O. A., McArthur, J. C., Royal, W. I., Updike, M. L., Nance-Sproson, T., Concha, M., Gordon, B., Solomon, L., & Vlahov, D. (1992). HIV-1 infection and intravenous drug use: Longitudinal neuropsychological evaluation of asymptomatic subjects. *Neurology, 42,* 1924–1930.

Sidtis, J. J., Gatsonis, C., Price, R. W., Singer, E. J., Collier, A. C., Richman, D. D., Hirsch, M. S., Schaerf, F. W., Fischl, M. A., Kieburtz, K., Simpson, D., Kocj, M. A., Feinberg, J., Dafini, U., & AIDS Clinical Trial Group. (1993). Zidovudine treatment of the AIDS dementia complex: Results of a placebo-controlled trial. AIDS Clinical Trials Group. *Annals of Neurology, 33,* 343–349.

Singer, E., Stoner, G., Singer, P., Tomiyasu, U., Licht, E., Fahy-Chandon, B., & Tourtellotte, W. (1994a). AIDS presenting as progressive multifocal leukoencephalopathy with clinical response to zidovudine. *Acta Neurologica Scandinavica, 90,* 443–447.

Singer, E. J., Syndulko, K., Fahy-Chandon, B., Kim, J., Conrad, A., Schmid, P., & Tourtellotte, W. W. (1994b). Cerebrospinal fluid p24 antigen levels and intrathecal immunoglobulin G synthesis are associated with cognitive disease severity in HIV-1. *AIDS, 8*(1), 29–37.

Singer, E. J., Syndulko, K., Fahy-Chandon, B., Kim, J., Conrad, A., Schmid, P., & Tourtellotte, W. W. (1994c). Intrathecal IgG synthesis and albumin leakage are increased in subjects with HIV-1 neurologic disease. *Journal of Acquired Immune Deficiency Syndromes, 7,* 265–271.

Snider, W. D., Simpson, D. M., Nielson, S., Gold, J. W. M., Metroka, C., & Posner, J. B. (1983). Neurological complications of acquired immune deficiency syndrome: Analysis of 50 patients. *Annals of Neurology, 14,* 403–418.

So, Y. T., Beckstead, J., & Davis, R. L. (1986). Primary CNS lymphoma in AIDS: A clinical and pathological study. *Annals of Neurology, 20,* S66–S72.

Stern, R., Silva, S., Chaisson, N., & Evans, D. (1996). Influence of cognitive reserve on neuropsychological functioning in asymptomatic human immunodeficiency virus-1 infection. *Archives of Neurology, 53,* 148–153.

Straus, D. (1997). Human immunodeficiency virus-associated lymphomas. *Medical Clinics of North America, 81,* 495–509.

Sugar, A., & Saunders, C. (1988). Oral fluconazole as suppressive therapy of disseminated cryptococcosis in patients with acquired immunodeficiency syndrome. *American Journal of Medicine, 85,* 481–489.

Tada, H., Rappaport, J., Lashgari, M., Amini, S., F, Wong-Staal, F. & Khalili, K. (1990). Trans-activation of the JC virus late promoter by the tat protein to type 1 human immunodeficiency virus in glial cells. *Proceedings of the National Academy of Sciences USA, 87,* 3479–3483.

Thomas, C., & Szabadi, E. (1987). Paranoid psychosis as the first presentation of a fulminating lethal case of AIDS. *British Journal of Psychiatry, 151,* 693–695.

Tozzi, V., Narciso, P., Galgani, S., Sette, P., Balestra, P., Gerace, C., Pau, F., Pigorini, F., Volpini, V., & Camporiondo, M. (1993). Effects of zidovudine in 30 patients with mild to end-stage AIDS dementia complex. *AIDS, 7,* 683–692.

Vago, L., Castagna, A., Lazzarin, A., Trabattoni, G., Cinque, P., & Costanzi, G. (1993). Reduced frequency of HIV-induced brain lesions in AIDS patients treated with zidovudine. *Journal of Acquired Immune Deficiency Syndromes, 6*(1), 42–45.

Vella, S., Floridia, M., Tomino, C., & et al. (1994). Zidovudine versus ddI in HIV-infected patients previously treated with zidovudine for at least six months: ISS 901 study. In *VIII National Conference on AIDS, Bologna, Italy.*

Vogel-Scibilia, S. E., Mulsant, B. H., & Keshavan, M. S. (1988). HIV infection presenting as psychosis: A critique. *Acta Psychiatrica Scandinavica, 78,* 652–656.

Weber, T., Turner, R., Frye, S., Luke, W., Kretzschmar, H., Luer, W., & Hunsmann, G. (1994). Progressive multifocal leukoencephalopathy diagnosed by amplification of JC virus-specific DNA from cerebrospinal fluid. *AIDS, 8,* 49–57.

Weiner, L. P., & Narayan, O. (1974). Progressive multifocal leukoencephalopathy. *Advances in Neurology, 6,* 87–92.

Zuger, A., Louie, E., Holzman, R. S., Simberkoff, M. S., & Rahal, J. J. (1986). Cryptococcal disease in patients with the acquired immunodeficiency syndrome: Diagnostic features and outcome of treatment. *Annals of Internal Medicine, 104*(2), 234–240.

Zurlo, J., O'Neill, D., Polis, M., Manischewitz, J., Yarchoan, R., Baseler, M., Lane, C., & Masur, H. (1993). Lack of clinical utility of cytomegalovirus blood and urine cultures in patients with HIV infection. *Annals of Internal Medicine, 118,* 12–17.

4

Neuropsychiatric Features of HIV Disease

ANDRÉS SCIOLLA
J. HAMPTON ATKINSON
IGOR GRANT

INTRODUCTION: CHANGE AS A CHALLENGE

HIV disease has not yet been fully described, and its history is being written—quite literally—together with these lines. The incidence and growth rate, geographic distribution, populations at highest risk, therapeutic practices and medications, prognosis and survival rates, and societal reactions to infected individuals have all changed significantly, if not dramatically, in the course of 15 years. These changes have two important consequences: First, observations made in the same population at points in the epidemic separated by only a few years may differ substantially; and, second, data collected in one population may not be generalizable to others. These consequences are discussed briefly here.

A remarkable change in psychological responses has been documented among white gay men in large U.S. cities along the years of the epidemic. For example, in a cohort study started in 1985 involving 746 gay men in New York City, both the occurrence and duration of bereavement effects are diminishing with time (J. L. Martin & Dean, 1993). Specifically, losses experienced in the early 1980s contributed to distress as long as 5 years later; after 1987, although the bereaved group continued to exhibit elevated levels of depression, traumatic stress, and sedative use, these differences were no longer statistically significant (J. L. Martin & Dean, 1993). Similarly, the WHO neuropsychiatric AIDS study indicated that in geographical areas where spreading of HIV infection is more recent and the social rejection of HIV-seropositive subjects is harsher, the symptomatic stages of the disease are associated with increased prevalence of both depressive symptoms and syndromal depression (Maj, 1996).

Most of the information on neuropsychiatric features of HIV disease contained in this chapter has been gathered in the population group where HIV disease was first described in North America and Western Europe—namely, white men who have sex with men (MSM).[1] Data available on newer risk groups (particularly women and people of color), and from other world regions, are preliminary, and methodological differences among studies make comparisons difficult at best. This situation has started to change, thanks to cross- and transcultural, multinational studies using internationally accepted nomenclature and standardized methods (Maj et al., 1991). Although some common themes are emerging, the clinical features of treatment strategies for, or prognoses of neuropsychiatric complications of HIV/AIDS are likely to differ among all populations currently at risk, given the psychosocial and socioeconomic differences among them (Gala et al., 1993).

For example, social support modulates stress and psychopathology in HIV-infected populations (Linn, Lewis, Cain, & Kimbrough, 1993; Patterson et al., 1993), and may also impact HIV disease progression. HIV-infected men reporting high levels of loneliness had significantly fewer CD4+ cells than did men reporting low levels of loneliness, regardless of disease stage (Straits-Tröster et al., 1994). Mental health practitioners working in large urban centers of the United States find a variety of helpful psychosocial resources in the community where they can refer gay men from the cultural majority. Women and members of ethnic minorities or socially disadvantaged groups, regardless of their HIV risk factors, may have lower levels of social support and experience significant barriers in access to psychosocial services. Data from the San Diego HIV Neurobehavioral Research Center (HNRC) cohort, for example, have shown that participants of color tended to

---

[1]For reasons other than misrepresentation (e.g., cultural), some men infected with HIV through sexual contact with other men do not define themselves as "gay," "homosexual," or "bisexual." The more descriptive term "men who have sex with men," albeit awkward, is used in this chapter to refer to that group whenever individuals have not self-identified as gay. Following other authors, we use the word "homosexual" as an adjective only, and not as a noun (Risman & Schwartz, 1988).

report less satisfaction with the support they received (Cherner et al., 1994) and psychosocial variables unique to women have been identified (Semple et al., 1996; Nannis, Patterson, & Semple, 1997).

Beneficial, or even life-transforming, aspects of HIV disease have been reported by mostly white, educated, high-functioning, middle-class HIV-positive gay men (Schwartzberg, 1994), and a positive outlook and strong morale after 3 years of an AIDS diagnosis (Rabkin, Remien, Katoff, & Williams, 1993b) was found in another study. In contrast, higher levels of depression among impoverished inner-city African-American gay men infected with HIV, as compared to data reported in the literature, have been reported (Cochran & Mays, 1994), and the additional psychosocial burdens experienced by African-American gay men have been underlined (Dowd, 1994). High levels of depression may also characterize other men, since one study did not find differences in depressive mood associated with HIV status or sexual orientation in a group of African-American gay, bisexual, and heterosexual men (Peterson, Folkman, & Bakeman, 1996).

Although it remains a controversial issue (Schmitt et al., 1988; Portegies, Epstein, Hung, de Gans, & Goudsmit, 1989; Day et al., 1992; McArthur et al., 1993), zidovudine use may have some protective effects on the brain against HIV, at least initially (Gulevich et al., 1993; Karlsen, Reinvang, & Froland, 1995). Some studies show that ethnic minorities are receiving antiretroviral agents at a later stage of the disease and are less likely to receive prophylactic treatment for opportunistic infections than are patients of the cultural majority (Easterbrook et al., 1991; Moore, Hidalgo, Bareta, & Chaisson, 1994). It is possible, then, that the incidence and severity of neurocognitive disorders in socially disadvantaged groups may be higher than in individuals of higher socioeconomic status.

Women infected with HIV through heterosexual transmission are currently the fastest-growing group of HIV patients in the United States. Studies have identified stressors unique to women (e.g., gynecological problems, future guardianship of children)—differences that may have implications for clinical management (Semple et al., 1993).

Compounding psychosocial factors, socioeconomic factors that make access to adequate health care difficult can hasten HIV disease progression and increase its neuropsychiatric complications. Recently, researchers have explained associations found in earlier studies between race/ethnicity, gender, drug use, or income level on the one hand, and HIV disease progression and survival on the other, as the result of varying adequacy of medical care (Chaisson, Keruly, & Moore, 1995). Note that race or ethnicity is not associated with a biological risk factor for HIV infection, just as homosexuality per se is not. Rather, individual differences or behaviors within the categories of race/ethnicity and sexual orientation may be associated with increased risk for HIV infection and transmission. These include younger age (Aral, 1994; Kelly et al., 1995b); female gender (Aral, Soskoline, Joesoef, & O'Reilly, 1991; Ehrhardt, 1992); immune function (Paxton et al., 1996); lower socioeconomic status, including barriers in access to health care (Aral, 1994; Sobo, 1993); less education (Kelly et al., 1995b); low self-esteem, including low gay self-acceptance (Perkins, Leserman, Murphy, & Evans, 1993b; Rotheram-Borus, Rosario, Reed, & Koopman, 1995; reported childhood sexual abuse (Allers, Benjack, White, & Rousey, 1993; Carballo-Diguez & Dolezal, 1995; Zierler et al., 1991; Holmes, 1997); mental disorders, including substance use disorders (Brooner, Greenfield, Schmidt, & Bigelow, 1993; Edlin et al., 1994; Ericksen & Trocki, 1992; Darke, Swift, & Hall, 1994; Ostrow, 1994; Perkins, Davidson, Leserman, Liao, & Evans, 1993a; Silberstein et al., 1994); personality traits (Kalichman et al., 1994a); coping (Beltrn, Ostriw, & Joseph, 1993; D. J. Martin, 1993); uncircumcised status (Kreiss & Hopkins, 1993); and exclusive preference for receptive anal intercourse (Weinrich, Grant, Jacobson, Robinson, & McCutchan, 1992).

The arrest of viral replication or even viral eradication resulting from the combination of antiretrovirals and the development of vaccines may not necessarily eradicate HIV. The main modes of HIV transmission are injection drug use (IDU) and unprotected sex—two highly complex behaviors with poorly understood motivations that cannot be easily modified. In fact, high risk in one behavior predicted high risk in the other among persons engaging in IDU (Booth, 1995). HIV disease may act as other sexually transmitted diseases (STDs) do. There are simple, effective, and relatively inexpensive treatment for syphilis and gonorrhea. In the United States, however, there are some geographic areas and large population groups with low levels of STDs, while others continue to experience an epidemic of STDs, particularly inner-city people of color (Piot & Islam, 1994). An association between the transmissions of syphilis and HIV has already been observed among heterosexual African-Americans in urban areas (Otten, Zaidi, Peterman, Rolfs, & Witte, 1994). An increase of gonorrhea cases among MSM by 74%, reported in several large U.S. cities from 1993 to 1996, signals an increase in high-risk encounters in this group that may precede another surge of cases of HIV disease (CDC, 1997). Therefore, a working knowledge of the medical, neurobehavioral, and psychosocial aspects of HIV disease will remain a necessity for mental health practitioners in the foreseeable future. In spite of the ever-changing nature of the HIV/AIDS epidemic, clinicians will feel compensated by working in one of today's most challenging yet rewarding professional fields. They may feel more effective whenever they face constant changes as motivations to acquire new knowledge and insights, as opposed to threats to their clinical skills or therapeutic abilities.

DIAGNOSTIC ISSUES:
HIV DISEASE AS A BRAIN DISEASE

HIV disease is best conceptualized as a brain disease for a number of reasons.[2] First, HIV infects lymphocytes and other cells having the cluster designation 4 (CD4) glycoprotein (McCutchan, 1994), a receptor present in monocytes and macrophages, which are the predominant cell types in the brain infected with HIV (Ho, Bredesen, Vinters, & Daar, 1989). Also, certain glycolipids that have been proposed as non-CD4 sources of HIV infection are found in oligodendroglia and neurons (Nathanson, Cook, Kolson, & Gonzalez-Scarano, 1994).

Second, brain function (behavior and cognition) may be altered as a direct result of this infection, as opposed to the individual's psychological reaction to the infection. HIV can be found in the cerebrospinal fluid (CSF) shortly after HIV enters the body (Goudsmit et al., 1986; Resnick, Berger, Shapshak, & Tourtellotte, 1988). In the central nervous system (CNS), the microglia and monocytes/macrophages are productively infected with HIV, while neurons, astrocytes, and oligodendrocytes are not infected (Wiley, 1994). Neuronal loss and reduced density of dendritic spines, the neuronal branches involved in cell-to-cell communication, are found in brains examined at postmortem (Masliah, Ge, & Mucke, in press).

Third, the conceptualization proposed may prevent misdiagnosis. Persons can react to events associated with HIV disease with anxiety and depression, social isolation for fear of stigmatization, and considerable stress stemming from financial problems and barriers to health care access. Common symptoms resulting from the myriad of challenges HIV-infected individuals face are low energy levels, apathy, withdrawal, sleep disturbance, loss of appetite, diminished libido, and problems with concentration and memory. Equally often, however, these kinds of symptoms result from systemic or CNS effects of HIV.

---

[2]This statement is not intended to downplay the contribution of psychological and social factors to mental disorders in HIV disease. In fact, as we have pointed out elsewhere (e.g., see Atkinson & Grant, 1997b), the fundamental tenet of modern psychiatry—namely, a biopsychosocial model of normal and abnormal behavior—is nowhere more clearly evident than in the neuropsychiatry of HIV.

Obviously, too, even these organic signs and symptoms are colored by individuals' psychological response.

By keeping in mind that HIV is a brain disease, clinicians will be compelled to assess the extent to which subjective complaints and objective features in each patient or client are psychological or organic. Feelings of guilt are highly prevalent among HIV-infected individuals; after all, HIV is a disease acquired in most cases through activities (sex and IDU) that characteristically break social taboos, which can result in shame or guilt. Increasingly, too, individuals who become infected know how to diminish the risk of HIV transmission. In such contexts HIV seroconversion may be perceived as a failure to protect oneself, and thus can be associated with feelings of inadequacy and powerlessness. Also, many individuals are aware of the relationship between the immune system and stress, anxiety, or depression. They may interpret evidence of further deterioration of their immunity as a personal failure to "do the right thing." Therefore, clinicians can remove from patients an undue burden and its impact on self-worth whenever they correctly attribute signs and symptoms to HIV. Most importantly, this correct attribution allows the possibility of effective treatment.

Fourth, after the lungs and the gastrointestinal tract, the CNS is the organ system most often involved in AIDS-associated diseases leading to death (Klatt, Nichols, & Noguchi, 1994). In addition, several lines of evidence suggest that symptomatic HIV infection of the CNS (e.g., neurocognitive impairment, psychosis) is associated with a poorer prognosis, including disease progression and survival rates (Mayeux et al., 1993; Stern et al., 1995; R. J. Ellis et al., 1997). Finally, a significant, albeit subclinical loss of visual function that is not the result of infectious retinopathy (Quiceno et al., 1992; Iragui et al., 1996; Plummer et al., 1996; Mueller et al., 1997), together with persistent hearing abnormalities described among HIV-infected individuals (Marra et al., 1996) are best understood in the context of a neurotrophic virus.

According to the *Diagnostic and Statistical Manual of Mental Disorders,* fourth edition (DSM-IV; American Psychiatric Association, 1994), mental disorders and neuropsychiatric syndromes in HIV-infected individuals can be divided into three groups: primary mental disorders (which have no specific etiology), substance-induced disorders, and mental disorders due to a general medical condition (HIV disease).[3] In addition to its heuristic value, the DSM-IV distinction allows a number of clinically useful generalizations. First, three of the population groups

---

[3]The present chapter follows DSM-IV nomenclature and diagnostic criteria, with the exception of neurocognitive disorders and HIV-associated sleep disturbance.

presenting with the highest risk for HIV—namely, gay men, women, and persons engaging in IDU—have higher prevalence rates of primary mental disorders prior to HIV infection, compared to the general population. Nevertheless, HIV disease itself does not seem to elevate such high premorbid rates significantly (i.e., before seroconversion). There are few new-onset primary mental disorders (i.e., after seroconversion) even in these psychopathologically vulnerable groups.

Second, the clinical features of primary mental disorders and substance-induced disorders do not change as a result of HIV disease (at least during the asymptomatic phase of the disease), and diagnosis remains straightforward in the majority of cases. In contrast, the diagnosis of mental disorders due to HIV disease is frequently difficult.

Third, each disease stage has a characteristic prevalence for each group of disorders. The prevalence of primary mental disorders remains stable over the course of the disease; mental disorders due to HIV disease tend to occur after the onset of immunodeficiency and are particularly prevalent in end-stage disease; and substance-induced disorders are uncommon in later stages, as many individuals "clean up their act" for health considerations or become physically unable to tolerate intoxication.

Fourth, the prognoses of primary mental disorders have less to do with HIV than with such factors as family history, personal medical and psychiatric history, coping and social support available, previous responses to therapy, and the like. Prognoses of substance-induced disorders depend on treating the underlying cause (i.e., substance abuse or dependence, exposure to toxins, side effects of a medication). In contrast, prognoses of disorders due to HIV disease are related to those of the underlying HIV infection.

Operationally defined neuropsychiatric disorders and syndromes constitute only a portion of the clinically significant phenomena that a mental health practitioner can encounter in dealing with HIV-infected individuals. Thus, adjustment disorders have been discussed, but what others have termed "acute stress reactions" (i.e., generally less severe and shorter-duration psychological responses to such stressors as diagnosis of infection and changes in the individual's clinical state; Maj, 1990) have been left out. The DSM-IV has introduced the diagnostic category of acute stress disorder, but little if any information is available about this disorder in the context of HIV disease. Maladaptive coping—a topic that may have a significant impact on the course of the disease—has not been covered, and the reader is referred to recent reviews of the subject (Chesney & Folkman, 1994; Kalichman & Sikkema, 1994). Topics of special interest, such as suicide, the "worried well," pain syndromes, and children/adolescents and the family, have been reviewed elsewhere (Atkinson & Grant, 1997b; Grant & Atkinson,

1995). Although anxiety and mood syndromes failing to meet full DSM-IV criteria (subsyndromal conditions) may be highly prevalent among HIV-infected persons, they are not discussed, since they are part of active research and their potential relevance to disease progression remains unclear.

The following is a discussion of the syndromes that have been the focus of most neuropsychiatric research—namely, the most common primary mental disorders and mental disorders due to HIV disease. Since the category of substance-induced disorders has been described only recently, no HIV-specific information is yet available. Also, in the context of HIV disease, they are more likely to be secondary to drugs of abuse (not medications or toxins), and their acute, transient nature makes research difficult. Therapeutic recommendations are provided in a later section.

Mood Disorders

Major Depressive Disorder

Epidemiology. Lifetime prevalence of major depressive disorder among men in the U.S. general population is 13% (Regier et al., 1988; Blazer, Kessler, McGonagle, & Swartz, 1994; Kessler et al., 1994), while among seropositive and seronegative gay men and men engaging in IDU it is 22–61% (Atkinson et al., 1988; G. R. Brown et al., 1992; Williams, Rabkin, Remien, Gorman, & Ehrhardt, 1991; Rosenberger et al., 1993; Bialer, Wallack, & Snyder, 1991) in seropositive and seronegative groups. In most cases, the first episode of major depression preceded seroconversion (Atkinson et al., 1988; Perry et al., 1990b; Williams et al., 1991; Rosenberger et al., 1993).

Although it has been usually assumed (e.g., Friedman & Downey, 1994) that the elevated rates among gay and bisexual men are related to sexual orientation, homosexuality is a complex category susceptible of subdivisions (Weinrich et al., 1993). Gay men who report high levels of gender nonconformity during their childhood (i.e., they displayed behaviors usually assumed by girls and women in our society) have increased rates of lifetime and current depression while individuals without gender dysphoria may have rates comparable to those of men in the general population (Weinrich, Atkinson, McCutchan, & Grant, 1995).

Most study sites sponsored by the World Health Organization (WHO; Bangkok, Thailand; Kinshasa, Zaire; Munich, Germany; and Nairobi, Kenya) found no significant elevation of either current or lifetime depression rates, among HIV-infected individuals. The one exception was the Sao Paulo, Brazil, site (current range, 0–5.5%;

lifetime range, 1.5–13.3%) (Maj et al., 1994a). Approximately half of the subjects at the Sao Paulo site were MSM, unlike subjects at the other sites, who were predominantly heterosexual individuals.

The point prevalence of major depression among gay men and men engaging in IDU has been in the range of 4–11% (Atkinson et al., 1988; G. R. Brown et al., 1992; Williams et al., 1991; Rosenberger et al., 1993), compared to the 3–4% rate among men in the general population (Robins & Regier, 1991; Blazer et al., 1994). Interestingly, these rates do not increase with HIV disease progression among ambulatory individuals (Satz et al., 1994; Lyketsos et al., 1996b), an observation that may be valid across several racial/ethnic, gender, educational, socioeconomic, and HIV risk groups (Maj et al., 1994a). Such similar prevalence rates of depression across disease stage, gathered in places where social support and other environmental factors are notably dissimilar, underline the resilience of individuals' resources. Hospitalized individuals with advanced HIV disease appear to have higher rates of depression (10%, Snyder et al., 1992; 32%, Alfonso et al., 1994; 30%, D. Ellis, Collis, & King, 1994), but these are consistent with a high prevalence of major depression in the hospitalized medically ill persons (Silverstone, 1996; Alexander, Dinesh, & Vidyasagar, 1993; Clarke, Minas, & Stuart, 1991; Koenig et al., 1991). Other researchers, who also found comparable lifetime rates of depressive, anxiety, and substance abuse disorders in HIV-seropositive men and seronegative counterparts at baseline, detected greater risk for the disorders among seropositive men at follow-up (Dew et al., 1997).

As in the general population, a gender difference in the prevalence of major depression has been reported in HIV-infected samples. Women who engage in IDU or have partners who do so have lifetime rates of major depression approaching 40% (Lipsitz et al., 1994), as compared to 21% among women in the general population (Robins & Regier, 1991; Blazer et al., 1994; Kessler et al., 1994). HIV per se does not seem to elevate the rates of new-onset depressive disorders significantly.

Etiology. HIV could be expected to be an "organic" cause of depressive symptoms or syndromal depression because (1) HIV infects the CNS, producing neuronal dysfunction and damage, which may involve neuronal circuits that regulate mood; (2) HIV may result in cognitive impairment and dementia that often have a "subcortical" pattern, subcortical dementia, more often than cortical dementia, is associated with depression; (3) interleukins, which are immunologically active chemicals that may influence mood, are markedly elevated in late HIV disease; and (4) HIV disease is associated with dysregulation of cortisol and testosterone, two hormones known to affect mood. In addition to these HIV-specific factors, nonspecific factors (e.g., increased prevalence of multiple and severe physical symptoms in advanced HIV disease and medication-induced depression) could also be at play, such as in other major chronic illnesses. Given these theoretical expectations, it is surprising that an association between HIV disease and depression has not been unequivocally and reliably documented thus far. Although several lines of evidence suggest an increased prevalence of depressive symptoms and syndromal depression in HIV disease, this assumption remains tentative and is likely to be clinically relevant only in late-stage illness (reviewed in Atkinson & Grant, 1997a).

Diagnosis. According to the DSM-IV, a primary major depressive episode must include the presence of either depressed mood or anhedonia (a pervasive loss of interest or pleasure in activities) for 2 weeks or more, and five (or more) of nine depressive symptoms. In addition, the symptoms must (1) cause clinically meaningful impairment or distress; (2) be unrelated to the physiological effects of a general medical condition or a substance; and (3) not occur within 2 months of the death of a loved one.

Although the diagnosis of major depression in HIV disease is straightforward in many if not most cases, HIV disease can be associated with poor appetite and weight loss, sleep disturbance, low energy levels, decreased libido, apathy, and cognitive difficulties. Paying close attention to phenomenology and actively engaging the cooperative and cognitively intact patient in the diagnostic process, however, help distinguish depressive from disease symptoms in the majority of cases. Clinicians should compare dates of onset for the depressive episode and for each of the symptoms under scrutiny and, in physically symptomatic persons, psychiatric interviewing should be combined with neuromedical evaluation and neuropsychological assessment (Grant & Atkinson, 1995). Further distinctions can be made according to the following guidelines:

• Depressed or sad mood should not be confused with the sense of feeling physically down.
• Lack of interest in things must be discriminated from difficulty in doing them because of fatigue, physical discomfort, or pain. Many patients can help with this distinction when asked whether they believe that their interest would be at a normal level if they physical well-being were improved.
• The sense of worthlessness of major depression is different from lowered self-esteem because of changes in body image or disappointment at not being able to perform at full capacity. Likewise, persisting guilt rumination must be distinguished from episodic guilt associated

with IDU or with having an STD, as well as from regret over lost opportunity (Grant & Atkinson, 1995).

• Thinking about death and dying in the context of a life-threatening illness, and thoughts, wishes, or plans to terminate one's life because of poor life quality, are almost universal at some point in HIV disease. These thoughts ought to be distinguished from self-destructiveness based on a morbid sense of failure, worthlessness, or past transgressions indicative of depression (Grant & Atkinson, 1995). The first types of thoughts are often ego-syntonic, while careful questioning often reveals an ego-dystonic quality in depressive thoughts of death and suicidal ideation.

• Since bedside examination of cognitive abilities is positive mostly when there is dementia, there are cases where full neuropsychological evaluation is necessary to make the differential diagnosis.

Some investigators have proposed that a burden of physical symptoms, including both general vegetative signs (e.g., fatigue) and specific symptoms (e.g., night sweats or diarrhea), is a useful indicator of a accompanying depressed mood, and that the fear of overlabeling such signs and symptoms as depressive is exaggerated (Belkin, Fleishman, Stein, Piette, & Mor, 1992). Others have stressed that if one seeks the cardinal symptoms and applies proper severity criteria, confounding by somatic symptoms does not affect diagnostic validity (Chochinov, Wilson, Enns, & Lander, 1994). One study suggested that the somatic complaints of seropositive individuals with subsyndromal depression were associated with scores of avoidant coping; these scores could discriminate the presence or absence of general fatigue, abdominal distress, chest pain or discomfort, and numbness or chills (Fukunishi et al., 1997). These results may reflect cultural differences in psychiatric disorders among the Japanese, but they also suggest that mental health practitioners could assess avoidant coping in these types of individuals and encourage the development of more adaptive coping.

Course. The course of primary depressive syndrome in the majority of HIV-infected individuals does not differ from that in noninfected individuals: an episode usually develops over days to weeks; the duration is variable, but an untreated episode typically lasts 6 months or longer. In most cases, symptoms remit completely and functioning returns to the premorbid level, but partial remission coupled with some disability or distress is not infrequent. Patients with a diagnosis of major depression are at higher risk for a subsequent episode than the general population. Most individuals have infrequent episodes spaced widely apart, but the rate of recurrence is highly variable among individuals, although rates within individuals can be more stable (some patients may even have predictable patterns of recurrence). Some studies indicate that the cumulative 2-year incidence of major depressive disorder in HIV-infected persons ranges between 10% and 25%; that it is equivalent across individuals with no symptoms, mild symptoms, or full-blown AIDS; and that the majority of these cases are "recurrent" rather than "new-onset" (Atkinson & Grant, 1994). Other studies, with longer longitudinal observation, have reported that both depressive symptoms and syndromal depression assessed semiannually 5 years before and 2 years after AIDS diagnosis showed a rise as high as 45% over prior stable levels beginning at 12–18 months and reaching a plateau 6 months before diagnosis. Although this finding remains as intriguing as unexplained, it could be predicted statistically by prior elevated depression scores, self-reported HIV symptoms, unemployment, and limited social support (Lyketsos et al., 1996a).

Attempted or completed suicide is the most serious consequence of major depression, and a high frequency of a psychiatric history, especially depression, in HIV-infected individuals who commit suicide has been reported (Pugh, O'Donell, & Catalan, 1993; Kalichman & Sikkema, 1994; Gala et al., 1992). Similarly, an association between HIV seropositivity on the one hand, and mood and substance use disorders on the other, has been noted in a general hospital population referred for psychiatric consultation because of suicidality (Alfonso et al., 1994). Moreover, a strong association between current suicidal ideation and depressive symptomatology, and physical symptoms of HIV disease as predictors of suicidal thoughts, have been noted (Belkin et al., 1992).

Other studies found current suicidality to be lower among sicker individuals (O'Dowd, Biderman, & McKegney, 1993). Furthermore, cases of suicide in the absence of a psychiatric diagnosis, but in the context of worsening physical illness from a fatal condition, have been documented (Pugh et al., 1993). These results suggest a complex relationship between suicide and HIV disease, in which disease progression may trigger different coping strategies in different individuals. Preliminary results from the San Diego cohort suggest that study participants who took their lives were less cognitively impaired overall than matched participants who died naturally, and had comparable (non-elevated) levels of depressive symptomatology and psychiatric diagnosis (Summers et al., 1995a).

Other investigators have noted that thoughts about death and wishes to die are frequent in AIDS patients, but that they are often context-specific, occurring almost exclusively at times of bereavement or during serious illness accompanied by severe pain (Rabkin, Remien, Katoff, & Williams, 1993a). In a study of 53 gay men with an AIDS diagnosis for at least 3 years, the investigators found that only 6% had current syndromal mood disorders, despite the protracted biological stress of a life-threatening illness and the psychological stress of living with AIDS (Rabkin et al., 1993a). In these men the dominant theme seemed to be survival, not suicide; their thoughts of death were not considered as suicidal, but as an adaptive coping method for retaining some sense of control in anticipated intolerable circumstances (Rabkin et al., 1993a). Distinguishing between rational suicidality stemming from quality-of-life considerations and suicidality stemming from clinical, treatable depression can be difficult in this population. (Burnell, 1995). The dilemmas faced by mental health practitioners in such contexts have not only legal aspects, but profound philosophical and spiritual connotations (Forstein, 1994; Block & Billings, 1995; Chochinov et al., 1995).

Bipolar Disorders

Epidemiology. Manic episodes appear to be rare in HIV infection, and informal estimates put the point prevalence at 0.01–1.5% (Schmidt & Miller, 1988). Anecdotal observation indicates that full-blown mania is uncommon, and that most episodes are hypomanic.

Etiology. Since manic episodes are frequently associated with uninhibited sexual behavior, a relative overrepresentation of bipolar disorder could be expected among HIV-infected individuals, and gp120-induced neurotoxicity via increased intracellular calcium might result in AIDS-related mania (el-Mallakh, 1991). Primary bipolar disorder and mood disorder due to HIV disease with manic features, nevertheless, appear to be rare (Grant & Atkinson, 1995). Substance-induced disorder with manic features, seems to be the most common diagnosis in HIV-infected populations. Steroids, zidovudine, and ganciclovir are the most frequently reported iatrogenic causes. Intoxication from alcohol, stimulants (e.g., cocaine, inhalants, hallucinogens, phencyclidine), sedatives, and hypnotics also produces manic symptoms. There are reports of manic syndromes in individuals without substance-induced mood disorder, and also without any previous personal or family history of mood disorder. In these cases the etiology is presumed to be HIV or associated opportunistic infections, along with concomitant adverse life circumstances (Atkinson & Grant, 1997b). Occasionally manic episodes are caused by HIV-related neurological conditions, such as stroke, meningitis, and tumor (Grant & Atkinson, 1995).

Diagnosis. DSM-IV requires a manic episode to consist of a 1-week period of abnormally expansive, elevated, or irritable mood (or of any duration if hospitalization is required because of the mood abnormality). In addition, three manic symptoms (four if the mood is merely irritable) need to be present during the period of mood disturbance. The symptoms must not meet criteria for a mixed episode (instances when criteria for both manic and major depression episodes are met), must cause meaningful impairment in functioning or require hospitalization, or must include psychotic features. If the symptoms are due to the direct effects of a substance (of abuse or therapeutic), the diagnosis of substance-induced mood disorder, with manic features, is made. If the symptoms are due to the HIV disease, the diagnosis of mood disorder due to HIV disease, with manic features, is made. In the last two diagnostic categories, the full criteria for a manic episode need not be met, but the diagnosis is not made if the mood disturbance occurs only during the course of a delirium.

Typical case reports involve individuals previously described as stable, who over a period of days or weeks undergo a change in personality (becoming pompous, belittling, or sexually inappropriate) and then progress into a fuller manic picture (Grant & Atkinson, 1995). Case reports in the literature assert that bedside mental status examinations do not disclose neurocognitive deficit, but detailed neuropsychological examinations have not been reported; therefore, mild neurocognitive disorder as a predisposing factor cannot be excluded (Atkinson & Grant, 1997b). In fact, a window of vulnerability to psychosis or mania occurring early in an HIV-dementing process has been proposed (el-Mallakh, 1992). So-called "secondary" mania and organic mood syndrome resulting from acute injury (e.g., stroke) or chronic (e.g., seizure disorder, dementia) brain injury have been reported in the literature. The neuromedical evaluation is generally unremarkable apart from findings expected for HIV disease, such as frontal release signs, antisaccadic eye movements, and diminished muscle strength (Buhrich, Cooper, & Freed, 1988).

Course. The majority of first episodes of primary mania occur in young adulthood. Manic episodes typically begin suddenly, with rapid escalation of symptoms over a few days, and are frequently preceded by psychosocial stressors. Episodes usually last from a few weeks to several months. Their onset and offset are more abrupt than those of major depressive episodes, and they occur immediately before or after a major depressive episode. The number of lifetime episodes for both bipolar I disorder (recurrent major depression and mania) and bipolar II disorder (recurrent depression and hypomania) tends to be higher than that for recurrent major depressive disorder. In mood disorder due to HIV disease, a manic episode frequently occurs once and does not recur. Although they can complicate any stage of HIV disease, manic or hypomanic episodes tend to occur in people exhibiting signs of immunodeficiency; in one series, death occurred within 6 months of the psychiatric presentation in nearly a quarter of the patients (el-Mallakh, 1991).

Substance-Related Disorders

Substance-related disorders are important for the mental health practitioner working with HIV disease for at least three reasons (Atkinson & Grant, 1997b). First, substance intoxication or withdrawal can significantly impair cognition and decision making, resulting in increased risk for HIV transmission (e.g., having unprotected sex in exchange for drugs or money drugs, sharing infected "works" with other drug users, sex with multiple anonymous partners, reduced use of condoms, etc.). Sex in exchange for drugs or money appears to be particularly prevalent among users of the highly addictive crack cocaine. This deadly intersection of two epidemics is affecting inner-city women in particular. In one study involving three large U.S. cities and almost 2,000 subjects who never injected drugs, the prevalence of HIV infection among women was as high as among MSM (i.e., over 40%; Edlin et al., 1994). Also, some individuals who knowingly avoid HIV infection otherwise may expose themselves to HIV during intoxication (e.g., a married man may have unprotected sex with anonymous male partners only when intoxicated with alcohol). Second, since they are associated with symptoms or abnormalities easily confused with HIV-associated neurocognitive disorders, substance intoxication or withdrawal can complicate the presentation of neuropsychiatric syndromes in the HIV-infected patient, leading to misdiagnosis and poor response to therapy. Third, substance-related disorders that remain untreated can complicate the course of other neuropsychiatric and medical syndromes, making clinical management extremely difficult (Atkinson & Grant, 1997b). In such cases, the deleterious impact on disease progression need not be emphasized.

Epidemiology

The estimated lifetime prevalence of alcohol dependence in the general population is 20% for men and 8% for women (Robins et al., 1984; Bronisch & Wittchen, 1992). Prevalence rates for nonalcohol substance dependence in the United States are 9% for men and 6% for women (Kessler et al., 1994). The lifetime rates of alcohol use disorders among

MSM and individuals engaging in IDU range from 20% to over 50% (Atkinson et al., 1988; G. R. Brown et al., 1992; Williams et al., 1991; Rosenberger et al., 1993). Some studies show higher rates of current (i.e., past-month) substance use disorders among seropositive MSM than among those from community samples (10–15%; Rosenberger et al., 1993), whereas others show roughly comparable or only slightly higher rates (i.e., 5%) (Atkinson et al., 1988; Perry et al., 1990b; G. R. Brown et al., 1992; Williams et al., 1991). With the exception of cocaine-related disorders (equally common among men and women) and sedative-, hypnotic-, and anxiolytic-related disorders (more common among women), substance-related disorders are significantly more frequent in men, with male–female ratios as high as 5:1.

Etiology

The etiology of substance-related disorders in those at risk for HIV infection is no better understood than it is for substance misuse generally. Although there is evidence for genetically determined differences among individuals in the doses required to produce alcohol intoxication (Whitfield & Martin, 1985; Reed, 1985), and for aggregation of substance-related disorders in families (Dinwiddie & Reich, 1993), some of this effect can be explained by the concurrent familial distribution of antisocial personality disorder (Hesselbrock & Hesselbrock, 1992). There are no data indicating that any particular race or ethnic group is biologically predisposed to substance-related disorders; however, individuals from ethnic minorities living in economically deprived areas have been overrepresented among persons with substance-related disorders. Since low educational level, unemployment, and lower socioeconomic status are associated with substance-related disorders, differences in use are most likely to reflect social factors. One study of 4,914 young Israel-born adults of European and North African background found that when socioeconomic status was held constant, rates of antisocial personality and substance use disorders were higher in males of North African background; this finding suggests social causation (increment of adversity attaching to disadvantaged ethnic status, producing increment in psychopathology), rather than social selection (downward mobility of the genetically predisposed) (Dohrenwend et al., 1992).

Although sparse and confounded by recruitment bias (e.g., inclusion of subjects recruited in gay bars), several studies have reported increased frequency of alcoholism and more frequent use of illicit drugs among lesbians and homosexual men as compared to their heterosexual counterparts (Friedman & Downey, 1994). These differences may stem from the developmental stresses of establishing an alternate sexual identity, and of negotiating this within the context of family expectations and stigmatization by society; substance use is seen as a way of mastering the distress arising from these stresses (Atkinson & Grant, 1997b).

Diagnosis

Both substance use disorders and substance-induced disorders are commonly diagnosed in HIV-infected populations, but the present discussion is centered around the two substance use disorders, substance abuse and substance dependence. Both DSM-IV diagnoses are based on qualitative features (how the substance is used) rather than quantitative ones (how *much* is used).

Most persons having a substance use disorder feel some degree of shame or guilt. Others simply deny the existence of problems derived from their pattern of substance use, and regularly offer more or less sensible explanations to reconcile conflicting information in this regard. The clinician, therefore, needs to convey trust and gather the information in a nonjudgmental manner, but she or he may need to rely as well on additional information provided by significant others, health care professionals, or professional records.

The main feature of substance dependence is a group of three or more behavioral, cognitive, and physiological symptoms indicating that the individual persists in using the substance despite meaningful problems linked to its use. The symptoms must occur at any time within the same 12-month period. The symptoms of dependence are similar across the various categories of substances, but for certain classes some symptoms are less salient or simply do not apply (e.g., withdrawal symptoms for hallucinogen dependence). Neither tolerance nor withdrawal is necessary or sufficient for a diagnosis of substance dependence. In the DSM-IV coding system, this situation is indicated by specifier (with/without physiological dependence).

The main feature of substance abuse is a dysfunctional pattern of substance use characterized by meaningful and recurring negative consequences. These problems must occur during the same 12-month period. The symptoms do not include tolerance, withdrawal, or compulsive use. Many individuals meet criteria for substance abuse when they start to use substances, but over time develop substance dependence. Once an individual has met criteria for substance dependence, the diagnosis of substance abuse is preempted, and the diagnosis of substance dependence with the appropriate specifier is made instead. Six course specifiers are available for substance dependence or abuse (i.e., early full remission, early partial remission, sustained full remission, sustained partial remission, on agonist therapy, and in a controlled environment). Since there are wide cultural variations in attitudes toward substance use, only symptoms that clearly differ from the individual's own cultural pattern should be considered as diagnostic criteria.

Both HIV and substance use can lead to neuropsychological impairment; therefore, the mental health practitioner may often need to differentiate these two sources of impairment when a person presents with cognitive deficits. Two kinds of considerations are worth bearing in mind in the differential diagnosis. First, a history of alcohol use, even if prolonged and heavy, is not necessarily associated with neuropsychological impairment. Furthermore, abstinence of a year or more is associated with normalization of cognitive functioning. Alcohol-associated impairment in HIV-seronegative individuals is restricted to learning and memory; verbal intelligence is generally preserved, and no significant reduction in psychomotor speed or attention has been noted (Løberg, 1986). Since this pattern differs from the profile of HIV-associated impairment (see "Neurocognitive Disorders," below), researchers have been able to distinguish HIV- and alcohol-associated neuropsychological impairment, at least in asymptomatic HIV-seropositive individuals (Bornstein et al., 1993).

Second, neuropsychological assessment should be postponed until some time after complete cessation of substance use, since deficits secondary to most drugs disappear with abstinence (Carlin, 1986). The only difference between the neuropsychological deficits of HIV-infected, abstinent individuals engaging in IDU and those of HIV-positive gay and bisexual men is severity, not pattern, which suggests that the effects of HIV on the CNS do not differ according to HIV risk factor (Handelsman et al., 1992).

Course

Data on the course of substance use disorders in HIV disease are currently available mostly for gay and bisexual men. Results from the San Diego cohort suggest that "incident" alcohol and nonalcohol substance use disorders represent relapses of disorders whose original onset preceded the likely date of seroconversion. Furthermore, seropositive and seronegative men were equally likely to experience an episode of the disorder within the follow-up period. Incident rates are generally less than 5% annually and are equivalent across asymptomatic and symptomatic groups, although those with frank AIDS have even lower rates (Atkinson & Grant, 1997b).

A review and summary (Ostrow, 1994) of data from the Chicago Multicenter AIDS Cohort Study (MACS) and the companion Coping and Change Study; the San Francisco Men's Health Study; the Boston

Partners Study; and a New York City community-based sample showed a sizeable decline in the rate of use of practically every substance studied during the first few years of the studies, followed by a stabilization of the rates. In another longitudinal study, a remission of substance use disorders stemming from health-related concerns was also noted (Remien et al., 1995). One notable exception is the use of volatile nitrites ("poppers"), which, in spite of a nationwide prohibition on sales, are increasingly available and continue to be used widely in sexual settings. The use of "poppers" has been shown to be associated with the highest risk for unprotected receptive anal intercourse in a number of studies (for a review, see Ostrow, 1994).

The remitting course of substance use disorders reported in gay and bisexual men seems remarkable given that most study participants had complicating psychiatric comorbidity. Since the course of substance use disorders varies also with the class of substance, route of administration, and other factors (e.g., chronicity of Axis I diagnosis, socioeconomic status), the course of these disorders in other HIV-infected populations may follow less favorable patterns. A number of recent studies have documented the interaction between other Axis I diagnoses and substance use disorders on the one hand, and increased risk for HIV transmission on the other, among HIV-seropositive and HIV-seronegative inner-city psychiatric outpatients (Silberstein et al., 1994), outpatients with chronic mental illness (Kalichman, Kelly, Johnson, & Bulto, 1994b), and homeless men with mental illness (Susser et al., 1995, 1996). With respect to Axis II, there may be a characteristic comorbidity of substance use disorders and borderline and histrionic personality disorders (Oldham et al., 1995). Recent studies in gay and bisexual men (Perkins et al., 1993a; Johnson, Williams, Rabkin, Goetz, & Remien, 1995) and individuals engaging in IDU (Brooner et al., 1993) underline the obstacles that personality disorders pose to HIV prevention and to health care of infected individuals. These underserved, dually diagnosed patients may be particularly challenging for the mental health practitioner.

Anxiety Disorders

Epidemiology

The rates of generalized anxiety disorder, panic disorder, and obsessive–compulsive disorder among HIV-infected individuals appear to have combined lifetime and current prevalences within the range expected from epidemiological studies in the general population (i.e., 1–2%; Robins & Regier, 1991; Kessler et al., 1994), and to be similar in prevalence across all disease stages (Atkinson & Grant, 1994). Studies that have found somewhat higher lifetime (10%) and current (6%) prevalence rates have also found no effect of disease progression; moreover, anxiety disorders were less likely than mood disorders to be precipitated by HIV-related events (Rosenberger et al., 1993).

Etiology

The neurobiological bases of major anxiety disorders are under intense investigation. The role of serotonergic mechanisms, with an emphasis on newer pharmacological agents, has been recently reviewed (Baldwin & Rudge, 1995). Interestingly, there are few data indicating that HIV infection of the brain produces a disorder with the features reminiscent of the "major" anxiety disorders (Fernández, 1989), although HIV may be the focus of the stated "content" of the anxiety (Atkinson & Grant, 1997b).

Diagnosis

The diagnosis of the major anxiety disorders is usually straightforward, and since these disorders are infrequent and are usually the object of specialized psychiatric treatment, their specific diagnosis is not reviewed here; instead, reference is made to standard psychiatric texts (e.g., Kaplan & Sadock, 1995). The main point often overlooked by clinicians is that symptoms of anxiety reflect an underlying depression, which should be the focus of therapeutic efforts (Atkinson & Grant, 1997b). Despite the low prevalence of DSM-IV anxiety disorders in HIV-infected individuals, *symptoms* of anxiety are highly prevalent in this population. In the San Diego cohort, up to 20% of study participants had episodes of symptomatic anxiety, which could last days, weeks, or months (Atkinson & Grant, 1994).

Course

Almost no data on the course and prognosis of anxiety disorders in HIV-infected populations are available, but probably they vary with each individual disorder. Very often the course is chronic, with waxing and waning symptomatology, and the prognosis is relatively benign.

Personality Disorders

Epidemiology

The DSM-IV regards personality disorders as persisting, inflexible, and dysfunctional patterns of viewing, interacting with and thinking about the environment and oneself. To meet diagnostic criteria, these patterns must be exhibited in a broad range of personal and social contexts, and must cause meaningful functional impairment or personal distress. Self-defeating and self-destructive behavior is frequent in Cluster B personality disorders (i.e., antisocial, borderline, histrionic, and narcissistic personality disorders). It is therefore theoretically possible that individuals with Cluster B personality disorders are at increased risk for HIV infection. Although a high incidence of personality vulnerability and personality disorders in a medical clinic caring for HIV-infected patients has been reported (Treisman et al., 1993), findings from systematic studies of personality disorders in HIV-infected populations have been inconsistent. These differences can be explained at least partly by differences in study design (i.e., cross-sectional or longitudinal), study population, and timing within the epidemic when they were conducted. Thus, early studies involving subjects who contracted HIV before the modes of HIV transmission were widely known may have found lower diagnostic rates than later studies with subjects who somehow became infected despite knowledge of risk-avoiding practices. Longitudinal studies, by their very nature, usually involve highly selective samples. In the HNRC cohort, for example, which initially excluded individuals with IDU, 9.6% of subjects had an Axis II diagnosis; however, no significant associations between HIV serostatus or disease stage and Axis II diagnosis, or between the latter and Axis I diagnosis, were found (S. J. Brown, Summers, Atkinson, McCutchan, & Grant, 1992). In contrast, another longitudinal study of non-IDU gay men using the Structured Clinical Interview for DSM-III-R Personality Disorders), found a significantly higher prevalence of personality disorder in the HIV-positive (33%) than in the HIV-negative (15%) subjects (Perkins et al., 1993a). Although Johnson et al. (1995), on the other hand, found an elevated rate of personality disorders (19%) in both HIV-seronegative and HIV-seropositive gay men followed longitudinally, 33% of HIV-positive men with personality disorders had current Axis I disorders, in comparison with 5% of the HIV-negative men without personality disorders. Also, seropositive men with personality disorders were more likely than either seropositive or seronegative men without personality disorders to have current Axis I disorders and lifetime anxiety disorders, and they were more likely than seronegatives without personality disorders to have current major depression (Johnson et al., 1995).

In another longitudinal study involving *only* individuals engaging in IDU, 44% of subjects met DSM-III-R criteria (assessed through the Alcohol Research Center Interview) for antisocial personality disorder; also, significantly more of the subjects with antisocial personality disorder (18%) than of the subjects without this disorder (8%) had HIV infection (Brooner et al., 1993). A retrospective study of HIV-infected outpatients (60% males, 72% with IDU), assessed through an unspecified semistructured instrument and diagnosed according to DSM-III-R criteria, found a 13% rate of personality disorders (Bellini et al., 1994).

Etiology

Anecdotal reports indicate that pure personality change due to HIV disease without cognitive deficits is relatively rare. On the other hand, antisocial and borderline personality disorders seem to be associated with a high risk for HIV transmission and are likely to be encountered by the mental health practitioner working with HIV-infected patients. For example, in one study antisocial personality disorder predicted sexual risk in both homosexually and heterosexually active men attending a genitourinary clinic (D. Ellis, Collis, & King, 1995). Adoption studies indicate that both genetic and environmental factors contribute to the risk of antisocial personality disorder (Cadoret, Yates, Troughton, Woodworth, & Stewart, 1995). In addition to early traumatic experiences (e.g., physical abuse, neglect, hostile conflict, and early parental loss or separation), recent studies have singled out reported childhood sexual abuse as a strong predictor of certain clinical features of borderline personality disorder (Brodsky, Cloitre, & Dulit, 1995; Silk, Lee, Hill, & Lohr, 1995). Importantly, some studies in MSM have found an association between childhood sexual abuse and risk for HIV transmission in men (Allers et al., 1993; Zierler et al., 1991), and that traumatic, but not nontraumatic, childhood sexual experiences were associated with unprotected anal sex (Carballo-Diguez & Dolezal, 1995).

Diagnosis

The DSM-IV diagnosis of personality disorder has a number of requirements. First, the persisting pattern of behavior and internal experience must deviate noticeably from what is expected in the individual's culture. Second, this pattern must be inflexible, must be exhibited in a wide range of social and personal situations, and must result in clinically meaningful distress or impaired functioning. Third, the pattern must be stable and long-lasting, starting in adolescence or early adulthood. The pattern may not be better described as a sign or result of another mental disorder, and may not be due to the physiological effects of a general medical condition or a substance. The need to evaluate the individual's long-term patterns of functioning across different situations, and to consider of the individual's ethnic, cultural, and social background, often makes it necessary to conduct more than one interview and to space these over time. Individuals may meet criteria for more than one personality disorder (and not necessarily ones from the same cluster), or may meet the general criteria, but not the criteria for any specific personality disorder (personality disorder not otherwise specified).

Given these challenges, it is not surprising that reviews of the literature have found that the reliability of unstandardized clinical evaluations is poor to fair, whereas joint-interview interrater reliability when standardized interviews are used is generally good to excellent (Zimmerman, 1994). As an interesting complement to Axis II diagnosis, the DSM-IV proposes a Defensive Functioning Scale among the axes for further study. In this scale, the clinician lists up to seven current defenses or coping styles and then indicates which of seven defense levels is predominantly exhibited by the individual.

Course

Little is known about the course of personality disorders in HIV-infected individuals. In HIV-negative populations, antisocial personality disorder has a chronic course but may become less evident or remit as the individual grows older, particularly by the fourth decade of life. The course of borderline personality disorder is characterized by chronic instability in early adulthood, episodes of serious affective and impulsive dyscontrol, high levels of use of mental health resources, and impairment and suicidal risk, which are greatest in the young adult years but gradually wane with advancing age. In one study of HIV-positive psychiatric inpatients, 14% were diagnosed with borderline personality disorder or traits, and all of them were admitted because of suicidal thoughts or attempts (Wiener, Schwartz, & O'Connell, 1994).

Adjustment Disorders

Epidemiology

Superimosed on background stressors, discrete points of psychological distress are common with HIV.[4] The ever-changing nature of the HIV epidemic is clearly reflected in the rates of adjustment disorders reported in HIV-infected populations; these vary widely according to study design, population studied, and the social context prevalent at

---

[4]For a discussion of a "transition model" accounting for psychiatric conditions in HIV, see Grant and Atkinson (1995). See also "Therapeutic Issues: Loss as a Crisis," below.

the time of the study. Thus, in military personnel who undergo mandatory testing or are examined within weeks or months of being informed of serostatus, rates of an adjustment disorder approach 15–39% (Prier, McNeil, & Burge, 1991). On the other hand, among gay men who have known their serostatus an average of at least 1 year after voluntary testing, rates of adjustment disorder are negligible (Atkinson et al., 1988) or not significantly different from the rates in controls (Rosenberg et al., 1993).

According to the WHO, up to 90% of subjects with a recent diagnosis of HIV infection present some form of "acute stress reaction" (Maj, 1990). A retrospective study in Spain of 107 HIV-infected patients (mostly males, almost all with IDU) referred to a psychiatric liaison service reported a 30% rate of adjustment disorders (Crespo-Hervs, Vincente Muelas, Ochoa Mangado, & del Pino Morales Socorro, 1992). A retrospective study in England comparing psychiatric diagnoses of 70 HIV-positive patients (mostly males, mostly gay) with 70 HIV-negative medical patients referred to a psychiatric liaison service found no significant difference in the rates of adjustment disorder (15.7% and 12.8%, respectively; D. Ellis et al., 1994). In Italy, a retrospective study of 53 HIV-positive outpatients (60% males, 72% with IDU) attending an infectious disease unit found very low rates for both adjustment disorder and major depression (1.9%; Bellini et al., 1994).

In a study of 42 newly admitted medical inpatients with AIDS (three-fourths males, mostly ethnic minorities, half MSM), 5 (12%) met criteria for adjustment disorder (Snyder et al., 1992). In 324 patients who visited an AIDS-related psychiatric outpatient clinic over a 3-year period (244 were HIV-positive; IDU or heterosexual transmission was the main risk factor in almost 80%; most were ethnic minorities, and half were women), adjustment disorder was the most common diagnosis in all stages of infection (average 70%; O'Dowd, Natali, Orr, & McKegney, 1991). In another study of 50 patients (mostly African-Americans, two-thirds males, one-third with IDU, and one-third MSM) who presented consecutively for medical care at an outpatient HIV clinic, 9 (18%) met criteria for some type of adjustment disorder (Lyketsos, Hanson, Fishman, McHugh, & Treisman, 1994). In a 5-year review of 91 HIV-infected psychiatric inpatients (80% males, half whites, 36% with IDU), 24% were diagnosed with adjustment disorder (Wiener et al., 1994).

Etiology

Few studies of specific factors associated with the diagnosis of adjustment disorder have been published. One study found that while HIV disease was not associated with a higher rate of adjustment disorder, in a small number of cases onset of adjustment disorder was associated with HIV-related stressful events (Rosenberger et al., 1993). Factors such as disease stage, socioeconomic status, coping patterns, and social support are likely to render an individual susceptible to develop an affective or behavioral response to an HIV-related stressor that is in excess of what would be expected or results in functional impairment. For example, in one study the use of more avoidance and less approach coping was significantly related to increased depressive symptomatology (Patterson et al., 1995). Degree of social support has been found to be associated with psychiatric morbidity in HIV-seropositive heterosexuals and HIV-seronegative controls (Pergami, Gala, Burgess, Invernizzi, & Catalan, 1994).

Diagnosis

The essential feature of an adjustment disorder is the development of clinically meaningful behavioral or affective symptoms in response to one or more identifiable psychosocial stressors (other than bereavement). The symptoms must arise within 3 months after the onset of the stressor(s), and the clinical importance is indicated either by distress beyond what would be expected from the nature of the stressor, or by functional impairment. The diagnosis is not made if the disturbance meets the criteria for another specific disorder. If there is a preexisting Axis I or II disorder, the diagnosis is made only if the preexisting condition does not account for the pattern of symptoms. According to the predominant symptoms, there are six different subtypes of adjustment disorder: with depressed mood, with anxiety, with mixed anxiety and depressed mood, with disturbance of conduct, with mixed disturbance of emotions and conduct, and unspecified (not classifiable as one of the other subtypes).

Course

By DSM-IV definition, symptoms last no longer than 6 months after the stressor or its effects have ceased (indicated by the "acute" specifier of duration of symptoms). If the stressor or its consequences endure (e.g., a chronic disabling condition), the disorder may also endure (indicated by the "chronic" specifier). HIV-related adjustment disorders usually follow a benign course and respond well to education and support, but an undetermined proportion of cases may evolve to meet full criteria for another mental disorder. Current anecdotal observation of gay and bisexual men indicates that testing seropositive is rarely accompanied by severe distress or suicidality.

Although not generalizable to other populations, this observation probably reflects subjective and societal changes in the perception of HIV disease, and the ever-improving prognosis as a result of scientific progress. Earlier in the epidemic, distress was elevated in subjects at perceived risk for infection, even before HIV testing. One study found suicidality in about 30% of one sample before HIV testing—a rate that remained basically unchanged after 1 week in subjects who tested seropositive, while the rate dropped substantially in those who tested seronegative. Two months after testing, nonetheless, the rates were comparable in both groups (Perry, Jacobsberg, & Fishman, 1990a).

Neurocognitive Disorders

HIV infection results in signs and symptoms reflecting dysfunction in both the CNS (meningoencephalitis, meningitis, vacuolar myelopathy, lymphoma, and opportunistic brain infections; Grant & Atkinson, 1995) and the peripheral nervous system (acute inflammatory demyelinating polyradiculoneuropathy, sensory polineuropathy, and myopathy). From a neuropsychiatric perspective, however, the most important of the neurobiological complications are the HIV-associated neurocognitive disorders. The cardinal feature of these disorders is impairment in cognitive functioning. Associated features include motor slowing or incoordination, and sometimes affective disturbances (Grant & Atkinson, 1995).

Mild Neurocognitive Disorder

Epidemiology. In contrast to dementia, the concept of mild neurocognitive disorder (the "HIV-associated minor cognitive/motor disorder" of the American Academy of Neurology [AAN] AIDS Task Force; AAN, 1991) has been articulated more recently. Therefore, comparable data on its prevalence are not available at this time. Most observers agree that symptomatic HIV infection is accompanied by increased rate of neuropsychological impairment (Grant & Martin, 1994). Exactly how much of an increased risk AIDS patients experience is not yet agreed upon. Studies have estimated rates of mild neuropsychological impairment ranging from 33% (reviewed in Grant, Heaton, Atkinson, & the HNRC Group, 1995) to 20% (Grant et al., 1995), although some studies have failed to detect differences between AIDS patients and controls (Riccio et al., 1993). A recent review study of AIDS patients found that the rate of neurocognitive impairment ranged from 12% to 87%, with a median of 53% (Heaton et al., in press).

With respect to the asymptomatic phase of HIV disease, initial reports indicated an increased prevalence of impairment (Grant et al., 1987), followed by reports indicating no differences in neuropsychological status between asymptomatic HIV-positive persons and controls (McArthur et al., 1989; E. N. Miller et al., 1990; Collier et al., 1992; McAllister et al., 1992; Riccio et al., 1993). Newer studies have again detected performance differences between asymptomatics and controls (Stern et al., 1991; Handelsman et al., 1992; E. M. Martin et al., 1992; Bornstein et al., 1993; Heaton, Kirson, Velin, Grant, & the HNRC Group, 1994a; Maj et al., 1994b), ranging from a low 9.1% in the WHO Neuropsychiatric AIDS Study (Maj et al., 1994b) to 30.5% in the San Diego HNRC cohort (Heaton et al., 1995). A review of 57 studies with data on rates of neuropsychological impairment in asymptomatic carriers and controls revealed a median rate of 12% among samples of HIV-seronegative controls (range 0–42%), 35% for asymptomatic HIV-seropositives (range 0–50%; D. A. White, Heaton, & Monsch, 1995), and that was more likely to be detected with larger, more comprehensive test batteries (D. A. White et al., 1995).

Etiology. Etiopathogenesis of all mental disorders due to HIV disease remains obscure. Only recently has mild cognitive disorder been operationally described, and it is presently unclear whether the disorder is a preamble to dementia. Perhaps as a result of this, no hypothesis on the pathogenesis of minor neurocognitive disorder has been put forward. Since clinical correlates for most neuropathological studies have been "neurocognitive impairment" or "dementia," both variously defined by different investigators, most of the relevant material reviewed is therefore discussed in the section on dementia.

HIV-associated pathological findings in the brain have been reported in postmortem examination of individuals who died in early phases of the disease, before the development of AIDS. Cerebral vasculitis, lymphocytic meningitis, myelin pallor with reactive astrocytosis, and microglial proliferation are significantly more frequent in these brains than in control brains (Gray et al., 1992).

HIV can be found in the CSF of infected individuals early in the course of the disease (Goudsmit et al., 1986; Resnick et al., 1988), and in a high proportion of persons with no overt neurological symptoms or neuropsychological dysfunction (Spector et al., 1993). Neuronal dysfunction, on the other hand, is suggested by reports of auditory P300 abnormalities detected in up to 30% of HIV-infected individuals without clinically evident neurological disease, some of whom have been infected for less than a year (Birdsall et al., 1994). Also one or more abnormal evoked potentials were abnormal in 14% of asymptomatic HIV-positive men and 43% of symptomatic men, as compared with 2% of seronegative controls (Iragui, Kalmijin, Thal, & Grant, 1994). Moreover, conduction was longer in symptomatic individuals, suggesting an increase in dysfunction with advanced disease (Iragui et al., 1994).

The increased prevalence of neurological symptoms across current Centers for Disease Control and Prevention (CDC) categories—coupled with a nonparallel rise in affective symptomatology—has also been interpreted as evidence of subtle, subclinical neurological involvement in early stages of HIV disease (Mehta et al., 1996).

MRI studies have shown progressive atrophy within both gray and white matter in the brain, which are evident in asymptomatic persons but most severe in advanced disease. Progressive volume loss within the gray matter was evident only in the caudate nucleus (Jernigan et al., 1993; Stout et al., in press).

Although no frank structural damage of the CNS has been observed in animals infected with simian immunodeficiency virus but showing only motor and/or cognitive impairment, neurochemical and neuropathological events have been found (da Cunha, Eiden, & Rausch, 1994).

Diagnosis. Although the *International Classification of Diseases* (ICD-10) currently lists "mild cognitive disorder" as a diagnosis, and this was proposed for inclusion in the DSM-IV (Gutierrez, Atkinson, & Grant, 1993), mild neurocognitive disorder is currently listed in the DSM-IV in the "Criteria Sets and Axes Provided for Further Study" (Appendix B). The essential feature of the disorder is the onset of cognitive impairment, which needs to be corroborated by neuropsychological testing or standardized bedside cognitive assessment, with a mild impact on day-to-day functioning. The disturbance does not meet criteria for dementia, delirium, or amnestic disorder, and is not accounted for better by another mental disorder.

"Neurocognitive disorder" refers to a disturbance in function resulting from presence of a neurocognitive impairment. "Neurocognitive (neuropsychological) impairment" is defined as a deficient performance in some area of cognitive functioning, such as attention/speed of information processing, verbal/language skills, abstracting (executive abilities), complex perceptual–motor abilities, psychomotor skills, sensory/perceptual ability, and memory functions (including learning and recall of information; Grant et al., 1995). To classify performance on a cognitive task as being "impaired," it is necessary for an investigator to establish a criterion outside which performance is considered to be abnormal (Grant et al., 1995).

According to the WHO, a disability exists when certain impairments interfere with a person's functioning. Thus, the term "disorder" (as in "neurocognitive disorder") should be reserved for those individuals who have neurocognitive impairments that are significant enough to produce disability—that is, by interfering with activities of daily living (Grant et al., 1995). Despite insufficient information on the implications of reliably determined neuropsychological impairment for day-to-day functioning (A. Martin, 1994a), Heaton et al. (1994b) found that the rate of unemployment of HIV-seropositive subjects with neuropsychological impairment was significantly higher (17.5% vs. 8%) than the rate of such subjects without impairment, and that neuropsychologically impaired individuals were more likely to report decreased job performance and worse performance on standardized work samples (Heaton et al., 1996b). These results suggest that the impairment of a subgroup of asymptomatic HIV-seropositive individuals may be clinically significant (i.e., such individuals are experiencing some degree of disability). It is not known how individual factors (e.g., motivation, educational level, and coping skills) and situational factors (e.g., job demands and eligibility for benefits) interact with neuropsychological impairment to produce disability.

An HIV-infected person experiencing mild neurocognitive disorder will typically report difficulty in concentrating, remembering, and mental fatigability, or a feeling of being mentally slowed down (Grant & Atkinson, 1995). One study, however, found that up to a fourth of subjects denied memory deficits evinced by testing (Hinkin et al., 1996). In the majority of cases, simple testing of cognitive functioning, such as the Mini-Mental State Examination, may not disclose gross deficits. The clinician, however, should always take complaints seriously; the need to request formal and comprehensive neuropsychological testing may arise in cases where there is a serious complaint and an unremarkable mental state examination. Before requesting such testing, however, the mental health practitioner should perform a thorough evaluation of possible psychiatric confounds, including substance use and mood and anxiety states. If such confounds are suspected, it is preferable to postpone the neuropsychological evaluation and pursue instead treatment of the psychiatric disorder. The clinician should document in objective terms the impact on daily functioning of the suspected cognitive impairment, because empirically informed clinical judgment will remain the golden rule for labeling a condition as a "disorder," as the relationship between neuropsychological tests and actual everyday performance in the world is complex at best and ambiguous at worst.

Neuropsychological testing usually reveals attentional problems, slowing of information processing, slowing of simple motor performance, and deficiencies in learning, difficulties with tasks involving problem solving, abstract reasoning, and decrement in verbal fluency, although verbal skills are in general less affected (Grant et al., 1995). Neurological examination of HNRC participants showed that both asymptomatic and symptomatic, neuropsychologically impaired HIV-seropositive men were significantly more likely to have an abnormality in the "central rating" (based upon signs such as hemiparesis or hemisensory loss, supranuclear gaze abnormality, myelopathy, and cognitive impairment), but not in the "peripheral rating," as compared to nonimpaired men (Heaton et al., 1995). Note the danger of overdiagnosis among ethnic minority individuals of dementia or minor cognitive disorder based on neuropsychological test performance that does not account for the confounding effect of acculturation. One study of HIV-infected individuals found that lower neuropsychological test performance of black as compared to white subjects became nonsignificant after accounting for acculturation (Manly et al., in press).

There is currently no laboratory marker in blood or CSF of minor neurocognitive disorder, although CSF levels of quinolinic acid, p24 antigen, immunoglobulin G synthesis rate, and quantitated polymerase chain reaction (PCR) levels of viral load are promising in this regard (Syndulko et al., 1994). One study, however, found CSF viral load assessed by PCR to be unrelated to HIV-associated cognitive impairment prior to the development of AIDS (R. J. Ellis et al., in press). In the HNRC cohort, no significant relationship between neuropsychological impairment and CD4+ cell count or serum ß-microglobulin was found (Heaton et al., 1995), although higher rates of impairment were seen in subjects with abnormal CSF ß-microglobulin (Heaton et al., 1995). Another finding that may be clinically useful and awaits further replication is the robust association of CD8+ lymphocyte count and neuropsychological impairment reported by Karlsen, Froland, and Reinvang (1994). Not only was a positive correlation between CD8+ counts and neuropsychological test results found in the total group, but the CD8+ cell count was the only immunological parameter that could significantly discriminate between AIDS patients with and without neuropsychological impairment.

Course. The progression of neurocognitive complications is poorly understood. Some investigators have found no evidence for cognitive decline in asymptomatic patients followed for approximately 2 years (Selnes et al., 1990), while others concluded that the seropositive subjects declined significantly over a year on neuropsychological tests as compared to seronegative controls (Dunbar, Perdices, Grunseit, & Cooper, 1992). In the HNRC series, a 2-year follow-up of over 150 participants found an annual rate of neuropsychological decline among seropositive individuals on the order of 20% (Grant et al., 1995). Moreover, subjects with minor cognitive disorder who survived were significantly more likely to present with worsening impairment at follow-up (median 2.4 years) (Heaton et al., 1996a). Although the risk of decline may not be strongly associated with stage of disease (neither CDC classification nor whether subjects progressed from one CDC category to the other was associated with likelihood of neurocognitive decline (Grant et al., 1995), an association seems to exist between likelihood of neuropsychological change and time elapsed since sero-conversion. Thus the annual hazard of neurocognitive impairment in the first 3 years after estimated date of seroconversion is on the order of 10% (Grant et al., 1994).

A more benign picture has been uncovered by other studies. In AIDS subjects followed for at least 2 years, a mild decline in fine motor skills with no significant change in other cognitive domains, no significant decline in cognitive functions before AIDS, unless overt dementia is present, and no decline in immunosuppressed subjects who have had no AIDS-defining illness have been reported (Selnes et al., 1995). In a group of 113 HIV-seropositive subjects followed over 4.5 years with semiannual neuropsychological testing, others found that improvement over time in tests of memory, executive function, language, and attention was attenuated or eliminated in patients with lower CD4 levels (below 200 cells/mm^3; Stern et al., 1995). In an analysis of 9 years of longitudinal data in Baltimore, one of the MACS sites, subjects with sustained psychomotor slowing, but not sustained cognitive decline, had an increased hazard of progression to dementia, AIDS, and death (Sacktor et al., 1996). These results suggest that a rather brief neuropsychological test battery that can assess psychomotor speed may be useful for early detection of individuals with poorer prognosis, who may benefit from more aggressive treatment to prevent dementia (Sacktor et al., 1996).

Of great interest are data suggesting that cognitive impairment is associated with higher mortality rates. In 111 HIV-seropositive gay men (both asymptomatic and symptomatic) followed over a 36-month period, the mortality risk ratio associated with poor neuropsychological test performance was significantly increased, and increased further when adjusted for factors associated with mortality (history of a disturbance in movement or gait, CD4 lymphocyte and red blood cell counts, and age; Mayeux et al., 1993). The rate of cognitive decline may also be associated with higher risk of death. In the 33 men who died in the study by Stern et al. (1995), there was a significantly more rapid decline in executive, language, and attentional test performance after

HIV disease severity was controlled for. HNRC data showed that both syndromic (minor cognitive/motor disorder) and nonsyndromic cognitive impairment (determined by neuropsychological testing) were associated with increased mortality, independently of baseline disease stage and CD4 T-cell count (R. J. Ellis et al., 1997).

HIV-Associated Dementia

Epidemiology. The more recent practice of using well-defined diagnostic criteria developed by the American Psychiatric Association (DSM), the WHO (ICD), or the AAN AIDS Task Force (all of these criteria sets have essential features in common) has led to more reliable and convergent estimates for the prevalence of dementia, both in the United States and internationally (Grant et al., 1995; Mussa et al., 1994). Using DSM-III criteria in a small series, Day et al. (1992) indicated an annual dementia incidence of 14% among symptomatic HIV-infected patients. Using DSM-III-R-like criteria, McArthur et al. (1993), reporting on data from the MACS, noted an annual incidence of 7.1%. Maj et al. (1994b), reporting on WHO data, found a prevalence among symptomatic HIV-infected persons ranging from 4.4% to 6.5% (DSM-III-R criteria) or 5.4% to 6.9% (ICD-10 criteria). In the past, failure to make distinctions among operationally defined minor cognitive disorder, dementia, and delirium led to widely differing estimates of "dementia" in HIV-infected persons (i.e., from 6.5%–66%; reviewed in Grant et al., 1995). In addition to HIV itself, a number of CNS opportunistic conditions may present with dementia.

As the epidemic matures and more people with profound immunosuppression live longer, the overall incidence of HIV-related neurological diseases can be expected to rise. In a comprehensive evaluation of the MACS experience between 1985 and 1992, an upward temporal trend in the incidence rate of toxoplasmosis and cryptococcal meningitis was found, in spite of protective trends due to antimicrobial prophylaxis (Bacellar et al., 1994). In the case of CMV infection, there are preliminary reports suggesting that although ganciclovir therapy may stabilize CMV retinitis, it does not appear to prevent the development of or to be effective in the treatment of CMV encephalitis (Berman & Kim, 1994).

Etiology. Although there are CNS neuropathological phenomena specifically related to or associated with HIV infection (Petito, 1988), earlier reviewers emphasized the variability of postmortem CNS abnormalities, and the fact that in a large proportion of cases findings were remarkably bland in relation to the clinical dysfunction (Navia et al.,

1986b). Both significant neuronal loss in cases of minor pathology
(Everall, Luthert, & Lantos, 1991) and absence of neuronal loss in cases
of well-diagnosed dementia have been reported (Seilhean et al., 1993).
It is important, however, to note that neuropathological changes may
include aberrant neuronal morphology as well (Masliah et al., 1992b)—
that involve specific subpopulations of neurons (i.e., pyramidal neurons
and interneurons; Masliah, Ge, Achim, Hansen, & Wiley, 1992a;
Masliah, Ge, et al., in press). In one study, the degree of neurocognitive
impairment was strongly related to the amount of dendritic simplifica-
tion (Masliah, Heaton, et al., in press).

The most characteristic neuropathological substrate of HIV dementia is termed "HIV encephalitis," an abundant infection and activation of brain macrophages (Achim & Wiley, 1996) and is highly
reproducible if defined in terms of viral burden (Wiley & Achim, 1994).
In one series, the abundance of HIV as assessed by PCR and the length
of time it was present in the CNS determined the severity of the
dementia (Wiley, Masliah, & Achim, 1994).

Since a discrepancy between the distribution and numbers of
virus-infected cells and concomitant brain tissue pathology has been
noted (Vazeux, 1991; Lipton, Yeh, & Dreyer, 1994), and the fact that
HIV cellular pathology in the brain is largely confined to cells other
than neurons (Wiley, Schrier, Nelson, Lampert, & Oldstone, 1986),
HIV has been considered neuroinvasive and not necessarily neuroviru-
lent. Also since the early report of HIV-infected cells releasing toxic
agents that destroyed cultured neurons (Giulian, Vaca, & Noonan,
1990), neuroscientists have investigated a number of neurotoxins (e.g.,
kynurenine metabolites, quinolinic acid, and tumor necrosis factor-α
[TNF–α]; Genis et al., 1992; Heyes et al., 1992; Lipton et al., 1994;
Sardar, Bell, & Reynolds, 1995).

In a recent, comprehensive model, HIV-infected macrophages and
microglia produce viral gp120, which can lead to release of neurotoxins
from uninfected macrophages and astrocytes. Macrophages respond to
gp120 with the production of TNF-α and interleukine-1ß (IL-1ß), which
increase voltage-dependent Ca^{2+} currents in neurons. Astrocytes respond to gp120 with glutamate efflux; glutamate and neurotoxins
produce Ca^{2+} efflux in neurons. Sustained, high levels of neurotoxins
is assured by macrophages, previously primed by HIV and activated by
proinflammatory cytokines, opportunistic infections, and tumor anti-
gens (Gendelman, Lipton, Tardieu, Bukrinsky, & Nottet, 1994). These
events ultimately result in glial proliferation and neuronal injury or
loss—two common postmortem neuropathological findings in brains of
HIV-seropositive persons. Neurotoxins also potentiate the *N*-methyl-D-
aspartate (NMDA) receptor, which is involved in the glutamate-medi-

ated neurotoxicity. Although astrocytes initially function as deactivators of macrophage-produced neurotoxins, they also respond directly to gp120 by enhanced glutamate efflux (Benos et al., 1994), which may ultimately lead to the breakdown of the homeostatic mechanism (Gendelman et al., 1994). The central role of astrocytes in pathogenesis of HIV infection of CNS has also been stressed by others (Blumberg, Gelbard, & Epstein, 1994; Saito et al., 1994).

The final common neuropathological pathway may be blocked by NMDA antagonists and Ca^{2+} channel or non-NMDA antagonists (Gendelman et al., 1994), although other glutamate receptor subtypes may also be involved (Gelbard et al., 1993). This opens the possibility of developing pharmacological interventions that may alleviate neuropsychological complications of HIV disease. However, neuronal damage in different regions of the CNS may be mediated by different pathogenic mechanisms (Fox, Alford, Achim, Malloty, & Masliah, 1997).

In another model, HIV infection of microglia is followed by excessive expression of IL-1ß, astrogliosis, and increased cytokine S100ß, ultimately leading to excessive expression of neuronal ß-amyloid precursor proteins, increased intraneuronal calcium levels, and abnormal growth of neurites, all of which contribute to progressive neuronal dysfunction and neuronal loss (Stanley et al., 1994). The most important implication of this model is that eradication of HIV infection may not prevent this cascade of neurodegenerative changes; additional interventions at the level of, for example, IL-1ß may be required to prevent neurodegenerative progression (Stanley et al., 1994).

Other factors not integrated in the previous models are apoptosis and free radicals (Lipton, 1997), monocytic endothelins (Coligan & Clouse, 1993), and cytomegalovirus (CMV), that can infect an HIV-infected cell (Belec et al., 1990). Based on postmortem observations in humans and in animal models, Buttini et al. (in press) proposed the expression of CD4 by mononuclear phagocytes as a mediator of indirect neuronal damage in infectious and immune-mediated CNS disease, whereby opportunistic infections, in the absence of HIV encephalitis, may induce neurodegeneration.

A recent *in vivo* model of HIV infection of the human brain (Achim & Wiley, 1994) and laboratory and animal model systems for HIV encephalitis and dementia (Persidsky & Gendelman, 1997) may allow further refinement in our understanding of HIV neuropathogenesis, and may ultimately promote development of effective therapies for both mild neurocognitive disorder and dementia. The reason why not all patients with HIV disease become demented continues to elude researchers, but it is likely that both viral strain and host mechanisms may be involved. Johnson et al. (1996) detected HIV by PCR, or viral RNA, or viral antigen in all brains studied, irrespective of the presence of dementia, suggesting that qualitative differences in virus strains, rather than the quantitative differences in viral load, are likely to be germane to the development of dementia. Another study (Pulliam, Gascon, Stubblebine, McGuire, & McGrath, 1997) found that patients with dementia were significantly more likely to have in their blood a particular subset of monocytes, and supernatants from cultures of these cells triggered apoptosis of human brain cells *in vitro*. Monocytes, unlike CD4+ lymphocytes, are infected by HIV in a chronic, nonlytic manner. Monocyte-derived macrophages are the cells predominantly infected in the brain, and most investigators agree that the mechanism responsible for cognitive dysfunction in HIV disease is indirect and associated with macrophages.

Diagnosis. There has been considerable confusion about the occurrence and features of the neurocognitive disorders. For example, one of the earliest terms was "HIV(-related) encephalopathy" (Britton & Miller, 1984; Snider et al., 1983). Another term was "AIDS dementia complex" (ADC), which suggested a constellation of cognitive, motor, affective, and behavioral complications (Navia et al., 1986b; Price & Brew, 1988), which many clinicians and investigators tended to use somewhat indiscriminately—not bearing in mind, for instance, that the term "dementia" connotes severe disability. This led to failure to recognize milder cognitive disorders, as well as underdiagnosing due to clinicians' reluctance to stigmatize a patient with an ADC label.

According to the DSM-IV, the dementias are disorders characterized by the onset of numerous cognitive deficits that include memory impairment and at least one of the following: apraxia, aphasia, agnosia, or disturbed executive functioning (clinical criteria). The deficits must cause impaired functioning, which must represent a decline from a previously higher level of functioning (disability criteria). The diagnosis is not made if the cognitive deficits occur only during a of delirium, although both diagnoses can be made if the diagnosis of dementia can be made at times when delirium is not present (exclusion criteria). Dementias may be due to multiple etiologies, to the enduring effects of a substance, or to the direct physiological effects of a general medical condition (such as HIV disease). In the latter case, an additional diagnostic criteria is required—namely, evidence from history, physical exam, or lab findings that the disturbance is the direct physiological result of the general medical condition.

A number of diverse conditions have been grouped together under the term "subcortical dementias" because they share a more or less generalized slowing of mentation. Clinical (Navia et al., 1986b), neuropsychological (Peavy et al., 1994; D. A. White et al., 1995), neuroradiological (Aylward et al., 1993), and neuropathological evidence (Navia et al., 1986a), has resulted in the conceptualization of dementia due to HIV disease as a subcortical dementia, although other subgroups may exist (reviewed in A. Martin, 1994b). In fact, preferential structural damage to the hippocampus has been noted (Reyes, Mohar, Mallory, Miller, & Masliah, 1994); therefore HIV dementia may be a predominantly but not exclusively subcortical process (Brew, 1991).

Typically, in milder cases patients complain of impaired concentration, comprehension difficulties, memory loss, apathy, and withdrawal; as the disease process evolves, global cognitive dysfunction is evident, and symptoms of varying degree of severity (e.g., psychomotor slowing, confusion, dysarthria or aphasia, ataxia, seizures, and incontinence) can appear. Delirium, mania- and depression-like states, psychosis, or socially inappropriate behavior often complicate the clinical picture (Ho et al., 1989).

Neurological examination is often normal in the early stages, but impairment of rapid eye and limb movements can be found, as well as diffuse hyperreflexia. Later, increased muscular tone develops (particularly in the lower extremities), accompanied by psychomotor slowing, tremor, clonus, diffuse release signs, and hyperactive reflexes. Signs and symptoms of concurrent HIV-related myelopathy or peripheral neuropathy are also common (McArthur, Selnes, Glass, Hoover, & Bacellar, 1994). Differential diagnosis can be difficult, particularly at early stages of dementia; neuropsychological examination and psychiatric or neurological consultation may be necessary in some cases. In addition, the diagnosis of dementia should be suspected even in asymptomatic phases of HIV disease whenever signs and symptoms of cognitive or motor impairment are present; in one series, over half of the 29 patients either survived for 5–16 months or died without exhibiting systemic manifestations of AIDS (Navia & Price, 1987).

Through detailed analysis of the neuropsychological data collected over 4 years, MACS researchers developed a neuropsychological battery that is sensitive to the earliest symptoms of HIV-induced cognitive impairment and takes approximately 45 minutes to complete, although more detailed cross-sectional workup of individual cases may be required (Selnes & Miller, 1994). The battery recommended by the National Institute of Mental Health (NIMH), for example, includes 25 different tests covering 10 separate cognitive domains, and requires an estimated 7–9 hours for administration (Butters et al., 1990). The recent development of a short quantitative scale for HIV dementia that is reliable and superior to other bedside tests (e.g., the Mini-Mental State Exam) is encouraging (Power, Selnes, Grim, & McArthur, 1995).

Controlled studies have not detected systematic interactions between age or education and serostatus, as long as age- and education-adjusted norms are applied to neuropsychological data (van Gorp et al., 1994). It is theoretically possible, however, that advancing age and lower education may decrease "cerebral reserve" (Satz et al., 1993) in HIV-seropositive persons, allowing subtle impairments to be detected more easily. Likewise, a history of substance use disorders does not seem to increase the likelihood of detecting impairment in HIV-seropositive asymptomatic individuals (D. A. White et al., 1995). In the HNRC cohort, reports of cumulative lifetime and current-year use of substances (expressed in milligrams per day) did not differ between neuropsychologically impaired and unimpaired persons (Heaton et al., 1995). This might not be generalizable to other populations, since the original cohort excluded individuals with IDU or with high levels of psychoactive substance consumption at the time of enrollment.

Most important, several studies have failed to detect a clinically significant association between mood disturbance and neuropsychological impairment in seropositive individuals (reviewed in Grant et al., 1995). Complaints with memory are prevalent in individuals with depressed mood, but subjective reports of memory problems in HIV-seropositive persons are just as likely to reflect underlying depressive mood as they are to signify neurocognitive disorder (Grant et al., 1995; Mapou et al., 1993).

On the other hand, in one study 14% of men with neurocognitive impairment had current, coexisting major depression, as compared to 5% of unimpaired men (Heaton et al., 1995). Thus, whereas depressed mood does not "explain" neurocognitive impairment in HIV, an individual with neurocognitive deficits is likely to be vulnerable to a major depression syndrome, which emphasizes the importance of a multidisciplinary approach to the diagnosis of dementia. In other dementias, it has been shown that psychiatrists' sensitivity rates for diagnosing dementia are low, whereas depression often goes unreported by neurologists (Verhey et al., 1993).

Although highly desirable clinically, a diagnostic laboratory test for HIV dementia remains elusive. Faster rates of decline in percentage of CD4 lymphocytes were related to poorer performance on measures of memory and reaction time in one study, but such a measure may be useful only when longitudinal data are available since the relationship was independent of stage of illness and CD4 level at the time of examination (Bornstein et al., 1991). Neopterin and interferon-γ (macrophage-produced substances presumed to reflect immune activation) are elevated in HIV-infected individuals with neurological disease (Griffin, McArthur, & Cornblath, 1991), and serum neopterin concentrations have been found to be negatively correlated with neurocognitive function (Karlsen et al., 1994). Others have observed irregular patterns of correlations between CSF abnormalities and severity of HIV infection of autopsied brains (Wiley et al., 1992), perhaps because opportunistic infections may alter immune-activation-associated factors and because CSF is inadequate as a marker of basal ganglia involvement in HIV encephalitis. Brew, Pemberton, Cunningham, and Law (1997) believe that PCR measurement of HIV viral load in CSF, but not in plasma, may be a tool in the diagnosis and monitoring of treatment of dementia, provided that opportunistic conditions such as cryptococcal meningitis are ruled out or treated. Importantly, one study showed that after the onset of AIDS, neuropsychological impairment was associated with significantly higher CSF viral load, although viral loads in plasma and CSF were not related (R. J. Ellis et al., in press).

MRI may be particularly sensitive to anatomical abnormalities in dementia (Aylward et al., 1995, but since abnormalities have not been observed in all patients with cognitive impairment (Kent et al., 1994), MRI can best aid differential diagnosis and contribute to the assessment of prognosis (Mundinger et al., 1992).

Course. In general, the mode of onset and subsequent course of dementia, including reversibility, are functions of the underlying pathology (i.e., HIV or opportunistic infections and malignancies) and the timely availability of treatment.

The course of dementia due to HIV disease is progressive, although some have noted temporary improvements after initiation of antiretroviral therapy (Portegies et al., 1993; Tozzi et al., 1993). There are few reports on the clinical course of HIV dementia diagnosed according to DSM, AAN, or ICD criteria. One of the likely reasons for this void of reliable information is the comparatively short survival time of individuals who develop dementia. Although dementia can appear in individuals without previous clinical indication of immunodeficiency, dementia tends to occur late in HIV disease (within the last few months of life), and may be more rapid in onset among those with the shortest survivals (McArthur et al., 1993). In one cohort study involving 492 gay men with AIDS, among the 64 subjects the median survival time was 6.0 months, compared with 7.8 months for nondemented subjects (McArthur et al., 1993). Other studies have reported survivals of about 12 months (Arendt et al., 1993) and 6.7 months (Portegies et al., 1993). If dementia is due to an opportunistic infection, the course will depend on the treatment response to the underlying cause.

HIV-Associated Delirium

Epidemiology. The prevalence and incidence of delirium in HIV disease are unknown, although it is generally one of the most frequent diagnoses made by neurology and psychiatric consultation services when evaluating hospitalized HIV patients (Dilley, Ochitill, Perl, & Volberding, 1985). It is likely that delirium is as underdiagnosed and undertreated in HIV populations as it is in others (Liptzin, Levkoff, Gottlieb, & Johnson, 1993).

Etiology. The combination of systemic illness, underlying neurocognitive impairment, and multiple medications with CNS effects is the recipe for delirium in patients with neurological diseases, including symptomatic HIV disease. Therapeutic agents likely to be associated with delirium are described in Table 4.1. Medications with anticholinergic properties, such as amitriptyline and chlorpromazine; antiemetic agents, such as scopolamine and prochlorperazine; and antihistamines and benzodiazepines are often implicated. Delirium has occasionally been reported as a complication of zidovudine and ganciclovir. Opportunistic or other infections, metabolic factors (hypoxemia, hypercapnia, electrolyte imbalances, hypoglycemia), hepatic and renal dysfunction, surgical intervention, and psychoactive intoxication and withdrawal can all contribute to the likelihood of delirium. *Pneumocystis carinii* pneumonia can be complicated by hypoxemia, which can lead to clouding of consciousness. Other causes of delirium in late-stage AIDS include severe nutritional deficiencies (e.g., vitamin B_{12}) and electrolyte imbalance (e.g., hyponatremia).

Diagnosis. The DSM-IV focuses on two cardinal symptoms: (1) lessened clarity of awareness of the environment and reduced ability to focus, shift, or sustain attention; and (2) a change in cognition (e.g., disorientation, memory deficit, language disturbance) or onset of perceptual disturbance (e.g., misinterpretations, illusions, hallucinations), not better explained by dementia. The disturbance arises over a short period of time (hours to days) and tends to vary over the course of the day. Evidence that the disturbance is caused by HIV disease (or substance intoxication or withdrawal, in the case of substance-induced delirium, or more than one etiology, in delirium due to multiple etiologies) from the history, physical exam, or lab findings must be present. In addition to lab findings that are characteristic of HIV disease, the electroencephalogram (EEG) is typically abnormal, showing either generalized slowing or fast activity, and is helpful in differentiating organic etiologies from psychiatric disorders (Brenner, 1991). The

TABLE 4.1. Neuropsychiatric Side Effects of Therapeutic Drugs for HIV

Agent	Effects
Anti-infective	
Acyclovir	Depressed mood, agitation, auditory and visual hallucinations, depersonalization, tearfulness, confusion, hyperaesthesia, hyperacusis, insomnia, thought insertion, headache
Amphotericin-B	Delirium
Azidothymidine (AZT)	Depressed mood, agitation, headache, myalgia, insomnia
Cephalosporins	Confusion, disorientation, paranoia
Cycloserine	Anxiety, confusion, depression, disorientation, hallucinations, paranoia, loss of appetite, fatigue
Dapsone	Agitation, hallucinations, insomnia
Ethambutol	Headache, dizziness, confusion, visual disturbances
Ethionamide	Depression, drowsiness, hallucinations, neuritis
5-Flucytosine	Delirium, headache, persisting neurocognitive impairment
Isoniazid	Depression, agitation, hallucinations, paranoia
Ketoconazole	Dizziness, headache, photosensitivity
Metronidazole	Depression, agitation, delirium, seizures
Pentamidine	Delirium, hallucinations
Rifampin	Headache, fatigue, loss of appetite
Sulfonamides	Headache, neuritis, insomnia, loss of appetite, photosensitivity
Thiabendazole	Hallucinations
Trimethoprim/ Sulfamethoxazole	Delirium, mutism, depression, loss of appetite, insomnia, apathy, headache, neuritis
Antineoplastic	
Methotrexate	Delirium
Procarbazine hydrochloride	Mania
Vinblastine sulfate	Depression, loss of appetite, headache, neuritis
Vincristine sulfate	Ataxia, headache, hallucinations, neuritis
Alpha interferon	Depression, weakness, anergic-apathetic states
Other	
Amantadine	Visual hallucinations
Barbiturates	Excitement, hyperactivity, hallucinations, depression
Benzodiazepines	Delirium, drowsiness, amnesia, excitement
Corticosteroids	Confusion, depression, hallucinations, mania, paranoia
Meperidine hydrochloride	Delirium
Metoclopramide hydrochloride	Depression, mania
Morphine sulfate	Delirium, agitation
Phenytoin sodium	Confusion, delirium, euphoria
Tricyclic antidepressants	Drowsiness, mania, delirium, insomnia

Note. From Kaplan and Sadock (1995). Copyright 1995 by Williams & Wilkins. Reprinted by permission.

combined contribution of organic and psychological factors to complex behavioral disorders increasingly common in HIV disease has been rightly emphasized (Freedman, O'Dowd, Wyszynski, Torres, & McKegney, 1994).

The disturbed sleep–wake cycle that was core criteria in the DSM-III-R is an "associated feature" in DSM-IV because it is heavily confounded in a hospital setting and does not add to the specificity of the diagnosis (Liptzin et al., 1993).

Memory impairment is a feature of both delirium and dementia, but a person with a dementia is alert and does not have the disturbed consciousness typical of delirium. Careful history taking, including information from family members or friends, may reveal a preexisting dementia, in which case the diagnosis of delirium superimposed on a dementia is made (e.g., dementia due to HIV disease, with delirium). In delirium, psychotic symptoms are shifting, fragmented, and unsystematic; occur in the context of disturbed consciousness; and are generally associated with EEG abnormalities. These features help in distinguishing delirium from brief psychotic disorder, schizophrenia, schizophreniform disorder, and mood disorder with psychotic features.

Course. The course and prognosis of delirium in the HIV patient appear to mimic those of delirium in other medical illnesses. There is a prodromal phase, which may be brief or of several days' duration; an acute phase when the diagnosis is made; and either rather prompt resolution or a more persisting subacute phase, which may last for several days or weeks or occasionally longer. If the underlying etiological factor is corrected (e.g., antibiotic treatment and supportive measures for pneumonia-induced hypoxemia) or is self-limited (e.g., substance intoxication), and there is no underlying dementia, recovery is more likely to be complete. Excess morbidity from delirium beyond its neuromedical etiology may result from suicide, falls from fleeing delusional dangers, or assault based on a paranoid perception of caretakers. If delirium is associated with an underlying HIV dementia, then the prognosis may be especially grave (Sewell et al., 1994a).

HIV-Associated Sleep Disturbance

In this section, the frequent occurrence of sleep disturbance as a direct result of HIV disease is emphasized. General medical and neurological conditions, use of a substance (drug of abuse or medication), delirium, dementia, and depressive or anxious syndromes can all be associated with sleep disturbance. These conditions are also likely to occur, at some point or another, during the course of HIV disease. Nevertheless, HIV-infected individuals frequently complain of sleep disturbance in the absence of any of these conditions. A disturbance that can cause distress or impaired functioning severe enough to merit clinical attention on its own is termed in the DSM-IV "sleep disorder due to HIV disease, insomnia type." The briefer "HIV-associated sleep disturbance" is preferred in this chapter.

Epidemiology

There are no studies on incidence of sleep disorders in HIV-infected populations in the absence of confounds. Using the three sleep items of the Hamilton Rating Scale for Depression, one study found that gay men with AIDS were significantly more likely to have sleep item scores above 0 (52%) than HIV-seronegative heterosexuals (11%), while total scores for the scale were not significantly different. Interpretation of the results was difficult, however, because sleep scores from gay controls and mildly symptomatic men were not different (S. J. Brown et al., 1991). In another study, 14% of HIV-infected individuals reported early awakening three or more times weekly, compared to 2% of controls. In addition, 28% of seropositives reported napping three or more times weekly, compared to 12% of controls. Both differences were statistically significant (Darko et al., 1992). Neither of these studies controlled for mood disturbance. Controlling for depression when studying HIV-associated sleep disturbance seems particularly critical in view of conflicting reports on the topic. Some have found an association between complaints of fatigue and insomnia and depression among asymptomatic seropositive men (Perkins et al., 1995). In contrast, an analysis of 4-year longitudinal data involving over 3,000 persons from the MACS showed that although there was no substantial increase in depressive symptomatology before AIDS, HIV-seropositive persons chronically reported more trouble sleeping, which was deemed a consequence of the viral infection rather than an indication of depressive disorders (Lyketsos et al., 1996b). In unpublished analyses (S. J. Brown, Sciolla, Nelson, Atkinson, & Grant, 1996) performed in a subsample of 355 subjects from the HNRC cohort without an Axis I diagnosis, seropositive men (46%) were significantly more likely to score 6 or above on the self-reported Pittsburgh Sleep Quality Index (indicating clinically significant sleep disturbance; Buysse, Reynolds, Monk, Berman, & Kupfer, 1989), as compared to seronegative controls (31%).

Etiology

Sleep disruption is very common in nondementing neurological disorders involving the brainstem, hypothalamus, and basal forebrain, which contain neuronal systems controlling wakefulness and sleep (Culebras, 1992) and in dementing neurological disorders (Bliwise, 1993). In addition, some viral and nonviral infectious diseases induce abnormalities in the sleep–wake cycle that are thought to involve immunopathological mechanisms (reviewed in Pollmacher, Mullington, Korth, & Hinze-Selch, 1995). Not surprisingly, HIV disease, which may result in neurodegeneration of basal ganglia, dementia, and immune function disruption, is commonly associated with sleep disturbance.

Although early reports suggested that zidovudine may cause sleep disturbance (Richman et al., 1987), later comparisons of sleep EEG data from zidovudine-treated and untreated HIV-infected men showed no significant differences (Moeller et al., 1992). Specific EEG abnormalities have been reported in HIV-infected asymptomatic subjects that could not be explained on the basis of underlying psychopathology (Norman et al., 1990; Norman et al., 1992). The increase in the percentage of slow-wave sleep in the later sleep cycles, observed by Norman et al., 1990, has been replicated in subjects from the San Diego cohort and remains one of the earliest and most consistently replicable neurobiological signs of HIV infection (J. L. White et al., 1995).

Interestingly, cats infected with feline immunodeficiency virus, a natural lentivirus pathogen of cats that produces an HIV-like immunodeficiency syndrome, exhibit sleep abnormalities similar to those previously described in AIDS patients (Prospero-Garcia et al., 1994). Moreover, infected cats exhibited no overt signs of systemic morbidity, such as fever or body weight loss (Philips et al., 1994).

Investigators from the HNRC originally proposed that immune dysregulation and excess production of certain somnogenic lymphokines may underlie sleep disturbance or fatigue (Darko et al., 1992). For example, IL-1α, IL-1ß, and TNF-α are somnogenic (Krueger et al., 1990), and are elevated in HIV-infected persons (Scott-Algara, Vuillier, Marasescu, de Saint Martin, & Dighiero, 1991). Recently, the degree of disruption of a previously unrecognized physiological coupling between TNF-α and sleep EEG delta amplitude fluctuations was shown to correlate with the number of days since seroconversion in HIV-seropositive men (Darko et al., 1995a). The relationship between altered cytokine concentrations and altered sleep has been also observed in a rat model (Opp et al., 1996).

HIV-associated sleep disturbance may also result from dysregulation of sleep–wake cycle and other circadian rhythms. Increased daytime napping, increased nocturnal awakening, and poor quality of sleep have been described in the healthy elderly (Bliwise, 1993). Sleep disturbance could result from HIV-associated premature "aging" of the brain, since changes in the elderly resemble the symptoms of HIV-associated sleep disturbance. Sleep changes in the elderly may stem from age-related changes in the circadian neural pacemaker in the suprachiasmatic nucleus of the hypothalamus (Swaab, Fliers, & Partiman, 1985) that result in phase-advanced and/or reduced-amplitude circadian rhythms in bodily functions (Brock, 1991). Disruption of the cyclic alternating pattern of sleep (Ferini-Strambi et al., 1995), abnormalities in circadian rhythms of circulating lymphocytes, plasma levels of adrenocorticotropic hormone, cortisol, and testicular hormones, in HIV-infected persons have been reported (Bourin et al., 1993; Malone et al., 1992; Martini et al., 1988; Swoyer et al., 1990; Vagnucci & Winkelstein, 1993; Villette et al., 1990). A disruption of the cyclic alternating pattern of sleep has also been reported (Ferini-Strambi et al., 1995).

The development of animal models that mimic aspects of HIV disease in the CNS provide an opportunity to investigate the mechanisms of sleep disturbance further and to develop therapeutic interventions (Darko, Mitler, & Henriksen, 1995b; Vitkovic, Stover, & Koslow, 1995).

Diagnosis

Although in the literature sleep disturbance and fatigue are often lumped together, it is clinically important, albeit difficult to distinguish these two symptoms, particularly daytime somnolence from fatigue. Whereas daytime sleepiness can occur at any stage of HIV disease; fatigue seems to be more prominent in later stages.

The most common symptoms are complaints of difficulty in maintaining sleep rather than initiating it, and of the need to take daytime naps. Typically, an individual reports frequent awakenings during the night, sometimes lasting an hour or more. This can be accompanied by early awakening and inability to fall back asleep. A feeling of not feeling refreshed upon awakening is common and sometimes can be the sole symptom. Daytime napping is also frequently reported, and increases with disease progression.

Careful history taking helps to rule out other causes (potentially treatable) of sleep disturbance, such as primary sleep disorders, medical or neurological conditions, mood or anxiety disorders, and substance-induced sleep disorders. Persons who complain of excessive daytime sleepiness (or their roommates or significant others) should be asked about the presence of snoring. They should be examined to rule out adenotonsillar hypertrophy, which can be caused by HIV disease. If hypertrophy is found, researchers have recommended that sleep evaluation be carried out to diagnose obstructive sleep apnea (Epstein et al., 1995). A DSM-IV diagnosis cannot be made in the presence of delirium, and requires clinically meaningful distress or impaired functioning.

Course

There are no reports on the course of HIV-associated sleep disturbance in the literature. Clinical and research experience indicate that symptoms may remit spontaneously after a few weeks or months, with no apparent relation to other events, and may recur similarly. Overall, sleep disturbance is more frequent in later stages of the disease, and symptoms tend to worsen over time. Some later-stage patients may have no regular sleep–wake pattern (i.e., one main episode of sleep every 24 hours); they move seemingly at random between short episodes of waking and sleeping (Sciolla et al., 1993). However, at later stages, the confounding effects of medications, opportunistic infections, delirium, and/or dementia are omnipresent.

Psychotic Disorders

Epidemiology

Large-scale surveys find a prevalence of 0.5% of psychotic disorder due to HIV disease, whereas chart review methods find frequencies ranging from 3% to 15% in persons for whom obvious causes (e.g., delirium) have been excluded (Harris, Jeste, Cleghorn, & Sewell, 1991; Sewell et al., 1994a). No estimates of substance-induced psychotic disorder in HIV-infected individuals are available.

Sex between men, IDU, and the compound effects of self-destructive behavior, sexual promiscuity, poor impulse control, and impaired appreciation of risks may characterize individuals with severe, chronic mental disorders. Elevated prevalence rates of primary psychotic disorders could therefore be expected among groups with HIV disease. In one study, nearly half of the sample of acute psychiatric patients reported a history of HIV-related risk behaviors during the previous 5 years, and one-fifth of them were at high risk for HIV infection (Sacks, Perry, Graver, Shindledecker, & Hall, 1990). In a subsequent study of patients voluntarily admitted to a psychiatric hospital in New York City over a period of 7 months, Sacks, Dermatis, Looser-Ott, Burton, and Perry (1992) found a 7.1% rate of HIV infection. In Africa, where HIV is transmitted mainly through heterosexual sex, one study of female psychiatric inpatients also noted a much higher HIV seroprevalence than the rest of the population (43.8% in patients of urban origin and 11.1% in patients or rural origin, vs. 21% in urban population and 1.7% in rural population; Bleyenheuft et al., 1992).

In a sample of chronically mentally ill inpatients and outpatients (half of them psychotic) admitted to a psychiatric hospital serving an inner-city area, the prevalence of HIV infection was 5.8% (Stewart, Zuckerman, & Ingle, 1994). While high HIV seroprevalence in black males and homeless patients was noted, female sex was independently associated with HIV infection; no difference in HIV seroprevalence by sexual orientation, inpatient–outpatient status, or psychiatric diagnosis was found (Stewart et al., 1994).

Among chronic psychiatric outpatients (over half of them psychotic), high rates of illicit drug use and frequent use of drugs or alcohol in association with sexual activity were found; 18% of the sample reported receiving money or drugs for sex in the previous year (Kalichman et al., 1994b). In addition, a substantial number of patients engaged in high-risk sexual behaviors with other patients in the context of unstable, often transient relationships and of misinformation about HIV transmission (Kalichman et al., 1994b). Other studies in similar populations have found 15% of the men reporting unprotected sex with male partners on 75% of occasions of sexual intercourse (Kelly et al., 1995a), and low-frequency but high-risk sex (without a condom and with nonmonogamous partners) (Susser et al., 1995). These authors also found that cocaine abuse or dependence was significantly associated with high-risk sexual behaviors (Susser et al., 1995). Also, the great majority of injection drug users in the sample had engaged in high-risk drug use behaviors (i.e., sharing needles and using "shooting galleries"), and had had unprotected sex with women or with men (Susser et al., 1996).

Etiology

For a discussion of etiology of primary psychotic disorders, see Kaplan and Sadock (1995). Both exposure to medications or drugs of abuse and HIV infection can result in psychotic signs and symptoms in HIV-infected individuals. In the latter case, psychosis has been attributed to direct effects of HIV in the brain, or to coinfection with other CNS viruses such as CMV or herpes simplex virus. The predilection of HIV for subcortical or temporal regions may be etiologically related to psychotic symptoms. A "window of vulnerability" has also been proposed that occurs relatively early in HIV dementing processes; psychosis is thought to remit with advancing dementia (el-Mallakh, 1992).

Diagnosis

In DSM-IV criteria for psychotic disorder due to a general medical condition and in substance-induced psychotic disorder, "psychotic" refers to delusions or only those hallucinations that are not accompanied by insight. When delusions develop only in the course of HIV-associated dementia, the diagnosis is dementia due to HIV disease, with delusions.

Psychotic states due to HIV disease are usually later-stage complications of HIV infection; they require immediate medical and neurological evaluation, and often require neuroleptic management.

The clinical presentation is extremely variable. The most prevalent symptom seems to be delusions (occurring in almost 90% of cases in some series) with persecutory, grandiose, or somatic components that can be quite elaborate. Delusions of thought insertion (thoughts being inserted into one's mind by outside forces), thought broadcasting (one's thoughts being audible to others), and physical acts controlled by aliens are also described. Most patients experience auditory hallucinations, with perhaps half of these also experiencing visual hallucinations. A majority of series also report disordered thought processes, including loose associations or frankly disorganized thinking (Sewell et al., 1994a). Disturbances of mood commonly coexist, with anxiety being the most prevalent symptom, followed by depressed mood, euphoria, or irritability, and mixed depressed and euphoric states. Lability, flatness, and inappropriate laughter or anger are also described. Disorganized and even bizarre behavior may be evident (Atkinson & Grant, 1997b).

Bedside examination reveals impairment in memory or other cognitive functions in up to one-third of patients with psychosis; more comprehensive and formal neuropsychological assessment would probably detect neurocognitive difficulties in a larger proportion of cases, but many psychotic individuals are unable to complete such examinations (Atkinson & Grant, 1997b). Other neurological findings are infrequent and nonspecific, usually consisting of ataxia, mild increases in motor tone, hyperreflexia, and tremor, but bizarre grimaces and posturing can be present. CSF is generally unremarkable, except for the mild pleocytosis common to HIV infection. Diffuse cortical slowing has been reported in about half of those cases where an EEG was obtained. Computerized tomography and MRI can reveal nonspecific cerebral atrophy in about half of cases. Rarely, focal abnormalities are evident, suggesting tumor, opportunistic infection, or vascular etiology (Atkinson & Grant, 1997b).

Course

The course and prognosis are highly variable and depend partly on whether specific complicating conditions coexist. For example, coexisting dementia indicates poor prognosis and rapid deterioration, with death often occurring within 6 months or less. On the other hand, when neurocognitive abnormalities are not detected or are mild, individuals have been followed for up to 2 years in a stable, treated course. Overall, there is some evidence that death occurs earlier in patients experiencing psychosis than in nonpsychotic patients who have similarly advanced HIV disease (Sewell et al., 1994a).

Complicated Bereavement

Epidemiology

HIV disease almost always affects more than one member of a family or a close-knit, informal group of individuals. In the case of heterosexual transmission, families may have one or more children and one or both parents infected. With IDU transmission, individuals often share more than drug injection paraphernalia; many of them form more or less loose networks of lovers, friends, and acquaintances, and interact not only in "shooting galleries" but in treatment programs. Perhaps nowhere else is this situation more clear than in the gay community of large urban centers. Here, the socializing and identity formation roles of families are played by closely intertwined webs of acquaintances, close friends, and lovers. In such community, deaths from AIDS have reached truly catastrophic proportions; in fact, much of the generation of sexually active gay males in large U.S. cities during the 1970s has been wiped out. Many survivors, HIV-infected or not, have seen dozens of members from their circle die one by one through the years of the epidemic. J. L. Martin and Dean (1993) have reported, in a cohort of 624 gay men, an average of 6.2 close deaths during the epidemic. Chronically bereaved men were more likely to be doing paid and volunteer work in HIV prevention (J. L. Martin & Dean, 1993). HIV-seropositive men and women, who are facing the possibility of premature death themselves, may be at particular risk for grief complications.

Etiology

Grief is often the most painful and disruptive experience a person ever endures. Immediately after the death of the loved one, the bereaved usually experiences a sense of shock and denial. This gives way to intense somatic and psychological distress (termed by some "separation distress" to distinguish it from the "separation anxiety" described in children), characterized by pangs of grief (self-limited 20 to 30-minute periods), searching behavior (which can include dreams, tactile or visual illusions, and frank hallucinations in some cases), preoccupation with and a sense of yearning for the deceased, and the full range of behavioral concomitants of sadness and anxiety. Distress usually comes in waves, with periods of serenity of variable duration interspersed between the pangs of grief. Grief is habitually accompanied by some degree of social and occupational disability. After a lapse of time (highly variable among individuals and cultures), the fruitless search gradually subsides, and the reality and irrevocability of the loss are accepted both emotionally and cognitively. Thus, bereaved individuals recognize what the loss has meant to them; they acknowledge that they have grieved, and that they now can resume old roles, acquire new ones as necessary, and reexperience pleasure in the companionship and love of others (Zisook, Shuchter, & Summers, 1995). This virtual universality of grief among humans of all cultures, and the resemblance of human grief and reactions to loss in several species of social animals, suggest that grief may be a basic "physiological" response to a loss (Jacobs, 1993).

Given the lack of a universally agreed-upon definition of "normal grief," it is not surprising to find difficulties in defining "pathological grief." Some consider all the clinical complications of bereavement as "pathological grief" in the broadest conceptual sense (Jacobs, 1993). Others have simply conceptualized "unresolved grief" as the nonresolution of the usual stages of the grief process. The unanswered question of why certain individuals find themselves in this maladaptive state is the subject of active research in the field. Individual factors such as gender, age, significant losses during childhood, the style of childhood attachment, and environmental factors (e.g., traumatic circumstances of the loss, social support) have been implicated in the development of psychiatric complications after a loss.

Knowing one's own HIV-positive status or AIDS diagnosis was the strongest, most consistent correlate of psychological distress found by 1993 in a large cohort study involving 746 gay men; the effect became increasingly severe with each passing calendar year (J. L. Martin & Dean, 1993). Work by the HNRC group suggests that self-control coping (strategies aimed at maintaining mastery over one's emotional response to a life stressor) may characterize HIV-infected or at-risk individuals meeting psychometric criteria (derived from the Texas Revised Inventory of Grief) for unresolved grief (Summers et al., 1992).

Diagnosis

Bereavement may be underdiagnosed and perhaps undertreated as well. In one study, bereavement was mentioned in only 28.2% of cases of HIV-positive persons referred for counseling by medical teams, although 43.1% of them had been bereaved, used bereavement counseling, and spontaneously commenced the session with bereavement issues (Sherr, Hedge, Steinhart, Davey, & Petrack, 1992). In the HNRC, up to 60% of the participants had experienced a loss within the previous 12 months, and 18% of them met criteria for unresolved grief (Summers et al., 1995b). Seropositive persons have been identified as at greater risk than their seronegative counterparts for complicated bereavement (J. L. Martin & Dean, 1993; Neugebauer et al., 1992; Summers et al., 1995b). Most individuals acknowledge signs and symptoms (e.g., depressed mood) arising in the context of grief and consider them as "normal." If they seek professional help, it is commonly only to obtain relief for associated symptoms such as insomnia. In the DSM-IV, the diagnosis of major depression is not given in the first 2 months after the death of a loved one, even if full criteria are present. Exceptionally, the diagnosis is made if any of the following symptoms is present: (1) guilt about things besides actions committed or omitted by the survivor at the time of death; (2) thoughts of death other than the survivor's wishing to be dead or to have died with the deceased person; (3) morbid concern with worthlessness; (4) pronounced psychomotor retardation; (5) extended and pronounced functional impairment; and (6) hallucinatory experiences other than the survivor's seeming to hear the voice or briefly see the image of the loved one.

In "normal grief" in North American culture, social and occupational functioning is markedly impaired only in the acute phase (first few days); separation distress subsides within 6 weeks of the loss; depressive symptoms are transient and usually peak in 4–6 months, anxiety symptoms are transient; and there is acceptance of the loss and improvement by 1 year. It is worthwhile to consider complicated bereavement and a therapeutic intervention every time a clear deviation from this pattern is encountered. Fear of losing control and anniversary reactions lasting more than a few days or causing marked impairment can be considered indicators of unresolved grief (Jacobs, 1993).

Course

Untreated complicated bereavement characteristically follows a protracted course, with frequent exacerbations associated with anniversaries or other environmental factors and subsequent partial remissions. Medical morbidity and mortality (Kemeny et al., 1995) and psychiatric morbidity have been reported to occur at some point in complicated bereavement and can thus shape its course (reviewed in Zisook et al., 1995). Particularly worrisome are reports of decreased NK cell activity among bereaved men at baseline and at 6-month follow-up (Godkin et al., 1996). In the HNRC cohort, men with unresolved grief were significantly more likely to be diagnosed with current major depression and panic disorder than were those with resolved grief, although lifetime diagnoses were not significantly different (Summers et al., 1995b). In a study of men who were caregivers until their partner's death from AIDS, unrelieved postbereavement depressive mood was associated with seropositive status, distancing and self-blame coping, and longer relationships (Folkman, Chesney, Collette, Boccellari, & Cooke, 1996). Clearly, in these cases the emergence of a psychiatric complication will compound the course of the bereavement process.

THERAPEUTIC ISSUES: LOSS AS A CRISIS

Because this chapter focuses on neuropsychiatric features of HIV disease and emphasizes their organic bases, the therapeutic approaches discussed in this section are mainly biological. Despite this, the subtitle of the section resets that emphasis in a broader and clinically more effective context.

Every therapeutic measure (biological or otherwise) delivered to an HIV-infected individual will be more effective when framed within the paradigm of "loss as a crisis." Most individuals will experience their HIV disease as an unrelenting succession of losses: It strips them of T cells, body image, partners and friends, financial status, normal bodily functions, and ultimately their very lives. It is a well-established fact that a loss is followed by a number of states of psychological distress, which can lead to a state of resolution and acceptance of the loss. In a more general sense, psychological crisis and situations of acute distress may very well lead eventually to improved psychological well-being and coping when an appropriate therapeutic intervention is carried out. In this light, it is clinically useful to conceptualize a crisis as a situation of danger and, at the same time, as an opportunity for favorable change. By considering the appearance of HIV disease-related signs and symptoms as correlates of some loss, and that loss as a crisis, and that crisis as a situation of danger and opportunity for growth, the mental health practitioner can act as a catalyzer of the best possible outcome. For example, a patient who always used to sleep soundly may be so frustrated over a new-onset sleep disturbance that he or she will find the side effects of a given sleep medication unacceptable. The physician then, while prescribing the appropriate medication, should also acknowledge the patient's emotions and validate them. When the clinician helps the patient work through his or her feelings over the loss of the habitual sleep pattern, the improved therapeutic alliance may ensure a better tolerance to the medication's side effects. Others have also pointed out that resisting the temptation to leave the Pandora's box of the patient's emotions closed is likely to foster better patient care and therapy compliance, in the context of pharmacotherapy of depression in HIV-infected patients (Markowitz, Rabkin, & Perry, 1994).

In a sense, this represents a refinement of our "transition model" presented elsewhere (Grant & Atkinson, 1995). The model proposes that psychological distress or mental disorders may be anticipated at key nodal points, such as discovery of seroconversion, initiation of antiretroviral treatment, onset of physical symptoms, advance in HIV disease stage, or an HIV-related loss; such distress or disorders reflect a compromised state of coping in the face of the stressor. Here we propose that the clinician's role is to identify the loss underlying an HIV-related "transition" and assess *and* address the corresponding grieving process.[5] Specific psychological interventions are discussed elsewhere in this book.

Much as in other chronic medical conditions and malignancies, depressed mood above cutoff points has been reported in as many as 42% of subjects in HIV samples (Belkin et al., 1992). Depressive symptoms have been found not to independently predict worse outcomes (Lyketsos et al., 1993), predict a more rapid decline in CD4 lymphocytes (Burack et al., 1993), greater mortality (Mayne et al., 1996), and be significantly associated with both quantitative and qualitative indicators of immune dysfunction (Kemeny et al., 1994). In the HNRC cohort, the interaction of life adversity and depressive symptoms at baseline predicted a decline in CD4+ percentage after 6 months (Patterson et al., 1995), while depressive symptoms predicted shorter longevity after controlling for symptoms and CD4+ cell counts (Patterson et al., 1996). In other similar cohorts, stress has been found to be associated with reductions in killer lymphocytes in HIV-positive men, but not in controls (Sahs et al., 1994)—a relationship not explained by confounding variables (greater depression in subjects with more stress,

---

[5]Naturally, any HIV-infected person can present with a state of psychological distress, behavioral maladjustment, or a mental disorder unrelated to HIV-related "transitions."

more advanced disease; Evans et al., 1995). A meta-analysis of studies
on the relations of stressors and depressive symptoms to HSV recurrence (n = 16) and HIV disease progression (n = 19) found that
depressive symptoms, but not stressors, are associated with increased
reporting of HIV-related symptoms, while stressors, especially popula-
tion-specific life events, are associated with numerical and functional
decrements in circulating NK cells (Zorrilla, McKay, Luborsky, &
Schmidt, 1996). A later study based on 2-year prospective data showed
that stress and depressive symptoms, especially when they occur jointly,
were associated with declines in CD8+ and NK cells (Leserman et al.,
1997). Although these findings should be replicated, followed longitudinally, and expanded to include quantitative *and* qualitative measures
of immune function, they are nonetheless consistent with the conceptualization of HIV disease as multifactorial (Fauci, 1993).

Given the likelihood that psychosocial factors influence the course
of HIV disease (Kemeny, 1994) as well as other viral illnesses (Zorrilla
et al., 1996), it seems wise to be particularly assertive and prompt in
initiating psychopharmacological treatment for neuropsychiatric disorders (especially mood and anxiety disorders) in individuals whose
immunity is already in jeopardy. Although such treatment should not
be offered *instead* of psychological treatment, which should always be
part of the therapeutic approach, there is no reason for keeping
patients presenting with psychiatric symptoms from receiving readily
available, safe, and effective psychotropic medication for any length of
time. On the other hand, these neuropsychoimmunological relationships should be considered vis-à-vis findings suggesting immunogeneti-
cally related individual differences (outside the individual's volition) in
responses to HIV infection (Paxton et al., 1996; Kaslow et al., 1996;
Michael et al., 1997) and viral opportunistic infection (Schrier, Freeman, Wiley, & McCutchan, 1995). Interestingly, in one study genetically
determined abilities to generate immune responses to HIV, CMV, and
herpes viruses were associated with lower risk to develop neurocognitive and neurological impairment but also higher risk for CD4+ cell
loss and death (Schrier, Wiley, Spina, McCutchan, & Grant, 1996). By
wisely emphasizing one of these relationships (i.e., psychosocial or
genetic contributions to disease progression), the mental health practitioner can alleviate excessive guilt in a person whose illness is
progressing in spite of his or her having the "right" attitude, or can
boost morale in another who is fatalistically convinced that nothing he
or she does will make a difference.

The psychopharmacological treatment of HIV-infected patients is
safe and effective, providing one uses the guidelines developed for the
use of psychotropic drugs in the medically ill and the elderly. The
experience to date indicates that for the most part standard psycho-

tropic drugs can be used safely in patients receiving antiretrovirals and that there are no adverse effects of psychotropic drugs on immunological function. Because there are so few data on the absorption, distribution, and metabolism of standard psychopharmacological agents in HIV-seropositive persons, or on drug interactions with agents used to treat HIV disease, psychiatrists must monitor their HIV patients more closely than the standards of practice based on non-HIV patients may dictate (Grant & Atkinson, 1995).

Mood Disorders

Studies have indicated that depression in all medically ill patients is both underdiagnosed and undertreated, which lowers the quality of life and increases disability for individuals who may already be experiencing poorer quality of life and disability as a consequence of HIV disease. In a study that examined the use of mental health services among seropositive gay men from San Francisco and Denver, only 40.3% of the depressed men had seen a mental health practitioner in the previous year, and only 6.3% were taking an antidepressant. It is likely that underdiagnosis and undertreatment of depression is even more common in more undeserved groups (Katz et al., 1996).

The usual therapeutic doses with standard agents are generally safe and effective in physically asymptomatic or moderately symptomatic individuals (Rabkin, Rabkin, Harrison, & Wagner, 1994a), although there are almost no data on maintenance treatment and longer-term follow-up. Some clinicians prefer customary first-line agents with low anticholinergic and other side effect profiles (e.g., desipramine), given their wide experience with these agents; other clinicians prefer newer drugs (e.g., fluoxetine, bupropion, or paroxetine) because of their even more favorable side-effect profiles (Rabkin et al., 1994b; Grassi, Gambini, Graghentini, Lazzarin, & Scarone, 1997). An open-label trial of SSRIs (sertraline, paroxetine, and fluoxetine) in depressed patients with symptomatic HIV disease or AIDS found significant reductions in both mood and somatic symptoms, although almost a third of subjects dropped out from the trial because of agitation, anxiety, and insomnia (Ferrando, Goldman, & Charness, 1997). Importantly, many of the somatic symptoms reported by the subjects had been attributed to the HIV disease before they were improved by antidepressants (Ferrando et al., 1997). In physically symptomatic individuals, the dictum "starting low, going slow" should be carefully observed. Starting dosages are usually about one-third or one-half those in customary psychiatric patients. The newer antidepressants may have specific disadvantages in the physically ill. Fluoxetine may be associated with insomnia and weight loss. Since symptomatic HIV individuals are at increased risk of seizure disorder related to HIV itself or to opportunistic infection or neoplasm, caution should also be used with bupropion (Atkinson & Grant, 1997b).

Physically asymptomatic individuals will show the best rates of response, and there may be somewhat reduced efficacy in patients with frank AIDS. The possibility of more limited efficacy in later-stage disease has also been related to loss of social support and the psychological burden of advancing physical illness (Atkinson & Grant, 1997b).

Physically ill patients with major depression who are unable to tolerate or do not respond to cyclic antidepressant regimens may respond to psychostimulants, such as methylphenidate, dextroamphetamine, or magnesium pemoline. Some clinicians prefer methylphenidate, since dextroamphetamine may produce severe tremor or a persisting movement disorder in later-stage patients (Fernández & Levy, 1994).

Monoamine oxidase inhibitors should be limited to patients with a history of successful use prior to HIV infection, particularly considering the potential interaction with zidovudine and the fact that patients' condition or dietary habits may render dietary restrictions impractical (Fernández & Levy, 1994).

Electroconvulsive therapy (ECT) is effective in patients whose depression requires urgent treatment, in those who have not responded to pharmacological therapies, or in those who have major depression with psychotic features. A neurological exam and brain imaging are necessary to rule out opportunistic brain disease and increased intracranial pressure before ECT is commenced (Atkinson & Grant, 1997b), although successful response has been reported even in cases with HIV-associated CNS and peripheral nervous system injury (Kessing, LaBianca, & Bolwig, 1994).

Mania or hypomania is adequately responsive to the available pharmacotherapeutic agents; however, late-stage disease patients may be more prone to experience dystonias, lithium encephalopathy, and neuroleptic malignant syndrome (el-Mallakh, 1991). Increased vigilance in toxicity monitoring when lithium carbonate is given to patients suffering from diarrhea or any form of fluid loss may be necessary (Fernández & Levy, 1994). Patients usually do not appear to require long-term, ongoing treatment, and recurrences have not been reported (el-Mallakh, 1991).

Substance-Related Disorders

Treatment of substance-related disorders in asymptomatic HIV-positive individuals should follow the same general guidelines as treatment recommended for those without the infection. A thorough review of the topic is beyond the scope of this chapter, but a combination of therapeutic approaches tailored to individual needs has been recommended, given the complexity of the biopsychosocial mechanisms involved in addiction (O'Brien, 1994). The interested reader is referred to comprehensive reviews of treatment for disorders of alcohol (Hodgson, 1994), stimulant (Schuckit, 1994), opiate (Johns, 1994), and benzodiazepine (Ashton, 1994) use. Reviews on therapeutic issues for specific populations, such as women (Hagan, Finnegan, & Nelson-Zlupko, 1994) and people of color (Finn, 1994), are also available.

By the time individuals reach later stages of HIV illness, the majority have ceased using psychoactive substances altogether, or have significantly cut down their use so that it is no longer clinically significant. Nevertheless, prompt and effective therapeutic interventions may be crucial in the medical and psychosocial management of HIV-infected persons. Survival and quality of life may be decreased not only directly by the physically deleterious effects of a substance, but, given the well-established association between substance use and risk for HIV infection or reinfection (Ostrow, 1994), indirectly by increasing the viral load within individuals or the infection with antiretroviral-resistant HIV strains. Furthermore, treatment of substance use disorders in HIV-positive individuals may help to contain the spread of the HIV epidemic.

Despite the failure of most "popper" users to meet DSM-IV criteria for substance abuse or dependence, mental health care practitioners should educate clients who use "poppers" regularly about the known associations between these substances and increased risk for HIV infection and transmission (reviewed in Ostrow, 1994).

It has been suggested that the reasons for combining substance use and high-risk sexual behaviors among disenfranchised MSM (e.g., low self-esteem and lack of access to community resources) may well differ from those already identified in cohort studies of gay-identified and largely well-educated majority men (Ostrow, 1994). This issue becomes particularly pressing, in light of the high prevalence of substance use disorders already noted among ethnic minority men. It has also been shown that ethnic minority men are overrepresented among MSM (Chu, Peterman, Doll, Buehler, & Curran, 1992) and men with IDU (Lewis & Watters, 1994) who do not identify themselves as gay despite behavioral bisexuality. The integration of HIV counseling and outreach activities into programs already providing social and health care services for vulnerable subpopulations of MSM engaging in both unprotected sex and substance use has been proposed as a more appropriate intervention for this population (Ostrow, 1994).

As discussed above, the presence of a personality disorder, especially antisocial personality disorder, has been associated with higher risk for HIV infection among injection drug users and with poorer treatment outcomes. Recently, one study of methadone maintenance clients found that benzodiazepine users were on higher methadone doses, more likely to relapse, and more likely to report IDU-related behaviors with high risk for HIV transmission. Benzodiazepine users also exhibited higher levels of psychopathology and social dysfunction (Darke et al., 1994). Clearly, these individuals constitute a dysfunctional subgroup and may pose additional problems for practitioners.

Anxiety Disorders

Symptomatic anxiety that does not meet criteria for a formal DSM-IV diagnosis is perhaps the most prevalent anxiety state in HIV-infected persons; it may arise episodically or may become a chronic feature of preoccupation with physical symptoms or illness. Restlessness, anxiousness, or inability to concentrate that impairs one's usual social relationships or functioning for a week or more may indicate a need for psychological or pharmacological therapy. Nonpharmacological treatments may be tried first, including supportive psychotherapy or the use of such stress and anxiety management approaches as relaxation training, education, and facilitating access to various social services (Grant & Atkinson, 1995).

Psychopharmacological treatment is usually conceptualized as brief (lasting no more than 2–6 weeks), with the view that most episodes of anxiety will remit within that time.

In general, evidence of a therapeutic effect should be expected within 1 week of starting treatment. Failure to improve means that the diagnosis should be reconsidered and that major depressive disorder or substance use disorder should be included in the differential diagnosis. Chronic anxiety states may be difficult to distinguish from hypochondriasis centered on HIV concerns. The latter tends to be treatment-resistant and extremely difficult to manage even with combined psychotherapeutic and pharmacological approaches, since obsessional or paranoid character structure may underlie symptomatology (Grant & Atkinson, 1995).

For individuals with recent histories of alcohol or other substance use disorders, the use of benzodiazepines may not be desirable. Buspirone hydrochloride or hydroxyzine is safe and effective. The delayed onset of therapeutic effect makes buspirone less suitable for cases of acute, severe anxiety (Grant & Atkinson, 1995).

Occasionally obsessive–compulsive disorder is evident, with HIV infection or AIDS as the focus of rumination and ritualistic behavior. The differential diagnosis should include major depressive disorder.

There are reports of such patients' responding well to standard antidepressant therapy. Agents that inhibit serotonin uptake, such as fluoxetine, fluvoxamine, sertraline, or clomipramine, should also be effective. In two open treatment studies, both fluoxetine (Rabkin et al., 1994a) and sertraline (Rabkin et al., 1994b) in standard doses were found to be effective and well tolerated among seropositive patients.

Similarly, panic disorder in physically asymptomatic or more symptomatic phases responds to standard therapy, which includes education, cognitive therapy, and pharmacological intervention (Grant & Atkinson, 1995).

Personality Disorders

There is little published information on therapeutic issues of personality disorders in the context of HIV disease. The reader is referred to reviews on treatment and management of borderline personality disorder (Higgitt & Fonagy, 1992; Searight, 1992) and personality disorders (Livesley, 1995).

Adjustment Disorders

Adjustment disorders unrelated to HIV-disease-associated stressors are not discussed here. During the first decade of the epidemic, feelings of hopelessness, anger, denial, and fear were widespread among gay men living with HIV and AIDS. With the advent of antiretroviral treatment and prophylaxis for opportunistic infections, as well as an overall improvement of psychosocial services and education regarding HIV disease in the general population, high levels of hope and resilience seem increasingly prevalent among HIV-infected persons over the last several years. Some gay men may even come to regard their HIV infection as a positive, or even transforming, experience in their lives (Schwartzberg, 1994). Although such attitudes have been observed mostly among white, well-educated, middle-class gay men living in large urban areas with well-established gay communities and access to social and health care services, they may provide a certain "gold standard" against which the overall adjustment and functioning of any HIV-infected individual can be compared.

A common "balancing act" that these well-adjusted individuals seem to negotiate successfully is maintaining a balance between control and surrender. In essence, they actively focus upon things amenable to change and let go of things that they cannot influence. This highly dynamic process recruits every resource available to an individual—spiritual, psychological, and environmental—and entails considerable amounts of cognitive flexibility. Health care professionals should help each person living with HIV that they provide for to move into such a process. Providing information in simple, clear terms that dispel false beliefs and correct misconceptions, and emphasizing rational decision making, are of paramount importance, and a considerable number of persons with adjustment disorders respond well to education and referrals to support services available in the community.

Specific therapeutic interventions should be tailored to the unique characteristics of each individual, and should therefore be preceded by an assessment of the stressor(s), disease stage, previous psychiatric history (including therapeutic interventions), and availability of formal health care and informal support (D. Miller & Riccio, 1990). Few studies comparing the effectiveness of psychological interventions have been published (e.g., Mulder et al., 1994; Markowitz et al., 1995), and there is a lack of outcome studies on treatment effectiveness that could inform a specific recommendation. The lack of controlled studies, however, contrasts with the richness and depth of observations informed by a variety of theoretical frameworks in the individual, family, or group modalities, gathered in clinical settings (see, e.g., Cadwell, Burnham, & Forstein, 1994).

Based on various theoretical frameworks, homogeneous, open-ended (Presberg & Kibel, 1994), anthropological (Brauer, 1994), Eriksonian (Tunnell, 1994), and psychodynamic (Baum & Fishman, 1994) group treatments, are particularly common and reportedly effective with gay and bisexual men (Cadwell, 1994). It is uncertain, however, whether such interventions can be relevant to other cultural groups (e.g., ethnic minority MSM). Regardless of modality, the overriding goal for all therapy with persons with HIV disease is to improve the quality of life (however the patients may define this) by increasing their understanding of maladaptive patterns, increasing their feelings of personal efficacy, and helping them to communicate needs, fears, and conflicts (Zegans, Gerhard, & Coates, 1994).

Adjustment disorders that do not respond readily to psychosocial interventions can be addressed with psychopharmacological agents. The same general guidelines outlined above for mood and anxiety disorders can be applied in these cases.

Neurocognitive Disorders

Delirium

Appropriate treatment for delirium stems from a thorough diagnostic process, since the etiology can involve more than one factor (i.e., HIV infection itself, another general medical condition, a drug of abuse, and/or medication or toxin exposure). Treatment of the underlying cause(s) is therefore the first step in the clinical management of delirium.

Nonspecific management can be effectively achieved with low doses of, preferably, high-potency agents such as haloperidol (0.25–5 mg once to three times daily) or, alternatively, low-potency neuroleptics such as chlorpromazine (10–25 mg once to three times daily) (Grant & Atkinson, 1995). An increased incidence of extrapyramidal symptoms associated with high-potency agents in advanced HIV disease, however, has been reported (Edelstein & Knight, 1987), and patients with underlying dementia due to HIV disease appear to be at highest risk for extrapyramidal side effects (Hriso, Kuhn, Masdeu, & Grundman, 1991). Extrapyramidal reactions in AIDS patients without dementia, even with low-potency neuroleptics used as antiemetics, have been reported (Swenson, Erman, Labelle, & Dimsdale, 1989). For patients who do not respond to low-dose oral therapy, excellent results have been reported with intravenous haloperidol given in individual boluses ranging from 2 to 10 mg every hour, or in extreme instances up to 150 mg daily. Some clinicians also have had good results with a combination of intravenous haloperidol and lorazepam, with an average daily intravenous dose of less than 50 mg of haloperidol and 10 mg of lorazepam (Fernández, Levy, & Mansell, 1989). In general, no serious adverse effects have been noted with these more aggressive intravenous regimens, although nearly half of the patients treated may have extrapyramidal symptoms (Fernández et al., 1989). Benzodiazepines alone (e.g., lorazepam) do not appear to be effective in delirious states and may accentuate confusion.

Dementia and Mild Neurocognitive Disorder

HIV dementia, and possibly mild neurocognitive disorder, is a treatable condition, and its deficits and functional impact are reversible in a proportion of patients. Numerous pharmacological agents are under investigation for management of HIV dementia. The most thoroughly investigated medication is zidovudine, with patients showing a decreased risk of developing dementia or improvement on neuropsychological, CSF, and neuropathological evaluations (Melton, Kirkwood, & Ghaemi, 1997). While the neuroprotective effects of antiretroviral monotherapy at standard doses are relatively limited, at higher doses, even severe dementia may respond. Currently, the recommended treatment for HIV dementia is zidovudine in the highest tolerable doses, and combination antiretroviral therapy with high-dose zidovudine plus dideoxyinosine for progressive encephalopathy, the equivalent of HIV dementia in children. Antiretroviral combination therapies and protease inhibitors can supress plasma HIV viral load by 2 log or greater. It can be reasonably expected that these treatments will result in larger and more sustained improvement of dementia symptoms as compared to those achieved with antiretroviral mono-therapy, either by inhibiting HIV replication in the brain or by reducing CNS seeding via suppression of systemic infection (reviewed in Sacktor & McArthur, 1997). Interestingly, there are a few reports indicating that these treatments may also alleviate dementia symptoms due to progressive multifocal leukoencephalopathy, which up to now was the only CNS opportunistic infection without effective prophylaxis or treatment.

Treatment of neurocognitive impairment in HIV can be both psychological and pharmacological. Ideally, it should involve family members, significant others, or close friends. The patient and these others should be informed of the strengths as well as the liabilities detected on neuropsychological testing; the clinician should emphasize that impairment in tests does not necessarily translate into disability in daily functioning, and that even when there is a disability, negative effects can be minimized. Advice should be given on simple measures such as adhering to a routine, keeping appointment books, doing one thing at a time, resting whenever necessary, and reducing external stimuli. Many HIV-infected individuals, particularly high-functioning and intelligent ones, know about and show concern about dementia. The clinician can assuage such fears in part by describing the current lack of evidence that minor cognitive impairments necessarily lead to dementia. A patient's safety is a high priority, and friends, family, and service organizations should be enlisted to assist with caretaking. At some point, it may be necessary to assess the patient's ability to drive motor vehicles. Some authors have also recommended the routine assessment of suicidal risk (Perry, 1990).

Health practitioners providing for persons with HIV-related im-pairment in attention/speed of information and verbal skills should be mindful of increased use of confrontive efforts to manage or regulate emotional responses to stressful situations in this group. It is possible that their difficulty sustaining attention to details or reduced ability to process verbal information leads to impulsive forms of coping because they are less able to assess the precise nature or extent of threat or harm posed by a stressful situation and the longer-term consequences of their coping (Manly et al., 1997).

Pharmacological intervention for neurocognitive impairment may involve the use of psychostimulants to improve attention, concentration, and psychomotor activity. A typical regimen in this group of patients might involve methylphenidate (2.5–5 mg twice a day with breakfast and at lunch), with slow increases up to 20 mg per day. Good results can be noted for many months, although doses may need to be increased (Fernández & Levy, 1994). Recent results from a large double-blind randomized placebo-controlled treatment trial of zidovudine showed beneficial effects of zidovudine on the CNS, regardless of degree of immune deficiency. The effects were demonstrated by both standardized neuropsychological testing (Baldeweg et al., 1995a) and quantitative EEGs (Baldeweg et al., 1995b). These clinical studies provide support for earlier neuropathological findings that both zidovudine and dideoxyinosine had effects on the occurrence of productive HIV infection of the brain (Gray et al., 1994; Portegies, 1995). These results should be replicated and expanded to include other antiretrovirals; they suggest, however, that clinicians may discuss with clients who present with neurocognitive impairment and are not receiving antiretrovirals the possibility of a therapeutic trial. Some authors have proposed that trials of medications to treat HIV-associated neurocognitive impairment should include patients with minor cognitive disorder, a more common syndrome with longer survival than HIV dementia (R. J. Ellis et al., 1997).

HIV-Associated Sleep Disturbance

No controlled studies of treatment of HIV-associated sleep disturbance have been published, and anecdotal experience shows that available therapy often provides only partial relief. More efficient and specific treatment is needed for immunocompromised individuals presenting with sleep disturbance. Besides the substantial contribution of disturbed sleep to disability (Darko et al., 1992), the relationships between the sleep–wake cycle and immune function make the development of effective treatment for sleep disturbance in the context of immune disruption more pressing. A positive correlation of total sleep time, sleep efficiency, and duration of slow-wave sleep with natural killer lymphocyte activity has been reported (Irwin, Smith, & Gillin, 1992).

Since sleep disturbance can be a chronic condition, benzodiazepines are not a first choice for treatment. Rather, antidepressants with sedative properties, such as trazodone, have been recommended in doses of 25–100 mg at bedtime. Anecdotal observation reveals that treatment response is variable, with many individuals experiencing only partial (if any), relief. Other general measures indicated in cases of insomnia (e.g., keeping a fixed schedule of activities and sleep, avoiding daytime naps, exercise in the early evening, staying out of bed when not sleeping, etc.) should always be tried (Sciolla, 1995). Promising results from a controlled trial of light treatment for HIV-associated sleep disturbance await replication (Sciolla, Brown, Summers, Atkinson, & Grant, 1997).

Psychotic Disorders

New-onset psychotic symptoms should be treated with neuroleptics. Both high-potency agents (haloperidol and bromperidol) and low-potency agents (thioridazine) reduce the overall level of psychosis and positive symptoms, but not that of negative symptoms (Perretta et al., 1992; Sewell et al., 1994b). Other clinicians advocate the use of molindone (10–15 mg daily) because of its lower likelihood of producing extrapyramidal syndromes (Fernández & Levy, 1993). Unfortunately, little has been published on the use of newer or atypical antipsychotics in HIV-infected persons. In the meantime, clinical guidelines provided for the use of this kind of drug in the elderly may help clinicians in the choice, dosage, and monitoring of side effects (Sciolla & Jeste, 1997).

The usual therapeutic dose of neuroleptics is one-tenth to one-third that used for most acute psychoses in psychiatric settings. It is unclear why lower-dose regimens are adequate, but it may be related to pharmacokinetic changes associated with chronic diseases, or to HIV-associated damage to subcortical limbic or basal ganglia structures. This latter explanation has also been thought to be the source of sensitivity of patients with HIV-associated psychosis to extrapyramidal side effects (Sewell et al., 1994b). Hriso et al. (1991) have reported that the risk of developing antipsychotic-induced extrapyramidal symptoms is 2.4 times higher in psychotic AIDS patients than in psychotic patients without AIDS. Moreover, an increased risk of tardive dyskinesia in this population has been suggested (Shedlack, Soldato-Couture, & Swanson, 1994). Movement disorders attributable to subcortical damage can appear in HIV-infected persons not taking neuroleptics; they include myoclonus, paroxysmal dystonia, parkinsonian features, essential tremors, hemiballism, and hemichorea (Nath, Jankovic, & Pettigrew, 1987; Nath & Jankovic, 1989). The reported development of neuroleptic malignant syndrome in AIDS patients (Breitbart, Marotta, & Call, 1988) is also not surprising: Brain-damaged patients seem to be at higher risk for developing the syndrome, due to reduction of dopamine in the hypothalamus and basal ganglia (Lazarus, 1992).

In general, extrapyramidal side effects can be managed with low doses of benztropine mesylate, although some authorities suggest substituting amantadine to avoid the anticholinergic properties of benztropine mesylate (Grant & Atkinson, 1995).

Complicated Bereavement

HIV-infected individuals experiencing an AIDS-related bereavement may be a subgroup particularly prone to seek professional psychological help. In one large cohort study of gay men, men who were bereaved sought treatment nearly four times as often as did the nonbereaved men (J. L. Martin & Dean, 1993).

There is a social stigma attached not only to a person living with AIDS, but also to a survivor of an AIDS-related death. Specialized support groups (as opposed to "nonspecific" support groups), in which the commonality of losing significant others to AIDS allows participants to discuss the stigma conferred by the larger community, have been found effective in alleviating symptoms of complicated bereavement (Summers et al., 1993). Feelings of guilt and shame stemming from forced silence about the loss are also best dealt with in these groups (Biller & Rice, 1990). Such groups may replace support systems that no longer function (e.g., family members of the deceased who turn against the survivor). Groups of seronegative individuals with specific bereavement issues that have been described include mothers whose sons died of AIDS (Longman, 1995) and the uninfected children of mothers who died of AIDS (Siegel & Gorey, 1994). Two issues that pose additional difficulties are the fact that survivors often provide some degree of care to many AIDS victims, and that the person who dies may not be the same person physically and mentally the survivor formed a relationship with prior to the decline (Biller & Rice, 1990). One of the most powerful therapeutic tools available to all practitioners is simply the discussion of events leading up to deaths; the healing powers of cathartic reactions triggered by such discussion in the context of an empathic atmosphere cannot be overemphasized. Practitioners can recommend their clients to engage actively in mourning rituals, particularly collective ones such as the AIDS quilt, since the beneficial effects of these are strongly supported on both theoretical (Shelby, 1994) and empirical grounds (Summers et al., 1995b).

In spite of demographic changes during the AIDS epidemic, the majority of new infections and AIDS cases still occur among gay men. Specific and unique characteristics of AIDS-related grief among gay men have been emphasized. These include (1) the adverse effect of multiple losses; (2) characteristics of the urban gay male subculture; (3) shortcomings of available grief models; and (4) the importance of finding meaning in ongoing adversity (Schwartzberg, 1992). These characteristics pose special challenges for practitioners providing psychological help to bereaved gay men. For these men, recovery or the closure of a grieving process may be unattainable in the traditional sense, given the ongoing and cumulative nature of AIDS-related loss. Also, gay men, particularly those identified with the urban gay subculture, have experienced the loss of an entire way of life (i.e., patterns of socializing, conducting relationships, and experiencing sexuality) as a result of the AIDS epidemic. The ultimate challenge to a grieving individual in this situation is to find some meaning or sense in AIDS, which becomes a focus of grieving for deaths and coping with life (Schwartzberg, 1992).

SUMMARY AND CONCLUSIONS

The facts that HIV disease is incurable and that no effective vaccine has been yet developed (despite the enormous progress made in slowing disease progression) are among the few facts that remain unchanged since the first cases were reported in the summer of 1981. Other epidemiological and clinical aspects of the disease have evolved, sometimes in striking ways, over the years. Against this backdrop of relentless drifts and shifts, this chapter has centered on two aspects that are unlikely to change in the foreseeable future. First, HIV is neuroinvasive; it is a disease of the brain as much as of the immune function. Second, because of its protracted course involving a gradual loss of key personal functions and characteristics, as well as the prospect of an early death, patients' resulting feelings need to be addressed by health care professionals, regardless of the specific services they deliver.

Because HIV invades the CNS early in the course of the disease and may induce functional and structural abnormalities, mental health practitioners should be cautious about ascribing psychological meanings or explanations to signs and symptoms in their clients. The possibility that biology may underlie clinical findings and complaints is higher in the terminal stage of the disease than in the asymptomatic phase (Cornblath et al., 1989), but HIV infection of the brain may result in clinically significant problems at any stage of the disease. In fact, experts now view the lack of symptoms not as a dormant phase, but a highly dynamic one entailing processes that are key to subsequent pathological developments.

The need for mental health practitioners to strive for competency in the field of HIV disease results directly from its mode of transmission. Persons who are infected with HIV or at higher risk for the infection have increased rates of psychiatric disorders predating infection, compared to the rest of the population. To illustrate this interaction consider, for example, substance use disorders and their well-established role in (non-HIV) STDs. Problem drinking among women more than quadruples the risk of STDs, independently of age, race, early age at first intercourse, and history of multiple partners; among men, problem drinking carries the same odds rate as a history of multiple sex partners (Ericksen & Trocki, 1992). In other words, mental health practitioners work with persons whose psychopathology increases their risk for HIV infection (and other STDs), and who, as a consequence, may present with neuropsychiatric complications of HIV disease.

Neurocognitive disorders, sleep disturbance, and psychosis (an uncommon but serious complication) are the most important neuropsychiatric syndromes caused by direct effects of HIV infection of the CNS. Psychosis is relatively rare and can be easily managed with neuroleptics, but is associated with high mortality. The two others are more common, but unfortunately the available therapy for sleep disturbance offers in many cases only partial relief. Effective treatment for mild neurocognitive disorder and dementia is almost completely lacking, although antiretroviral agents are showing some promise in this regard. Significant advances in elucidating the pathogenic mechanisms underlying these disorders offer hope that appropriate treatment may be developed. Besides obvious clinical challenges, the presence of cognitive impairment may pose additional constraints to psychotherapeutic goals—goals that are generally made modest in the first place by the shorter life expectancy of HIV-positive persons. Psychopharmacological treatment for other disorders diagnosed in HIV-infected individuals is effective and safe, provided that general guidelines for the medically ill are observed.

The second aspect of HIV/AIDS that this chapter has focused on is the psychological issue of loss. Needless to say, among the multiple psychological challenges posed by HIV disease, this is not the main or the most common theme in every person at all times. However, its centrality in the overall disease process, and the wealth of knowledge amassed on the psychotherapeutic aspects of loss, make it a paradigm with both heuristic and clinical value. If a clinician looks at neuropsychiatric disorders or syndromes through the prism of this paradigm, an accompanying loss or losses can almost always be identified. Identification of the loss should lead at the very least to facilitating catharsis and acknowledgment of feelings. This simple therapeutic action may result in clinically useful outcomes. By strengthening the rapport and trust between client and clinician, it may provide a sound basis for correct diagnosis and improve the client's compliance with therapeutic measures, biological or otherwise.

This practical, efficiency-oriented approach should not be misconstrued as an imposition of theoretical models on the rich diversity of individuals infected with HIV. For mental health professionals, HIV disease is as much of a lesson in flexibility and humility as it is for those living with it. Patients themselves, not books, are often the best source of information. Truly listening to their stories of despair, hope, anger, love, fear, and courage can only make clinicians more efficient and responsive in their work; this can yield truly rewarding results in the times of this epidemic.

REFERENCES

Achim, C. L., & Wiley, C. A. (1994). *In vivo* model of HIV infection of the human brain. *Advances in Neuroimmunology, 4*(3), 261–264.

Achim, C. L., & Wiley, C. A. (1996). Immflamation in AIDS and the role of the macrophage in brain pathology. *Current Opinion in Neurology, 9*(3), 221–225.

Albert, M. L., Feldman, R. G., & Willis, A. L. (1974). The "subcortical dementia" of progressive supranuclear palsy. *Journal of Neurology, Neurosurgery, and Psychiatry, 37,* 121–130.

Alexander, P. J., Dinesh, N., & Vidyasager, M. S. (1993). Psychiatric morbidity among cancer patients and its relationship with awareness of illness and expectations about treatment outcome. *Acta Oncologica, 32*(6), 623–626.

Alfonso, C. A., Cohen, M. A. A., Aladjem, A. D., Morrison, F., Powell, D. R., Winters, R. A., & Orlowski, B. K. (1994). HIV seropositivity as a major risk factor for suicide in the general hospital. *Psychosomatics, 35*(4), 368–373.

Allers, C. T., Benjack, K. J., White, J., & Rousey, J. T. (1993). HIV vulnerability and the adult survivor of childhood sexual abuse. *Child Abuse and Neglect, 17*(2), 291–298.

American Academy of Neurology (AAN). (1991). Nomenclature and research case definitions for neurologic manifestations of human immunodeficiency virus-type 1 (HIV-1) infection: Report of a working group of the American Academy of Neurology AIDS Task Force. *Neurology, 41*(6), 778–785.

American Psychiatric Association. (1987). *Diagnostic and statistical manual of mental disorders* (3rd ed., rev.). Washington, DC: Author.

American Psychiatric Association. (1994). *Diagnostic and statistical manual of mental disorders* (4th ed.). Washington, DC: Author.

Aral, S. O. (1994). Sexual behavior in sexually transmitted disease research: An overview. *Sexually Transmitted Diseases, 21*(Suppl. 2), S59–S64.

Aral, S. O., Soskoline, V., Joesoef, R. M., & O'Reilly, K. R. (1991). Sex partner recruitment as risk factor for STD: Clustering of risky modes. *Sexually Transmitted Diseases, 18*(1), 10–17.

Arendt, G., Hefter, H., Neuen-Jacob, E., Wist, S., Kuhlmann, H., Strohmeyer, G., & Freund, H. J. (1993). Electrophysiological motor testing, MRI findings and clinical course in AIDS patients with dementia. *Journal of Neurology, 240*(7), 439–445.

Ashton, H. (1994). The treatment of benzodiazepine dependence. *Addiction, 89*(11), 1535–1541.

Atkinson, J. H., & Grant, I. (1994). Natural history of neuropsychiatric manifestations of HIV disease. *Psychiatric Clinics of North America, 17*(1), 17–33.

Atkinson, J. H., & Grant, I. (1997a). Mood disorders due to human immunodeficiency virus: Yes, no, or maybe? *Seminars in Clinical Neuropsychiatry 2*(4), 276–284.

Atkinson, J. H., & Grant, I. (1997b). Neuropsychiatry of human immunodeficiency virus infection. In J. R. Berger & R. M. Levy (Eds.), *AIDS and the nervous system* (2nd ed., pp. 419–449). Philadelphia: Lippincott-Raven.

Atkinson, J. H., Jr., Grant, I., Kennedy, C. J., Richman, D. D., Spector, S. A., & McCutchan, J. A. (1988). Prevalence of psychiatric disorders among men infected with human immunodeficiency virus: A controlled study. *Archives of General Psychiatry, 45*(9), 859–864.

Aylward, E. H., Brettschneider, P. D., McArthur, J. C., Harris, G. J., Schlaepfer, T. E., Henderer, J. D., Barta, P. E., Tien, A. Y., & Pearlson, G. D. (1995). Magnetic resonance imaging measurement of gray matter volume reductions in HIV dementia. *American Journal of Psychiatry, 152*(7), 987–994.

Aylward, E. H., Henderer, J. D., McArthur, J. C., Brettschneider, P. D., Harris, G. J., Barta, P. E., & Pearlson, G. D. (1993). Reduced basal ganglia volume in HIV-1-associated dementia: Results from quantitative neuroimaging. *Neurology, 43*(10), 2099–2104.

Bacellar, H., Munoz, A., Miller, E. N., Cohen, B. A., Besley, D., Selnes, O. A., Becker, J. T., & McArthur, J. C. (1994). Temporal trends in the incidence of HIV-1-related neurologic diseases: Multicenter AIDS Cohort Study, 1985–1992. *Neurology, 44*(10), 1892–1900.

Baldeweg, T., Catalan, J., Lovett, E., Gruzelier, J., Riccio, M., & Hawkins, D. (1995a). Long-term zidovudine reduces neurocognitive deficits in HIV-1 infection. *AIDS, 9*(6), 589–596.

Baldeweg, T., Riccio, M., Gruzelier, J., Hawkins, D., Burgess, A., Irving, G., Stygall, J., Catt, S., & Catalan, J. (1995b). Neurophysiological evaluation of zidovudine in asymptomatic HIV-1 infection: A longitudinal placebo-controlled study. *Journal of the Neurological Sciences, 132*(2), 162–169.

Baldwin, D., & Rudge, S. (1995). The role of serotonin in depression and anxiety. *International Clinical Psychopharmacology, 9*(Suppl. 4), 41–45.

Baum, M., & Fishman, J. (1994). AIDS sexual compulsivity and gay men: A group treatment approach. In S. A. Cadwell, R. A. Burnham, & M. Forstein (Eds.), *Therapists on the front line: Psychotherapy with gay men in the age of AIDS* (pp. 255–274). Washington, DC: American Psychiatric Press.

Belec, L., Gray, F., Mikol, J., Scaravilli, F., Mhiri, C., Sobel, A., & Poirier, J. (1990). Cytomegalovirus (CMV) encephalomyeloradiculitis and human immunodeficiency virus (HIV) encephalitis: Presence of HIV and CMV co-infected multinucleated giant cells. *Acta Neuropathologica, 81*(1), 99–104.

Belkin, G. S., Fleishman, J. A., Stein, M. D., Piette, J., & Mor, V. (1992). Physical symptoms and depressive symptoms among individuals with HIV infection. *Psychosomatics, 33*(4), 416–427.

Bellini, M., Bruschi, C., Babini, P., Capannini, D., Scaramelli, A. R., Taruschio, G., Raise, E., Cannella, B., De Marco, P., Orsini, N., et al. (1994). [Diagnosis of major depression in HIV-infected patients]. *Minerva Psichiatrica, 35*(3), 129–138.

Beltrán, E. D., Ostrow, D. G., & Joseph, J. G. (1993). Predictors of sexual behavior change among men requesting their HIV-1 antibody status: The Chicago MACS/CCS cohort of homosexual/bisexual men, 1985–1986. *AIDS Education and Prevention, 5*(3), 185–195.

Benos, D. J., Hahn, B. H., Bubien, J. K., Ghosh, S. K., Mashburn, N. A., Chaikin, M. A., Shaw, G. M., & Benveniste, E. N. (1994). Envelope glycoprotein gp120 of human immunodeficiency virus type 1 alters ion transport in astrocytes: Implications for AIDS dementia complex. *Proceedings of the National Academy of Sciences USA, 91*(2), 494–498.

Berman, S. M., & Kim, R. C. (1994). The development of cytomegalovirus encephalitis in AIDS patients receiving ganciclovir. *American Journal of Medicine, 96*(5), 415–419.

Bialer, P. A., Wallack, J. J., & Snyder, S. L. (1991). Psychiatric diagnosis in HIV-spectrum disorders. *Psychiatric Medicine, 9*(3), 361–375.

Biller, R., & Rice, S. (1990). Experiencing multiple loss of persons with AIDS: Grief and bereavement issues. *Health and Social Work, 15*(4), 283–290.

Birdsall, H. H., Ozluoglu, L. N., Lew, H. L., Trial, J., Brown, D. P., Wofford, M. J., Jerger, J. F., & Rossen, R. D. (1994). Auditory P300 abnormalities and leukocyte activation in HIV infection. *Otolaryngology and Head and Neck Surgery, 110*(1), 53–59.

Blazer, D. G., Kessler, R. C., McGonagle, K. A., & Swartz, M. S. (1994). The prevalence and distribution of major depression in a national community sample: The National Comorbidity Survey. *American Journal of Psychiatry, 151*(7), 979–986.

Bleyenheuft, L., Janne, P., Reynaert, C., Munyandamutsa, N., Verhoeven, F., Muremyangango, B., & Cassiers, L. (1992). [Prevalence of human immunodeficiency virus infection in a psychiatric population in Central Africa]. *Acta Psychiatrica Belgica, 92*(2), 99–108.

Bliwise, D. L. (1993). Sleep in normal aging and dementia. *Sleep, 16*(1), 40–81.

Block, S. D., & Billings, J. A. (1995). Patient requests for euthanasia and assisted suicide in terminal illness: The role of the psychiatrist. *Psychosomatics, 36*(5), 445–457.

Blumberg, B. M., Gelbard, H. A., & Epstein, L. G. (1994). HIV-1 infection of the developing nervous system: Central role of astrocytes in pathogenesis. *Virus Research, 32*(2), 253–267.

Booth, R. E. (1995). Gender differences in high-risk sex behaviors among heterosexual drug injectors and crack smokers. *Journal of Drug and Alcohol Abuse, 21*(4), 419–432.

Bornstein, R. A., Fama, R., Rosenberger, P., Whitacre, C. C., Para, M. F., Nasrallah, H. A., & Fass, R. J. (1993). Drug and alcohol use and neuropsychological performance in asymptomatic HIV infection. *Journal of Neuropsychiatry and Clinical Neurosciences, 5,* 254–259.

Bornstein, R. A., Nasrallah, H. A., Para, M. F., Fass, R. J., Whitacre, C. C., & Rice, R. R., Jr. (1993). Rate of CD4 decline and neuropsychological performance in HIV infection. *Archives of Neurology, 48*(7), 704–707.

Bourin, P., Mansour, I., Doinel, C., Roue, R., Rouger, P., & Levi, F. (1993). Circadian rhythms of circulating NK cells in healthy and human immunodeficiency virus-infected men. *Chronobiology International, 10*(4), 298–305.

Brauer, S. B. (1994). HIV-infected men: Group work as a rite of passage. In S. A. Cadwell, R. A. Burnham, & Forstein, M. (Eds.), *Therapists on the front line: Psychotherapy with gay men in the age of AIDS* (pp. 223–236). Washington, DC: American Psychiatric Press.

Breitbart, W., Marotta, R. F., & Call P. (1988). AIDS and neuroleptic malignant syndrome [Letter]. *Lancet, ii,* 1488–1489.

Brenner, R. P. (1991). Utility of EEG in delirium: Past views and current practice. *International Psychogeriatrics, 3*(2), 211–229.

Brew, B. J. (1991). Neuronal loss in frontal cortex in HIV infection [Letter]. *Lancet, 338,* 129–130.

Brew, B. J., Pemberton, L., Cunnigham, P., & Law, M. G. (1997). Levels of human immunodeficiency virus type 1 RNA cerebrospinal fluid correlate with AIDS dementia stage. *Journal of Infectious Diseases, 175*(4), 963–966.

Bridge, T. P. (1988). AIDS and HIV CNS disease: A neuropsychiatric disorder. In T. P. Bridge, A. F. Mirsky, & F. K. Goodwin (Eds.), *Advances in biochemical psychopharmacology: Vol. 44. Psychological, neuropsychiatric, and substance abuse aspects of AIDS* (pp. 1–13). New York: Raven Press.

Britton, C. B., & Miller, J. R. (1984). Neurologic complications in acquired immunodeficiency syndrome (AIDS). *Neurologic Clinics, 2*(2), 315–339.

Brock, M. A. (1991). Chronobiology and aging. *Journal of the American Geriatrics Society, 39*(1), 74–91.

Brodsky, B. S., Cloitre, M., & Dulit, R. A. (1995). Relationship of dissociation to self-mutilation and childhood abuse in borderline personality disorder. *American Journal of Psychiatry, 152*(12), 1788–1792.

Bronisch, T., & Wittchen, H. U. (1992). Lifetime and 6-month prevalence of abuse and dependence of alcohol in the Munich Follow-Up Study. *European Archives of Psychiatry and Clinical Neuroscience, 241*(5), 273–282.

Brooner, R. K., Greenfield, L., Schmidt, C. W., & Bigelow, G. E. (1993). Antisocial personality disorder and HIV infection among intravenous drug abusers. *American Journal of Psychiatry, 150*(1), 53–58.

Brown, G. R., Rundell, J. R., McManis, S. E., Kendall, S. N., Zachary, R., & Temoshok, L. (1992). Prevalence of psychiatric disorders in early stages of HIV infection. *Psychosomatic Medicine, 54*(5), 588–601.

Brown, S. J., Mitler, M., Atkinson, J. H., Malone, J., Chandler, J. L., McCutchan, J. A., & Grant, I. (1991). Correlation of subjective complaints, absolute T-4 cell number and anxiety in HIV illness. *Sleep Research, 20,* 363.

Brown, S. J., Summers, J., Atkinson, J. H., McCutchan, A., & Grant, I. (1992, March–April). *Prevalence of personality disorders in men at high risk for HIV.*

Paper presented at the 50th Annual Meeting of the American Psychosomatic Society, New York.

Brown, S. J., Sciolla, A., Nelson, J. A., Atkinson, J. H., & Grant, I. (1996). *Napping is increased in asymptomatic HIV disease in absence of psychiatric diagnosis.* Unpublished analyses.

Buhrich, N., Cooper, D. A., & Freed, E. (1988). HIV infection associated with symptoms indistinguishable from functional psychosis. *British Journal of Psychiatry, 152,* 649–653.

Burack, J. H., Barrett, D. C., Stall, R. D., Chesney, M. A., Ekstrand, M. L., & Coates, T. J. (1993). Depressive symptoms and CD4 lymphocyte decline among HIV-infected men. *Journal of the American Medical Association, 270*(21), 2568–2573.

Burnell, G. M. (1995). Psychiatric assessment of the suicidal terminally ill. *Hawaii Medical Journal, 54*(4), 510–513.

Butters, N., Grant, I., Haxby, J., Judd, L. L., Martin, A., McClelland, J., Pequegnat, W., Schacter, D., & Stover, E. (1990). Assessment of AIDS-related cognitive changes: Recommendations of the NIMH Workshop on Neuropsychological Assessment Approaches. *Journal of Clinical and Experimental Neuropsychology, 12*(6), 963–978.

Buttini, M., Westland, C. E., Masliah, E., Yafeh, A. M., Wyss-Coray, T., & Mucke, L. (in press). Novel role of human CD4 molecule identified in neurodegeneration. *Nature Medicine.*

Buysse, D. J., Reynolds, C. F., III, Monk, T. H., Berman, S. R., & Kupfer, D. J. (1989). The Pittsburgh Sleep Quality Index: A new instrument for psychiatric practice and research. *Psychiatry Research, 28*(2), 193–213.

Cadoret, R. J., Yates, W. R., Troughton, E., Woodworth, G., & Stewart, M. A. (1995). Genetic–environmental interaction in the genesis of aggressivity and conduct disorders. *Archives of General Psychiatry, 52*(11), 916–924.

Cadwell, S. A. (1995). Twice removed: The stigma suffered by gay men with AIDS. In S. A. Cadwell, R. A. Burnham, & Forstein, M. (Eds.), *Therapists on the front line: Psychotherapy with gay men in the age of AIDS* (pp. 3–24). Washington, DC: American Psychiatric Press.

Cadwell, S. A., Burnham, R. A., & Forstein, M. (Eds.). (1995). *Therapists on the front line: Psychotherapy with gay men in the age of AIDS.* Washington, DC: American Psychiatric Press.

Carballo-Dieguez, A., & Dolezal, C. (1995). Association between history of childhood sexual abuse and adult HIV-risk sexual behavior in Puerto Rican men who have sex with men. *Child Abuse and Neglect, 19*(5), 595–605.

Carlin, A. S. (1986). Neuropsychological consequences of drug abuse. In I. Grant & K. M. Adams (Eds.), *Neuropsychological assessment of neuropsychiatric disorders* (pp. 478–497). New York: Oxford University Press.

Centers for Disease Control. (1997, September 26). Gonorrhea among men who have sex with men—Selected sexually transmitted disease clinics, 1993–1996. *Morbidity and Mortality Weekly Report, 64*(38).

Chaisson, R. E., Keruly, J. C., & Moore, R. D. (1995). Race, sex, drug use, and porgression of human immunodeficiency virus disease. *New England Journal of Medicine, 333*(12), 751–756.

Cherner, M., Patterson, T., Semple, S., Koch, W., Manly, J., Atkinson, J. H., Grant, I., & the HNRC Group. (1994). Ethnic differences in depression, coping, and social support among HIV-infected men. *Annals of Behavioral Medicine, 16*(Suppl. 181).

Chesney, M. A., & Folkman, S. (1994). Psychological impact of HIV disease and implications for intervention. *Psychiatric Clinics of North America, 17*(1), 163–182.

Chochinov, H. M., Wilson, K. G., Enns, M., & Lander, S. (1994). Prevalence of depression in the terminally ill: Effects of diagnostic criteria and symptom threshold judgments. *American Journal of Psychiatry, 151*(4), 537–540.

Chochinov, H. M., Wilson, K. G., Enns, M., Mowchun, N., Lander, S., Levitt, M., & Clinch, J. J. (1995). Desire for death in the terminally ill. *American Journal of Psychiatry, 152*(8), 1185–1191.

Chu, S. Y., Peterman, T. A., Doll, L. S., Buehler, J. W., & Curran, J. W. (1992). AIDS in bisexual men in the United States: Epidemiology and transmission to women. *American Journal of Public Health, 82*(2), 220–224.

Clarke, D. M., Minas, I. H., & Stuart, G. W. (1991). The prevalence of psychiatric morbidity in general hospital inpatients. *Australian and New Zealand Journal of Psychiatry, 25*(3), 322–329.

Cochran, S. D., & Mays, V. M. (1994). Depressive distress among homosexually active African American men and women. *American Journal of Psychiatry, 151*(4), 524–529.

Coligan, J. E., & Clouse, K. A. (1993). Potent stimulation of monocytic endothelin-1 production by HIV-1 glycoprotein 120. *Journal of Immunology, 150*(10), 4601–4609.

Collier, A. C., Marra, C., Coombs, R. W., Claypoole, K., Cohen, W., Longstreth, W. T., Jr., Townes, B. D., Maravilla, K. R., Critchlow, C., Murphy, V. L., et al. (1992). Central nervous system manifestations in human immunodeficiency virus infection without AIDS. *Journal of Acquired Immune Deficiency Syndromes, 5*(3), 229–241.

Cornblath, D. R., Chmiel, J. S., Wang, M. C., et al. (1989). Low prevalence of neurological and neuropsychological abnormalities in otherwise healthy HIV-1 infected individuals: Results from the Multicenter AIDS Cohort Study. *Annals of Neurology, 26*(5), 601–611.

Crespo-Hervás, M. D., Vicente Muelas, N., Ochoa Mangado, E., & del Pino Morales Socorro, M. (1992). [Findings in HIV infected patients in a psychiatry unit]. *Actas Luso-Espanolas de Neurologia, Psiquiatria y Ciencias Afines, 20*(4), 168–174.

Culebras, A. (1992). Neuroanatomic and neurologic correlates of sleep disturbances. *Neurology, 42*(7, Suppl. 6), 19–27.

da Cunha, A., Eiden, L. E., & Rausch, D. M. (1994). Neuronal substrates for SIV encephalopathy. *Advances in Neuroimmunology, 4*(3), 265–271.

Darke, S., Swift, W., & Hall, W. (1994). Prevalence, severity and correlates of psychological morbidity among methadone maintenance clients. *Addiction, 89*(2), 211–217.

Darko, D. F., McCutchan, J. A., Kripke, D. F., Gillin, J. C., & Golshan, S. (1992).

Fatigue, sleep disturbance, disability, and indices of progression of HIV infection. *American Journal of Psychiatry, 149*(4), 514–520.

Darko, D. F., Miller, J. C., Gallen, C., White, J., Koziol, J., Brown, S. J., Hayduk, R., Atkinson, J. H., Assmus, J., Munnell, D. T., et al. (1995a). Sleep electroencephalogram delta-frequency amplitude, night plasma levels of tumor necrosis factor alpha, and human immunodeficiency virus infection. *Proceedings of the National Academy of Sciences USA, 92*(26), 12080–12084.

Darko, D. F., Mitler, M. M., & Henriksen, S. J. (1995b). Lentiviral infection, immune response peptides and sleep. *Advances in Neuroimmunology, 5*(1), 57–77.

Day, J. J., Grant, I., Atkinson, J. H., Brysk, L. T., McCutchan, J. A., Hesselink, J. R., Heaton, R. K., Weinrich, J. D., Spector, S. A., & Richman, D. D. (1992). Incidence of AIDS dementia in a two-year follow-up of AIDS and ARC patients on an initial phase II AZT placebo-controlled study: San Diego cohort. *Journal of Neuropsychiatry and Clinical Neurosciences, 4*(1), 15–20.

Dew, M. A., Becker, J. T., Sanchez, J., Caldararo, R., Lopez, O. L., Wess, J., Dorst, S. K., & Banks, G. (1997). Prevalence and predictors of depressive, anxiety, and substance use disorders in HIV-infected and uninfected men: A longitudinal evaluation. *Psychological Medicine, 27*(2), 395–409.

Dilley, J. W., Ochitill, H. N., Perl, M., & Volberding, P. A. (1985). Findings in psychiatric consultations with patients with acquired immune deficiency syndrome. *American Journal of Psychiatry, 142*(1), 82–86.

Dinwiddie, S. H., & Reich, T. (1993). Genetic and family studies in psychiatric illness and alcohol and drug dependence. *Journal of Addictive Diseases, 12*(3), 17–27.

Dohrenwend, B. P., Levav, I., Shrout, P. E., Schwartz, S., Naveh, G., Link, B. G., Skodol, A. E., & Stueve, A. (1992). Socioeconomic status and psychiatric disorders: The causation-selection issue. *Science, 255*(5047), 946–952.

Dowd, S. A. (1994). African-American gay men and HIV and AIDS: Therapeutic challenges. In S. A. Cadwell, R. A. Burnham, & Forstein, M. (Eds.), *Therapists on the front line: Psychotherapy with gay men in the age of AIDS* (pp. 319–337). Washington, DC: American Psychiatric Press.

Dunbar, N., Perdices, M., Grunseit, A., & Cooper, D. A. (1992). Changes in neuropsychological performance of AIDS-related complex patients who progress to AIDS. *AIDS, 6*(7), 691–700.

Easterbrook, P. J., Keruly, J. C., Creagh-Kirk, T., Richman, D. D., Chaisson, R. E., & Moore, R. D. (1991). Racial and ethnic differences in outcome in zidovudine-treated patients with advanced HIV disease. Zidovudine Epidemiology Study Group. *Journal of the American Medical Association, 266*(19), 2713–2718.

Edelstein, H., & Knight, R. T. (1987). Severe parkinsonism in two AIDS patients taking prochlorperazine [Letter]. *Lancet, ii,* 341–342.

Edlin, B. R., Irwin, K. L., Faruque, S., McCoy, C. B., Word, C., Serrano, Y., Inciardi, J. A., Bowser, B. P., Schilling, R. F., Holmberg, S. D., et al. (1994). Intersecting epidemics: Crack cocaine use and HIV infection among inner-city young adults. *New England Journal of Medicine, 331*(21), 1422–1427.

Ehrhardt, A. A. (1992). Trends in sexual behavior and the HIV pandemic [Editorial, comment]. *American Journal of Public Health, 82*(11), 1459–1461.

el-Mallakh, R. S. (1991). Mania in AIDS: Clinical significance and theoretical considerations. *International Journal of Psychiatry in Medicine, 21*(4), 383–391.

el-Mallakh, R. S. (1992). AIDS dementia-related psychosis: Is there a window of vulnerability? *AIDS Care, 4*(4), 381–387.

Ellis, D., Collis, I., & King, M. A. (1994). A controlled comparison of HIV and general medical referrals to a liaison psychiatry service. *AIDS Care, 6*(1), 69–76.

Ellis, D., Collis, I., & King, M. (1995). Personality disorder and sexual risk taking among homosexually active and heterosexually active men attending a genito-urinary medicine clinic. *Journal of Psychosomatic Research, 39*(7), 901–910.

Ellis, R. J., Deutsch, R., Heaton, R. K., Marcotte, T. D., McCutchan, J. A., Nelson, J. A., Abramson, I., Thal, L. J., Atkinson, J. H., Wallace, M. R., & Grant, I. (1997). Neurocognitive impairment is an independent risk factor for death in HIV. *Archives of Neurology, 54*(4), 416–424.

Ellis, R. J., Hsia, K., Spector, S. A., Nelson, J. A., Heaton, R. K., Wallace, M. R., Abramson, I., Atkinson, J. H., Grant, I., McCutchan, J. A., & the HNRC Group (in press). Cerebrospinal fluid human immunodeficiency virus type 1 RNA levels are elevated in neurocognitively impaired individuals with acquired immunodeficiency syndrome. *Annals of Neurology.*

Epstein, L. J., Strollo, P. J., Jr., Donegan, R. B., Delmar, J., Hendrix, C., & Westbrook, P. R. (1995). Obstructive sleep apnea in patients with human immunodeficiency virus (HIV) disease. *Sleep, 18*(5), 368–376.

Ericksen, K. P., & Trocki, K. F. (1992). Behavioral risk factors for sexually transmitted diseases in American households. *Social Science and Medicine, 34*(8), 843–853.

Evans, D. L., Leserman, J., Perkins, D. O., Stern, R. A., Murphy, C., Tamul, K., Liao, D., van der Horst, C. M., Hall, C. D., Folds, J. D., et al. (1995). Stress-associated reductions of cytotoxic T lymphocytes and natural killer cells in asymptomatic HIV infection. *American Journal of Psychiatry, 152*(4), 543–550.

Everall, I. P., Luthert, P. J., & Lantos, P. L. (1991). Neuronal loss in the frontal cortex in HIV infection. *Lancet, 337*(8750), 1119–1121.

Fauci, A. S. (1993). Multifactorial nature of human immunodeficiency virus disease: Implications for therapy. *Science, 262*(5136), 1011–1018.

Ferini-Strambi, L., Oldani, A., Tirloni, G., Zucconi, M., Castagna, A., Lazzarin, A., & Smirne, S. (1995). Slow wave sleep and cyclic alternating pattern (CAP) in HIV-infected asymptomatic men. *Sleep, 18*(6), 446–450.

Fernández, F. (1989). Anxiety and the neuropsychiatry of AIDS. *Journal of Clinical Psychiatry, 50*(Suppl.), 9–14.

Fernández, F., & Levy, J. K. (1993). The use of molindone in the treatment of psychotic and delirious patients infected with the human immunodeficiency virus. Case reports. *General Hospital Psychiatry, 15*(1), 31–35.

Fernández, F., & Levy, J. K. (1994). Psychopharmacology in HIV spectrum disorders. *Psychiatric Clinics of North America, 17*(1), 135–148.

Fernández, F., Levy, J. K., & Mansell, P. W. (1989). Management of delirium in terminally ill AIDS patients. *International Journal of Psychiatry in Medicine, 19*(2), 165–172.

Ferrando, S. J., Goldman, J. D., & Charness, W. E. (1997). Selective serotonin reuptake inhibitor treatment of depression in symptomatic HIV infection and AIDS. Improvements in affective and somatic symptoms. *General Hospital Psychiatry, 19*(2), 89–97.

Finn, P. (1994). Addressing the needs of cultural minorities in drug treatment. *Journal of Substance Abuse Treatment, 11*(4), 325–337.

Folkman, S., Chesney, M., Collette, L., Boccellari, A., & Cooke, M. (1996). Postbereavement depressive mood and its prebevereavement predictors in HIV+ and HIV- men. *Journal of Personality and Social Psychology, 70*(2), 336–348.

Forstein, M. (1994). Suicidality in HIV in gay men. In S. A. Cadwell, R. A. Burnham, & M. Forstein (Eds.), *Therapists on the front line: Psychotherapy with gay men in the age of AIDS* (pp. 111–146). Washington, DC: American Psychiatric Press.

Fox, L., Alford, M., Achim, C., Mallory, M., & Masliah, E. (1997). Neurodegeneration of somatostatin-immunoreactive neurons in HIV encephalitis. *Journal of Neuropathology and Experimental Neurology, 56*(4), 360–368.

Freedman, J. B., O'Dowd, M. A., Wyszynski, B., Torres, J. R., & McKegney, F. P. (1994). Depression, HIV dementia, delirium, posttraumatic stress disorder (or all of the above) [Clinical conference]. *General Hospital Psychiatry, 16*(6), 426–434.

Friedman, R. C., & Downey, J. I. (1994). Homosexuality. *New England Journal of Medicine, 331*(14), 923–930.

Fukunishi, I., Hayashi, M., Matsumoto, T., Negishi, M., Hosaka, T., & Moriya, H. (1997). Liaison psychiatry and HIV infection (I): Avoidance coping responses associated with depressive symptoms accompanying somatic complaints. *Psychiatry and Clinical Neurosciences, 51*(1), 1–4.

Gala, C., Pergami, A., Catalan, J., Durbano, F., Musicco, M., Riccio, M., Baldewag, T., & Invernizzi, G. (1993). The psychosocial impact of HIV infection in gay men, drug users, and heterosexuals: Controlled investigation. *British Journal of Psychiatry, 163*, 651–659.

Gala, C., Pergami, A., Catalan, J., Riccio, M., Durbano, F., Musicco, M., Baldewag, T., & Invernizzi, G. (1992). Risk of deliberate self-harm and factors associated with suicidal behavior among asymptomatic individuals with human immunodeficiency virus infection. *Acta Psychiatrica Scandinavica, 86*(1), 70–75.

Gelbard, H. A., Dzenko, K. A., DiLoreto, D., del Cerro, C., del Cerro, M., & Epstein, L. G. (1993). Neurotoxic effects of tumor necrosis factor alpha in primary human neuronal cultures are mediated by activation of the glutamate AMPA receptor subtype: Implications for AIDS neuropathogenesis. *Developmental Neuroscience, 15*(6), 417–422.

Gendelman, H. E., Lipton, S. A., Tardieu, M., Bukrinsky, M. I., & Nottet, H. S. (1994). The neuropathogenesis of HIV-1 infection. *Journal of Leukocyte Biology, 56*(3), 389–398.

Genis, P., Jett, M., Bernton, E. W., Boyle, T., Gelbard, H. A., Dzenko, K., Keane,

R. W., Resnick, L., Mizrachi, Y., Volsky, D. J., et al. (1992). Cytokines and arachidonic metabolites produced during human immunodeficiency virus (HIV)-infected macrophage–astroglia interactions: Implications for the neuropathogenesis of HIV disease. *Journal of Experimental Medicine, 176*(6), 1703–1718.

Giulian, D., Vaca, K., & Noonan, C. A. (1990). Secretion of neurotoxins by mononuclear phagocytes infected with HIV-1. *Science, 250*(4987), 1593–1596.

Goodkin, K., Feaster, D. J., Tuttle, R., Blaney, N. T., Kumar, M., Baum, M. K., Shapshak, P., & Fletcher, M. A. (1996). Bereavement is associated with time-dependent decrements in cellular immune function in asymptomatic human immunodeficiency virus type 1–seropostive homosexual men. *Clinical and Diagnositic Laboratory Immunology, 3*(1), 109–118.

Goudsmit, J., de Wolf, F., Paul, D. A., Epstein, L. G., Lange, J. M., Krone, W. J., Speelman, H., Wolters, E. C., Van der Noordaa, J., Oleske, J. M., et al. (1986). Expression of human immunodeficiency virus antigen (HIV-Ag) in serum and cerebrospinal fluid during acute and chronic infection. Lancet, *ii*(8500), 177–180.

Grant, I., & Atkinson, J. H. (1995). Psychobiology of HIV infection. In H. I. Kaplan & B. J. Sadock (Eds.), *Comprehensive textbook of psychiatry* (6th ed.). Baltimore: Williams & Wilkins.

Grant, I., & Martin, A. (1994). Introduction: Neurocognitive disorders associated with HIV-1 infection. In I. Grant & A. Martin (Eds.), *Neuropsychology of HIV infection* (pp 3–19). New York: Oxford University Press.

Grant, I., Atkinson, J. H., Hesselink, J. R., Kennedy, C. J., Richman, D. D., Spector, S. A., & McCutchan, J. A. (1987). Evidence for early central nervous system involvement in the acquired immunodeficiency syndrome (AIDS) and other human immunodeficiency virus (HIV) infections: Studies with neuropsychologic testing and magnetic resonance imaging. *Annals of Internal Medicine, 107*(6), 828–836. (Published erratum appears in same journal, 1988, *108*(3), 496.)

Grant, I., Heaton, R. K., Atkinson, J. H., & the HNRC Group. (1995). Neurocognitive disorder in HIV-1 infection. In M. B. A. Oldstone & L. Vitkovic (Eds.), *Current topics in microbiology and immunology: HIV and dementia.* Berlin: Springer-Verlag.

Grant, I., Heaton, R. K., Deutsch, R., McCutchan, J. A., Atkinson, J. H., & Chandler, J. (1994, August). *Risk of neuropsychological impairment steadily rises from date of seroconversion: HNRC experience.* Paper presented at the Tenth International Conference on AIDS, Yokohama, Japan.

Grassi, B., Gambini, O., Garghentini, G., Lazzarin, A., & Scarone, S. (1997). Efficacy of paroxetine for the treatment of depression in the context of HIV infection. *Pharmacopsychiatry, 30*(2), 70–71.

Gray, F., Belec, L., Keohane, C., De Truchis, P., Clair, B., Durigon, M., Sobel, A., & Gherardi, R. (1994). Zidovudine therapy and HIV encephalitis: A 10-year neuropathological survey. *AIDS, 8*(4), 489–493.

Gray, F., Lescs, M. C., Keohane, C., Paraire, F., Marc, B., Durigon, M., & Gherardi, R. (1994). Early brain changes in HIV infection: Neuropathological study of 11 HIV seropositive, non-AIDS cases. *Journal of Neuropathology and Experimental Neurology, 51*(2), 177–185.

Griffin, D. E., McArthur, J. C., & Cornblath, D. R. (1991). Neopterin and interferon-gamma in serum and cerebrospinal fluid of patients with HIV-associated neurologic disease. *Neurology, 41*(1), 69–74.

Gulevich, S. J., McCutchan, J. A., Thal, L. J., Kirson, D., Durand, D., Wallace, M., Mehta, P., Heyes, M. P., & Grant, I. (1993). Effect of antiretroviral therapy on the cerebrospinal fluid of patients seropositive for the human immunodeficiency virus. *Journal of Acquired Immune Deficiency Syndromes, 6*(9), 1002–1007. (Published erratum appears in same journal, 1994, 7(9), 994.)

Gutierrez, R., Atkinson, J. H., & Grant, I. (1993). Mild neurocognitive disorder: Needed addition to the nosology of cognitive impairment (organic mental) disorders. *Journal of Neuropsychiatry and Clinical Neurosciences, 5*(2), 161–177. (Published erratum appears in same journal, 1994, 6(1), 75–86.)

Hagan, T. A., Finnegan, L. P., & Nelson-Zlupko, L. (1994). Impediments to comprehensive treatment models for substance-dependent women: Treatment and research questions. *Journal of Psychoactive Drugs, 26*(2), 163–171.

Handelsman, L., Aronson, M., Maurer, G., Wiener, J., Jacobson, J., Bernstein, D., Ness, R., Herman, S., Losonczy, M., Song, I. S., et al. (1992). Neuropsychological and neurological manifestations of HIV-1 dementia in drug users. *Journal of Neuropsychiatry and Clinical Neurosciences, 4*(1), 21–28.

Harris, M. J., Jeste, D. V., Gleghorn, A., & Sewell, D. D. (1991). New-onset psychosis in HIV-infected patients. *Journal of Clinical Psychiatry, 52*(9), 369–376.

Heaton, R. K., Grant, I., Butters, N., White, D. A., Kirson, D., Atkinson, J. H., McCutchan, J. A., Taylor, M. J., Kelly, M. D., Ellis, R. J., Wolfson, T., Velin, R., Marcotte, T. D., Hesselink, J. R., Jerningan, T. L., Chandler, J., Wallace, M., Abramson, I., & the HNRC Group. (1995). The HNRC 500: Neuropsychology of HIV infection at different disease stages. *Journal of the International Neuropsychological Society, 1,* 231–251.

Heaton, R. K., Kirson, D., Velin, R. A., Grant, I., & the HNRC Group. (1994a). The utility of clinical ratings for detecting cognitive change in HIV infection. In I. Grant & A. Martin (Eds.), *Neuropsychology of HIV infection* (pp. 188–206). New York: Oxford University Press.

Heaton, R. K., Marcotte, T. D., Ellis, R. J., Deutsch, R., Abramson, I., Grant, I., & the HNRC Group (1996a). Neuropsychological profile and prognostic significance of minor motor cognitive/motor disorder. *Journal of Neurovirology, 2,* 39.

Heaton, R. K., Marcotte, T. D., White, D. A., Ross, D., Meredith, K., Taylor, M. J., Kaplan, R., & Grant, I. (1996b). Nature and vocational significance of neuropsychological impairment associated with HIV infection. *The Clinical Neuropsychologist, 10*(1), 1–14.

Heaton, R. K., Velin, R. A., Atkinson, J. H., Gulevich, S. J., McCutchan, J. A., Hesselink, J. R., Chandler, J. L., Grant, I., & the HNRC Group. (in press). Neuropsychological impairment in an HIV-positive male cohort. In M. Stein & A. Baum (Eds.), *Perspective in behavioral medicine.* Hillsdale, NJ: Erlbaum.

Heaton, R. K., Velin, R. A., McCutchan, J. A., Gulevich, S. J., Atkinson, J. H.,

Wallace, M. R., Godfrey, H. P., Kirson, D. A., & Grant, I. (1994b). Neuro-psychological impairment in human immunodeficiency virus-infection: Implications for employment. HNRC Group, HIV Neurobehavioral Research Center. *Psychosomatic Medicine, 56*(1), 8–17.

Hesselbrock M. N., & Hesselbrock V. M. (1992). Relationship of family history, antisocial personality disorder and personality traits in young men at risk for alcoholism. *Journal of Studies on Alcohol, 53*(6), 619–625.

Heyes, M. P., Brew, B. J., Saito, K., Quearry, B. J., Price, R. W., Lee, K., Bhalla, R. B., Der, M., & Markey, S. P. (1992). Inter-relationships between quinolinic acid, neuroactive kynurenines, neopterin and beta 2-microglobulin in cerebrospinal fluid and serum of HIV-1-infected patients. *Journal of Neuroimmunology, 40*(1), 71–80.

Higgitt, A., & Fonagy, P. (1992). Psychotherapy in borderline and narcissistic personality disorder. *British Journal of Psychiatry, 161*, 23–43.

Hinkin, C. H., van Gorp, W. G., Satz, P., Marcotte, T., Durvasula, R. S., Wood, S., Campbell, L., & Baluda, M. R. (1996). Actual versus self-reported cognitive dysfunction in HIV-1 infection: Memory-metamemory dissociations. *Journal of Clinical and Experimental Neuropsychology, 18*(3), 431–443.

Ho, D. D., Bredesen, D. E., Vinters, H. V., & Daar, E. S. (1989). The acquired immunodeficiency syndrome (AIDS) dementia complex [Clinical conference]. *Annals of Internal Medicine, 111*(5), 400–410.

Hodgson, R. (1994). Treatment of alcohol problems. *Addiction, 89*(11), 1529–1534.

Holmes, W. C. (1997). Association between a history of childhood sexual abuse and subsequent, adolescent psychoactive substance use disorder in a sample of HIV seropositive men. *Journal of Adolescent Health, 20*(6), 414–419.

Hriso, E., Kuhn, T., Masdeu, J. C., & Grundman, M. (1991). Extrapyramidal symptoms due to dopamine-blocking agents in patients with AIDS encephalopathy. *American Journal of Psychiatry, 148*(11), 1558–1561.

Iragui, V. J., Kalmijn, J., Plummer, D. J., Sample, P. A., Trick, G. L., & Freeman, W. R. (1996). Pattern electroretinograms and visual evoked potentials in HIV infection: Evidence of asymptomatic retinal and postretinal impairment in the absence of infectious retinopathy. *Neurology, 47*(6), 1452–1456.

Iragui, V. J., Kalmijn, J., Thal, L. J., & Grant, I. (1994). Neurological dysfunction in asymptomatic HIV-1 infected men: Evidence from evoked potentials. HNRC Group. *Electroencephalography and Clinical Neurophysiology, 92* (1), 1–10.

Irwin, M., Smith, T. L., & Gillin, J. C. (1992). Electroencephalographic sleep and natural killer activity in depressed patients and control subjects. *Psychosomatic Medicine, 54*(1), 10–21.

Jacobs, S. (1993). *Pathologic grief: Maladaptation to loss.* Washington, DC: American Psychiatric Press.

Jernigan, T. L., Archibald, S., Hesselink, J., Atkinson, J. H., Velin, R. A., McCutchan, J., Chandler, J. L., Grant, I., & the HNRC Group. (1993). Magnetic resonance imaging morphometric analysis of cerebral volume loss in human immunodeficiency virus infection. *Archives of Neurology, 50,* 250–255.

Johns, A. (1994). Opiate treatments. *Addiction, 89*(11), 1551–1558.

Johnson, J. G., Williams, J. B., Rabkin, J. G., Goetz, R. R., & Remien, R. H. (1995). Axis I psychiatric symptoms associated with HIV infection and personality disorder. *American Journal of Psychiatry, 152*(4), 551–554.

Johnson, R. T., Glass, J. D., McArthur, J. C., & Chesebro, B. W. (1996). Quantitation of human immunodeficiency virus in brains of demented and nondemented patients with acquired immunodeficiency syndrome. *Annals of Neurology, 39*(3), 392–395.

Kalichman, S. C., & Sikkema, K. J. (1994). Psychological sequelae of HIV infection and AIDS: Review of empirical findings. *Clinical Psychology Review, 14*(7), 611–632.

Kalichman, S. C., Johnson, J. R., Adair, V., Rompa, D., Multhauf, K., & Kelly, J. A. (1994a). Sexual sensation seeking: Scale development and predicting AIDS-risk behavior among homosexually active men. *Journal of Personality Assessment, 62*(3), 385–397.

Kalichman, S. C., Kelly, J. A., Johnson, J. R., & Bulto, M. (1994b). Factors associated with risk for HIV infection among chronic mentally ill adults. *American Journal of Psychiatry, 151*(2), 221–227.

Kaplan, H. I., & Sadock, B. J. (Eds.). (1995). *Comprehensive textbook of psychiatry* (6th ed.). Baltimore: Williams & Wilkins.

Karlsen, N. R., Froland, S. S., & Reinvang, I. (1994). HIV-related neuropsychological impairment and immunodeficiency. CD8+ lymphocytes and neopterin are related to HIV-encephalopathy. *Scandinavian Journal of Psychology, 35*(3), 230–239.

Karlsen, N. R., Reinvang, I., & Froland, S. S. (1995). A follow-up study of neuropsychological functioning in AIDS-patients: Prognostic significance and effect of zidovudine therapy. *Acta Neurologica Scandinavica, 91*(3), 215–221.

Kaslow, R. A., Carrington, M., Apple, R., Park, L., Munoz, A., Saah, A. J., Goedert, J. J., Winkler, C., O'Brien, S. J., Rinaldo, C., et al. (1996). Influence of combinations of human major histocompatibility complex genes on the course of HIV-1 infection. *Nature Medicine, 2*(4), 55–111.

Katz, M. H., Douglas, J. M., Bolan, G. A., Marx, R., Sweat, M., Park, M. S., & Buchbinder, S. P. (1996). Depression and use of mental health services among HIV-infected men. *Aids Care, 8*(4), 433–442.

Kelly, J. A., Murphy, D. A., Sikkema, K. J., Somlai, A. M., Mulry, G. W., Fernandez, M. I., Miller, J. G., & Stevenson, L. Y. (1995a). Predictors of high and low levels of HIV risk behavior among adults with chronic mental illness. *Psychiatric Services, 46*(8), 813–818.

Kelly, J. A., Sikkema, K. J., Winett, R. A., Solomon, L. J., Roffman, R. A., Heckman, T. G., Stevenson, L. Y., Perry, M. J., Norman, A. D., & Desiderato, L. J. (1995b). Factors predicting continued high-risk behavior among gay men in small cities: Psychological, behavioral, and demographic characteristics related to unsafe sex. *Journal of Consulting and Clinical Psychology, 63*(1), 101–107.

Kemeny, M. E. (1994). Psychoneuroimmunology of HIV infection. *Psychiatric Clinics of North America, 17*(1), 55–68.

Kemeny, M. E., Weiner, H., Duran, R., Taylor, S. E., Visscher, B., & Fahey, J. L. (1995). Immune system changes after the death of a partner in HIV-positive gay men. *Psychosomatic Medicine, 57*(6), 547–545.

Kemeny, M. E., Weiner, H., Taylor, S. E., Schneider, S., Visscher, B., & Fahey, J. L. (1994). Repeated bereavement, depressed mood, and immune parameters in HIV seropositive and seronegative gay men. *Health Psychology, 13*(1), 14–24.

Kent, T. A., Gelman, B. B., Casper, K., Langsjoen, H. A., Harvey, S. L., & Hillman, G. R. (1994). Neuroimaging in HIV infection: Neuropsychological and pathological correlation. In I. Grant & A. Martin (Eds.), *Neuropsychology of HIV infection* (pp. 260–275). New York: Oxford University Press.

Kessing, L., LaBianca, J. H., & Bolwig, T. G. (1994). HIV-induced stupor treated with ECT. *Convulsive Therapy, 10*(3), 232–235.

Kessler, R. C., McGonagle, K. A., Zhao, S., Nelson, C. B., Hughes, M., Eshleman, S., Wittchen, H. U., & Kendler, K. S. (1994). Lifetime and 12-month prevalence of DSM-III-R psychiatric disorders in the United States: Results from the National Comorbidity Survey. *Archives of General Psychiatry, 51*(1), 8–19.

Klatt, E. C., Nichols, L., & Noguchi, T. T. (1994). Evolving trends revealed by autopsies of patients with the acquired immunodeficiency syndrome: 565 autopsies in adults with the acquired immunodeficiency syndrome, Los Angeles, Calif., 1982–1993. *Archives of Pathology and Laboratory Medicine, 118*(9), 884–890. (Published erratum appears in same journal, 1994, *118*(12), 1200.)

Koenig, H. G., Meador, K. G., Shelp, F., Goli, V., Cohen, H. J., & Blazer, D. G. (1991). Major depressive disorder in hospitalized patients: An examination of young and elderly male veterans. *Journal of the American Geriatrics Society, 39*(9), 881–890.

Kreiss, J. K., & Hopkins, S. G. (1993). The association between circumcision status and human immunodeficiency virus infection among homosexual men. *Journal of Infectious Diseases, 168*(6), 1404–1408.

Krueger, J. M., Obal, F., Jr., Opp, M., Toth, L., Johannsen, L., & Cady, A. B. (1990). Somnogenic cytokines and models concerning their effects on sleep. *Yale Journal of Biology and Medicine, 63*(2), 157–172.

Lazarus, A. (1992). Neuroleptic malignant syndrome and preexisting brain damage. *Journal of Neuropsychiatry and Clinical Neurosciences, 4*(2), 185–187.

Leserman, J., Petitto, J. M., Perkins, D. O., Folds, J. D., Golden, R. N., & Evans, D. L. (1997). Severe stress, depressive symptoms, and changes in lymphocyte subsets in human immunodeficiency virus-infected men: A 2-year follow-up study. *Archives of General Psychiatry, 54*(3), 279–285.

Lewis, D. K., & Watters, J. K. (1994). Sexual behavior and sexual identity in male injection drug users. *Journal of Acquired Immune Deficiency Syndromes, 7,* 190–198.

Linn, J. G., Lewis, F. M., Cain, V. A., & Kimbrough, G. A. (1993). HIV-illness, social support, sense of coherence, and psychosocial well-being in a sample of help-seeking adults. *AIDS Education and Prevention, 5*(3), 254–262.

Lipsitz, J. D., Williams, J. B., Rabkin, J. G., Remien, R. H., Bradbury, M., el Sadr,

W., Goetz, R., Sorrell, S., & Gorman, J. M. (1994). Psychopathology in male and female intravenous drug users with and without HIV infection. *American Journal of Psychiatry, 151*(11), 1662–1668.

Lipton, S. A. (1997). Neuropathogenesis of acquired immunodeficiency syndrome dementia. *Current Opinion in Neurology, 10*(3), 247–253.

Lipton, S. A., Yeh, M., & Dreyer, E. B. (1994). Update on current models of HIV-related neuronal injury: Platelet-activating factor, arachidonic acid and nitric oxide. *Advances in Neuroimmunology, 4*(3), 181–188.

Liptzin, B., Levkoff, S. E., Gottlieb, G. L., & Johnson, J. C. (1993). Delirium. *Journal of Neuropsychiatry and Clinical Neurosciences, 5*(2), 154–160.

Livesley, W. J. (Ed.). (1995). *The DSM-IV personality disorders.* New York: Guilford Press.

Løberg, T. (1986). Neuropsychological findings in the early and middle phases of alcoholism. In I. Grant & K. M. Adams (Eds.), *Neuropsychological assessment of neuropsychiatric disorders* (pp. 415–440). New York: Oxford University Press.

Longman, A. J. (1995). Connecting and disconnecting: Bereavement experiences of six mothers whose sons died of AIDS. *Health Care for Women International, 16*(1), 85–95.

Lyketsos, C. G., Hanson, A., Fishman, M., McHugh, P. R., & Treisman, G. J. (1994). Screening for psychiatric morbidity in a medical outpatient clinic for HIV infection: The need for a psychiatric presence. *International Journal of Psychiatry in Medicine, 24*(2), 103–113.

Lyketsos, C. G., Hoover, D. R., Guccione, M., Dew, M. A., Wesch, M. A., Bing, E. G., & Treisman, G. J. (1996a). Changes in depressive symptoms as AIDS develops. The Multicenter AIDS Cohort Study. *American Journal of Psychiatry, 153*(11), 1430–1437.

Lyketsos, C. G., Hoover, D. R., Guccione, M., Dew, M. A., Wesch, J., Bing, E. G., & Treisman, G. J. (1996b). Depressive symptoms over the course of HIV infection before AIDS. *Social Psychiatry and Psychiatric Epidemiology, 31,* 212–219.

Lyketsos, C. G., Hoover, D. R., Guccione, M., Senterfitt, W., Dew, M. A., Wesch, J., VanRaden, M. J., Treisman, G. J., & Morgenstern, H. (1993). Depressive symptoms as predictors of medical outcomes in HIV infection: Multicenter AIDS Cohort Study. *Journal of the American Medical Association, 270*(21), 2563–2567.

Maj, M. (1990). Psychiatric aspects of HIV-1 infection and AIDS. *Psychological Medicine, 20*(3), 547–563.

Maj, M. (1996). Depressive syndromes and symptoms in subjects with human immunodeficiency virus (HIV) infection. *British Journal of Psychiatry*(Suppl. 30), 117–122.

Maj, M., Janssen, R., Satz, P., Zaudig, M., Starace, F., Boor, D., Sughondhabirom, B., Bing, E. G., Luabeya, M. K., Ndetei, D., et al. (1991). The World Health Organization's cross-cultural study on neuropsychiatric aspects of infection with the human immunodeficiency virus 1 (HIV-1): Preparation and pilot phase. *British Journal of Psychiatry, 159,* 351–356.

Maj, M., Janssen, R., Starace, F., Zaudig, M., Satz, P., Sughondhabirom, B.,

Luabeya, M. A., Riedel, R., Ndetei, D., Calil, H. M., et al. (1994a). WHO Neuropsychiatric AIDS Study, Cross-Sectional Phase I: Study design and psychiatric findings. *Archives of General Psychiatry, 51*(1), 39–49.

Maj, M., Satz, P., Janssen, R., Zaudig, M., Starace, F., D'Elia, L., Sughondhabirom, B., Mussa, M., Naber, D., Ndetei, D., et al. (1994b). WHO Neuropsychiatric AIDS Study, Cross-Sectional Phase II: Neuropsychological and neurological findings. *Archives of General Psychiatry, 51*(1), 51–61.

Malone, J. L., Oldfield, E. C., III, Wagner, K. F., Simms, T. E., Daly, R., O'Brian, J., & Burke, D. S. (1992). Abnormalities of morning serum cortisol levels and circadian rhythms of CD4+ lymphocyte counts in human immunodeficiency virus type 1-infected adult patients [Letter]. *Journal of Infectious Diseases, 165*(1), 185–186.

Manly, J. J., Miller, S. W., Heaton, R. K., Byrd, D., Reilly, J., Velasquez, R. J., Saccuzzo, D. P., Grant, I., & the HNRC Group. (in press). The effect of African American acculturation on neuropsychological test performance in normal and HIV positive individuals. *Journal of the International Neuropsychological Society.*

Manly, J. J., Patterson, T. L., Heaton, R. K., Semple, S. J., White, D. A., Velin, R. A., Atkinson, J. H., McCutchan, J. A., Chandler, J. L., Grant, I., & the HNRC Group. (1997). The relationship between neuropsychological functioning and coping activity among HIV-positive men. *AIDS and Behavior, 1*(2), 81–91.

Mapou, R. L., Law, W. A., Martin, A., Kampen, D., Salazar, A. M., & Rundell, J. R. (1993). Neuropsychological performance, mood, and complaints of cognitive and motor difficulties in individuals infected with the human immunodeficiency virus. *Journal of Neuropsychiatry and Clinical Neurosciences, 5*(1), 86–93.

Markowitz, J. C., Klerman, G. L., Clougherty, K. F., Spielman, L. A., Jacobsberg, L. B., Fishman, B., Frances, A. J., Kocsis, J. H., & Perry, S. W. (1995). Individual psychotherapies for depressed HIV-positive patients. *American Journal of Psychiatry, 152*(10), 1504–1509.

Markowitz, J. C., Rabkin, J. G., & Perry, S. W. (1994). Treating depression in HIV-positive patients [Editorial]. *AIDS, 8*(4), 403–412.

Marra, C. M., Longstreth, W. T., Handsfield, H. H., Townes, B. D., Coombs, R. W., Murphy, V. L., Collier, A. C., Maxwell, C. L., Claypoole, K. H., Maravilla, K. R., Sloan, R., Cohen, W. A., & Ross, S. B. (1996). Neurologic manifestations of HIV infection without AIDS: Follow-up of a cohort of homosexual and bisexual men. *Journal of Neuro-AIDS 1*(2), 41–65.

Martin, A. (1994a). Clinically significant cognitive dysfunction in medically asymptomatic human immunodeficiency virus-infected (HIV+) individuals? [Editorial, comment]. *Psychosomatic Medicine, 56*(1), 18–19.

Martin, A. (1994b). HIV, cognition, and the basal ganglia. In I. Grant & A. Martin (Eds.), *Neuropsychology of HIV infection* (pp. 234–259). New York: Oxford University Press.

Martin, D. J. (1993). Coping with AIDS and AIDS-risk reduction efforts among gay men. *AIDS Education and Prevention, 5*(2), 104–120.

Martin, E. M., Robertson, L. C., Edelstein, H. E., Jagust, W. J., Sorensen, D. J.,

San Giovanni, D., & Chirurgi, V. A. (1992). Performance of patients with early HIV-1 infection on the Stroop task. *Journal of Clinical and Experimental Neuropsychology, 14*(5), 857–868.

Martin, J. L., & Dean, L. (1993). Effects of AIDS-related bereavement and HIV-related illness on psychological distress among gay men: A 7-year longitudinal study, 1985–1991. *Journal of Consulting and Clinical Psychology, 61*(1), 94–103.

Martini, E., Muller, J. Y., Gastal, C., Doinel, C., Meyohas, M. C., Roquin, H., Frottier, J., & Salmon, C. (1988). [Early anomalies of CD4 and CD20 lymphocyte cycles in human immunodeficiency virus]. *Presse Medicale, 17*(41), 2167–2168, 2171–2172.

Masliah, E., Ge, N., & Mucke, L. (in press). Pathogenesis of HIV-1 associated neurodegeneration. *Critical Reviews in Neurobiology.*

Masliah, E., Ge, N., Achim, C. L., Hansen, L. A., & Wiley, C. A. (1992a). Selective neuronal vulnerability in HIV encephalitis. *Journal of Neuropathology and Experimental Neurology, 51*(6), 585–593.

Masliah, E., Ge, N., Achim, C. L., & Wiley, C. A. (1994). Cytokine receptor alterations during HIV infection in the human central nervous system. *Brain Research, 663*(1), 1–6.

Masliah, E., Ge, N., Achim, C. L., & Wiley, C. A. (1995). Differential vulnerability of calbindin-immunoreactive neurons in HIV encephalitis. *Journal of Neuropathology and Experimental Neurology, 54*(3), 350–357.

Masliah, E., Ge, N., Morey, M., DeTeresa, R., Terry, R. D., & Wiley, C. A. (1992b). Cortical dendritic pathology in human immunodeficiency virus encephalitis. *Laboratory Investigation, 66*(3), 285–291.

Masliah, E., Ge, N., & Mucke, L. (in press). Pathogenesis of HIV-1 associated neurodegeneration, *Critical Reviews in Neurobiology.*

Masliah, E., Heaton, R. K., Marcotte, T. D., Ellis, R. J., Wiley, C. A., Mallory, M., Achim, C. L., McCutchan, J. A., Nelson, J. A., Atkinson, J. H., Grant, I., & the HNRC Group (in press). Dendritic injury is a pathologic substrate for HIV-related cognitive disorders. *Annals of Neurology.*

Mayeux, R., Stern, Y., Tang, M. X., Todak, G., Marder, K., Sano, M., Richards, M., Stein, Z., Ehrhardt, A. A., & Gorman, J. M. (1993). Mortality risks in gay men with human immunodeficiency virus infection and cognitive impairment. *Neurology, 43*(1), 176–182.

Mayne, T. J., Vittinghoff, E., Chesney, M. A., Barret, D. C., & Coates, T. J. (1996). Depressive affect and survival among gay and bisexual men infected with HIV. *Archives of Internal Medicine, 156*(19), 2233–2238.

McAllister, R. H., Herns, M. V., Harrison, M. J., Newman, S. P., Connolly, S., Fowler, C. J., Fell, M., Durrance,, P., Manji, H., Kendall, B. E., et al. (1992). Neurological and neuropsychological performance in HIV seropositive men without symptoms. *Journal of Neurology, Neurosurgery and Psychiatry, 55*(2), 143–148.

McArthur, J. C., Cohen, B. A., Selnes, O. A., Kumar, A. J., Cooper, K., McArthur, J. H., Soucy, G., Cornblath, D. R., Chmiel, J. S., Wang, M. C., et al. (1989). Low prevalence of neurological and neuropsychological abnormalities in otherwise healthy HIV-1-infected individuals: Results from the Multicenter AIDS Cohort Study. *Annals of Neurology, 26*(5), 601–611.

McArthur, J. C., Hoover, D. R., Bacellar, H., Miller, E. N., Cohen, B. A., Becker, J. T., Graham, N. M., McArthur, J. H., Selnes, O. A., Jacobson, L. P., et al. (1993). Dementia in AIDS patients: Incidence and risk factors. Multicenter AIDS Cohort Study. *Neurology, 43*(11), 2245–2252.

McArthur, J. C., Selnes, O. A., Glass, J. D., Hoover, D. R., & Bacellar, H. (1994). HIV dementia: Incidence and risk factors. In R. W. Price & S. Perry III (Eds.), *Research publications of the Association for Research in Nervous and Mental Disease: Vol. 72. HIV, AIDS and the brain* (pp. 251–272). New York: Raven Press.

McCutchan, J. A. (1994). Virology, immunology, and clinical course of HIV infection. In I. Grant & A. Martin(Eds.), *Neuropsychology of HIV infection* (pp. 23–40). New York: Oxford University Press.

Mehta, P., Gulevich, S. J., Thal, L. J., Jin, H., Olichney, J. M., McCutchan, J. A., Heaton, R. K., Kirson, D., Kaplanski, G., Nelson, J., Atkinson, J. H., Wallace, M. R., Grant, I., & the HNRC Group (1996). Neurological symptoms, not signs, are common in early HIV infection. *Journal of Neuro-AIDS, 1*(2), 67–85.

Melton, S. T., Kirkwood, C. K., Ghaemi, S. N. (1997). Pharmacotherapy of HIV dementia. *The Annals of Pharmacotherapy 31*(4), 457–473.

Melton, S. T., Kirkwood, C. K., & Ghaemi, S. N. (1997). Pharmacotherapy of HIV dementia. *Annals of Pharmacotherapy, 31*(4), 457–473.

Michael, N. L., Louie, L. G., & Rohrbaugh, A. L. (1997). The role of CCR5 and CCR2 polymorphisms in HIV-1 transmission and disease progression. *Nature Medicine, 3* (10), 1160.

Miller, D., & Riccio, M. (1990). Non-organic psychiatric and psychosocial syndromes associated with HIV-1 infection and disease. *AIDS, 4*(5), 381–388.

Miller, E. N., Selnes, O. A., McArthur, J. C., Satz, P., Becker, J. T., Cohen, B. A., Sheridan, K., Machado, A. M., van Gorp, W. G., & Visscher, B. (1990). Neuropsychological performance in HIV-1-infected homosexual men: The Multicenter AIDS Cohort Study (MACS). *Neurology, 40*(2), 197–203.

Mirsky, A. F. (1988). Neuropsychological manifestations and predictors of HIV disease in vulnerable persons. In T. P. Bridge, A. F. Mirsky, & F. K. Goodwin (Eds.), *Advances in biochemical psychopharmacology: Vol. 44. Psychological, neuropsychiatric, and substance abuse aspects of AIDS* (pp. 1–13). New York: Raven Press.

Moeller, A. A., Wiegand, M., Oechsner, M., Krieg, J. C., Holsboer, F., & Emminger, C. (1992). Effects of zidovudine on EEG sleep in HIV-infected men [Letter]. *Journal of Acquired Immune Deficiency Syndromes, 5*(6), 636–637.

Moore, R. D., Hidalgo, J., Bareta, J. C., & Chaisson, R. E. (1994). Zidovudine therapy and health resource utilization in AIDS. *Journal of Acquired Immune Deficiency Syndromes, 7*(4), 349–354.

Mueller, A. J., Plummer, D. J., Dua, R., Taskintuna, I., Sample, P. A., Grant, I., & Freeman, W. R. (1997). Analysis of visual dysfunctions in HIV-positive patients without retinitis. *American Journal of Ophthalmology, 124*(2), 158–167.

Mulder, C. L., Emmelkamp, P. M., Antoni, M. H., Mulder, J. W., Sandfort, T. G.,

& de Vries, M. J. (1994). Cognitive-behavioral and experiential group psychotherapy for HIV-infected homosexual men: A comparative study. *Psychosomatic Medicine, 56*(5), 423–431.

Mundinger, A., Adam, T., Ott, D., Dinkel, E., Beck, A., Peter, H. H., Volk, B., & Schumacher, M. (1992). CT and MRI: Prognostic tools in patients with AIDS and neurological deficits. *Neuroradiology, 35*(1), 75–78.

Mussa, M., Naber, D., Ndetei, D., et al. (1994). WHO Neuropsychiatric AIDS Study, Cross-Sectional Phase II: Neuropsychological and neurological findings. *Archives of General Psychiatry, 51*(1), 51–61.

Nannis, E. D., Patterson, T. L., & Semple, S. J. (1997). Coping with HIV disease among seropositive women: Psychosocial correlates. *Women and Health, 25*(1), 1–22.

Nath, A., & Jankovic, J. (1989). Motor disorders in patients with human immunodeficiency virus infection. *Progress in AIDS Pathology, 1,* 159–166.

Nath, A., Jankovic, J., & Pettigrew, L. C. (1987). Movement disorders and AIDS. *Neurology, 37*(1), 37–41.

Nathanson, N., Cook, D. G., Kolson, D. L., & Gonzalez-Scarano, F. (1994). Pathogenesis of HIV encephalopathy. Annals of the New York Academy of *Sciences, 724,* 87–106.

Navia, B. A., & Price, R. W. (1987). The acquired immunodeficiency syndrome dementia complex as the presenting or sole manifestation of human immunodeficiency virus infection. *Archives of Neurology, 44*(1), 65–69.

Navia, B. A., Cho, E. S., Petito, C. K., & Price, R. W. (1986a). The AIDS dementia complex: II. Neuropathology. *Annals of Neurology, 19*(6), 525–535.

Navia, B. A., Jordan, B. D., & Price, R. W. (1986b). The AIDS dementia complex: I. Clinical features. *Annals of Neurology, 19*(6), 517–524.

Neugebauer, R., Rabkin, J. G., Williams, J. B., Remien, R. H., Goetz, R., & Gorman, J. M. (1992). Bereavement reactions among homosexual men experiencing multiple losses in the AIDS epidemic. *American Journal of Psychiatry, 149*(10), 1374–1379.

Norman, S. E., Chediak, A. D., Freeman, C., Kiel, M., Mendez, A., Duncan, R., Simoneau, J., & Nolan, B. (1992). Sleep disturbances in men with asymptomatic human immunodeficiency (HIV) infection. *Sleep, 15*(2), 150–155.

Norman, S. E., Chediak, A. D., Kiel, M., & Cohn, M. A. (1990). Sleep disturbances in HIV-infected homosexual men. *AIDS, 4*(8), 775–781.

O'Brien, C. P. (1994). Overview: The treatment of drug dependence. *Addiction, 89*(11), 1565–1569.

O'Dowd, M. A., Biderman, D. J., & McKegney, F. P. (1993). Incidence of suicidality in AIDS and HIV-positive patients attending a psychiatric outpatient program. *Psychosomatics, 34*(1), 33–40.

O'Dowd, M. A., Natali, C., Orr, D., & McKegney, F. P. (1991). Characteristics of patients attending an HIV-related psychiatric clinic. *Hospital and Community Psychiatry, 42*(6), 615–619.

Oldham, J. M., Skodol, A. E., Kellman, H. D., Hyler, S. E., Doidge, N., Rosnick, L., & Gallaher, P. E. (1995). Comorbidity of Axis I and Axis II disorders. *American Journal of Psychiatry, 152*(4), 571–8.

Opp, M. R., Rady, P. L., Hughes, T. K., Cadet, P., Tyring, S. K., & Smith, E. M.

(1996). Human immunodeficiency virus envelop glycoprotein 120 alters sleep and induces cytokin mRNA expression in rats. *American Journal of Physiology, 270* (5 Pt. 2), R963–970.

Ostrow, D. G. (1994). Substance abuse and HIV infection. *Psychiatric Clinics of North America, 17*(1), 69–89.

Otten, M. W., Jr., Zaidi, A. A., Peterman, T. A., Rolfs, R. T., & Witte, J. J. (1994). High rate of HIV seroconversion among patients attending urban sexually transmitted disease clinics. *AIDS, 8*(4), 549–553.

Patterson, T. L., Semple, S. J., Temshok, L. R., Atkinson, J. H., McCutchan, J. A., Straits-Tröster, K. A., Chandler, J. L., Grant, I., & the HNRC Group. (1993). Depressive symptoms among HIV-positive men: Life stress, coping, and social support. *Journal of Applied Biobehavioral Research, 7,* 64–87.

Patterson, T. L., Semple, S. J., Temshok, L. R., Atkinson, J. H., McCutchan, J. A., Straits-Tröster, K. A., Chandler, J. L., Grant, I., & the HNRC Group. (1995). Stress and depressive symptoms prospectively predict immune change among HIV-seropositive men. *Psychiatry: Interpersonal and Biological Processes, 58,* 315–328.

Patterson, T. L., Shaw, W. S., Semple, S. J., Cherner, M. McCutchan, J. A., Atkinson, J. H., Grant, I., Nannis, E., & the HNRC Group. (1996). Relationship of psychosocial factors to HIV disease progression. *Annals of Behavioral Medicine 18*(1), 30–39.

Paxton, W. A., Martin, S. R., Tse, D., O'Brien, T. R., Skurnick, J., VanDevanter, N. L., Padian, N., Braun, J. F., Kotler, D. P., Wolinsky, S. M., et al. (1996). Relative resistance to HIV-1 infection of CD4 lymphocytes from persons who remain uninfected despite multiple high-risk sexual exposure. *Nature Medicine, 2*(4), 412–417.

Peavy, G., Jacobs, D., Salmon, D. P., Butters, N., Delis, D. C., Taylor, M., Massman, P., Stout, J. C., Heindel, W. C., Kirson, D., et al. (1994). Verbal memory performance of patients with human immunodeficiency virus infection: Evidence of subcortical dysfunction. The HNRC Group. *Journal of Clinical and Experimental Neuropsychology, 16*(4), 508–523.

Pergami, A., Gala, C., Burgess, A., Invernizzi, G., & Catalan, J. (1994). Heterosexuals and HIV disease: A controlled investigation into the psychosocial factors associated with psychiatric morbidity. *Journal of Psychosomatic Research, 38*(4), 305–313.

Perkins, D. O., Davidson, E. J., Leserman, J., Liao, D., & Evans, D. L. (1993a). Personality disorder in patients infected with HIV: A controlled study with implications for clinical care. *American Journal of Psychiatry, 150*(2), 309–315.

Perkins, D. O., Leserman, J., Murphy, C., & Evans, D. L. (1993b). Psychosocial predictors of high-risk sexual behavior among HIV-negative homosexual men. *AIDS Education and Prevention, 5*(2), 141–152.

Perkins, D. O., Leserman, J., Stern, R. A., Baum, S. F., Liao, D., Golden, R. N., & Evans, D. L. (1995). Somatic symptoms and HIV infection: Relationship to depressive symptoms and indicators of HIV disease. *American Journal of Psychiatry, 152*(12), 1776–1781.

Perretta, P., Nisita, C., Zaccagnini, E., Scasso, A., Nuccorini, A., Santa, M. D., & Cassano, G. B. (1992). Diagnosis and clinical use of bromperidol in HIV-related psychoses in a sample of seropositive patients with brain damage. *International Clinical Psychopharmacology, 7*(2), 95–99.

Perry, S. W. (1990). Organic mental disorders caused by HIV: Update on early diagnosis and treatment. *American Journal of Psychiatry, 147*(6), 696–710.

Perry, S., Jacobsberg, L. B., Fishman, B., Frances, A., Bobo, J., & Jacobsberg, B. K. (1990b). Psychiatric diagnosis before serological testing for the human immunodeficiency virus. *American Journal of Psychiatry, 147*(1), 89–93.

Perry, S., Jacobsberg, L., & Fishman, B. (1990b). Suicidal ideation and HIV testing. *Journal of the American Medical Association, 263*(5), 679–682.

Persidsky, Y., & Gendelman, H. E. (1997). Development of laboratory and animal model systems for HIV-1 encephalitis and its associated dementia. *Journal of Leukocyte Biology, 1997, 62*(1): 100–106.

Peterson, J. L., Folkman, S., & Bakeman, R. (1996). Stress, coping, HIV status, psychosocial resources, and depressive mood in African American gay, bisexual, and heterosexual men. *American Journal of Community Psychology, 24*(4), 461–487.

Petito, C. K. (1988). Review of central nervous system pathology in human immunodeficiency virus infection. *Annals of Neurology, 23*(Suppl.), S54–S57.

Peyser, C. E., & Folstein, S. E. (1990). Huntington's disease as a model for mood disorders. *Molecular and Chemical Neuropathology, 12,* 99–119.

Philips, T. R., Prospero-Garcia, O., Puaoi, D. L., Lerner, D. L., Fox, H. S., Olmsted, R. A., Bloom, F. E., Henriksen, S. J., & Elder, J. H. (1994). Neurological abnormalities associated with feline immunodeficiency virus infection. *Journal of General Virology, 75*(Pt. 5), 979–987.

Piot, P., & Islam, M. Q. (1994). Sexually transmitted diseases in the 1990s: Global epidemiology and challenges for control. *Sexually Transmitted Diseases, 21*(2, Suppl.), S7–S13.

Plummer, D. J., Sample, P. A., Arevalo, J. F., Grant, I., Quiceno, J. I., Dua, R., & Freeman, W. R. (1996). Visual field loss in HIV-positive patients without infectious retinopathy. *American Journal of Ophthalmology, 122*(4), 542–549.

Pollmacher, T., Mullington, J., Korth, C., & Hinze-Selch, D. (1995). Influence of host defense activation on sleep in humans. *Advances in Neuroimmunology, 5*(2), 155–169.

Portegies, P. (1995). Review of antiretroviral therapy in the prevention of HIV-related AIDS dementia complex (ADC). *Drugs, 49*(Suppl. 1), 25–31; discussion, 38–40.

Portegies, P., Enting, R. H., de Gans, J., Algra, P. R., Derix, M. M., Lange, J. M., & Goudsmit, J. (1993). Presentation and course of AIDS dementia complex: 10 years of follow-up in Amsterdam, The Netherlands. *AIDS, 7*(5), 669–675.

Portegies, P., Epstein, L. G., Hung, S. T., de Gans, J., & Goudsmit, J. (1989). Human immunodeficiency virus type 1 antigen in cerebrospinal fluid: Correlation with clinical neurologic status. *Archives of Neurology, 46*(3), 261–264. (Published erratum appears in same journal, 1989, *46*(11), 1174.)

Power, C., Selnes, O. A., Grim, J. A., & McArthur, J. C. (1995). HIV Dementia Scale: A rapid screening test. *Journal of Acquired Immune Deficiency Syndromes and Human Retrovirology, 8*(3), 273–278.

Presberg, B. A., & Kibel, H. D. (1994). Confronting death: Group psychotherapy with terminally ill individuals. *Group, 18*(1), 19–28.

Price, R. W., & Brew, B. J. (1988). The AIDS dementia complex. *Journal of Infectious Diseases, 158*(5), 1079–1083.

Prier, R. E., McNeil, J. G., & Burge, J. R. (1991). Inpatient psychiatric morbidity of HIV-infected soldiers. *Hospital and Community Psychiatry, 42*(6), 619–623.

Prospero-Garcia, O., Herold, N., Phillips, T. R., Elder, J. H., Bloom, F. E., & Henricksen, S. J. (1994). Sleep patterns are disturbed in cates infected with feline immunodeficiency virus. *Proceedings of the National Academy of Sciences USA, 91*(26), 12947–12951.

Pugh, K., O'Donell, I., & Catalan, J. (1993). Suicide and HIV disease. *AIDS Care, 5*(4), 391–400.

Pulliam, L., Gascon, R., Stubblebine, M., McGuire, D., & McGrath, M. S. (1997). Unique moncyte subset in patients with AIDS dementia. *Lancet, 349,* 692–695.

Quiceno, J. I., Capparelli, E., Sadun, A. A., Munguia, D., Grant, I., Listhaus, A., Crapotta, J., Lambert, B., & Freeman, W. R. (1992). Visual dysfunction without retinitis in patients with acquired immunodeficiency syndrome. *American Journal of Ophthalmology, 113*(1), 8–13.

Rabkin, J. G., Rabkin, R., Harrison, W., & Wagner, G. (1994a). Effect of imipramine on mood and enumerative measures of immune status in depressed patients with HIV illness. *American Journal of Psychiatry, 151*(4), 516–523.

Rabkin, J. G., Remien, R., Katoff, L., & Williams, J. B. (1993a). Suicidality in AIDS long-term survivors: What is the evidence? *AIDS Care, 5*(4), 401–411.

Rabkin, J. G., Remien, R., Katoff, L., & Williams, J. B. (1993b). Resilience in adversity among long-term survivors of AIDS. *Hospital and Community Psychiatry, 44*(2), 162–167. (Published erratum appears in same journal, 1993, *44*(4), 371.)

Rabkin, J. G., Wagner, G., & Rabkin, R. (1994b). Effects of sertraline on mood and immune status in patients with major depression and HIV illness: An open trial. *Journal of Clinical Psychiatry, 55*(10), 433–439.

Reed, T. E. (1985). Ethnic differences in alcohol use, abuse, and sensitivity: A review with genetic interpretation. *Social Biology, 32*(3–4), 195–209.

Regier, D. A., Boyd, J. H., Burke, J. D., Jr., Rae, D. S., Myers, J. K., Kramer, M., Robins, L. N., George, L. K., Karno, M., & Locke, B. Z. (1988). One-month prevalence of mental disorders in the United States. Based on five Epidemiologic Catchment Area sites. *Archives of General Psychiatry, 45*(11), 977–986.

Remien, R. H., Goetz, R., Rabkin, J. G., Williams, J. B., Bradbury, M., Ehrhardt, A. A., & Gorman, J. M. (1995). Remission of substance use disorders: Gay men in the first decade of AIDS. *Journal of Studies on Alcohol, 56*(2), 226–232.

Resnick, L., Berger, J. R., Shapshak, P., & Tourtellotte, W. W. (1988). Early penetration of the blood–brain barrier by HIV. *Neurology, 38*(1), 9–14.

Reyes, E., Mohar, A., Mallory, M., Miller, A., & Masliah, E. (1994). Hippocampal involvement associated with human immunodeficiency virus encephalitis in Mexico. *Archives of Pathology and Laboratory Medicine, 118*(11), 1130–1134.

Riccio, M., Pugh, K., Jadresic, D., Burgess, A., Thompson, C., Wilson, B., Lovett, E., Baldeweg, T., Hawkins, D. A., & Catalan, J. (1993). Neuropsychiatric aspects of HIV-1 infection in gay men: Controlled investigation of psychiatric, neuropsychological and neurological status. *Journal of Psychosomatic Research, 37*(8), 819–830.

Richman, D. D., Fischl, M. A., Grieco, M. H., Gottlieb, M. S., Volberding, P. A., Laskin, O. L., Leedom, J. M., Groopman, J. E., Mildvan, D., Hirsch, M. S., et al. (1987). The toxicity of azidothymidine (AZT) in the treatment of patients with AIDS and AIDS-related complex: A double-blind, placebo-controlled trial. *New England Journal of Medicine, 317*(4), 192–197.

Risman, B., & Schwartz, P. (1988). Sociological research on male and female homosexuality. *Annual Review of Sociology, 14,* 125–147.

Robins, L. N., & Regier, D. A. (Eds.). (1991). *Psychiatric disorders in America.* New York: Free Press.

Rosenberger, P. H., Bornstein, R. A., Nasrallah, H. A., Para, M. F., Whitaker, C. C., Fass, R. J., & Rice, R. R., Jr. (1993). Psychopathology in human immunodeficiency virus infection: Lifetime and current assessment. *Comprehensive Psychiatry, 34*(3), 150–158.

Rotheram-Borus, M. J., Rosario, M., Reid, H., & Koopman, C. (1995). Predicting patterns of sexual acts among homosexual and bisexual youths. *American Journal of Psychiatry, 152*(4), 588–595.

Sacks, M., Dermatis, H., Looser-Ott, S., Burton, W., & Perry, S. (1992). Undetected HIV infection among acutely ill psychiatric inpatients. *American Journal of Psychiatry, 149*(4), 544–545.

Sacks, M. H., Perry, S., Graver, R., Shindledecker, R., & Hall, S. (1990). Self-reported HIV-related risk behaviors in acute psychiatric inpatients: A pilot study. *Hospital and Community Psychiatry, 41*(11), 1253–1255.

Sacktor, N., & McArthur, J. (1997). Prospects for therapy of HIV-associated neurologic diseases. *Journal of Neurovirology 3,* 89–101.

Sacktor, N. C., Bacellar, H, Hoover, D. R., Nance-Sproson, T. E., Selnes, O. A., Miller, E. N., Dal Pan, G. J., Kleeberger, C., Brown, A., Saah A., et al. (1996). Psychomotor slowing in HIV infection: A predictor of dementia, AIDS, and death. *Journal of Neurovirology, 2*(6), 404–410.

Sahs, J. A., Goetz, R., Reddy, M., Rabkin, J. G., Williams, J. B., Kertzner, R., & Gorman, J. M. (1994). Psychological distress and natural killer cells in gay men with and without HIV infection. *American Journal of Psychiatry, 151*(10), 1479–1484.

Saito, Y., Sharer, L. R., Epstein, L. G., Michaels, J., Mintz, M., Louder, M., Golding, K., Cvetkovich, T. A., & Blumberg, B. M. (1994). Overexpression of *nef* as a marker for restricted HIV-1 infection of astrocytes in postmortem pediatric central nervous tissues. *Neurology, 44*(3, Pt. 1), 474–481.

Sardar, A. M., Bell, J. E., & Reynolds, G. P. (1995). Increased concentrations of the neurotoxin 3-hydroxykynurenine in the frontal cortex of HIV-1-positive patients. *Journal of Neurochemistry, 64*(2), 932–935.

Satz, P., Morgenstern, H., Miller, E. N., Selnes, O. A., McArthur, J. C., Cohen, B. A., Wesch, J., Becker, J. T., Jacobson, L., D'Elia, L. F., et al. (1993). Low education as a possible risk factor for cognitive abnormalities in HIV-1:

Findings from the Multicenter AIDS Cohort Study (MACS). *Journal of Acquired Immune Deficiency Syndromes, 6*(5), 503–511.

Satz, P., Ostrow, D. G., Bing, E. G., Harker, J., Maj, M., Myers, H., Evans, G., & Fawzy, F. I. (1994). Depression and HIV-1: A review. In *Psychopharmacology in the HIV-spectrum.* New York: Plenum Press.

Schmidt, U., & Miller, D. (1988). Two cases of hypomania in AIDS. *British Journal of Psychiatry, 152,* 839–842.

Schmitt, F. A., Bigley, J. W., McKinnis, R., Logue, P. E., Evans, R. W., & Drucker, J. L. (1988). Neuropsychological outcome of zidovudine (AZT) treatment of patients with AIDS and AIDS-related complex. *New England Journal of Medicine, 319*(24), 1573–1578.

Schrier, R. D., Freeman, W. R., Wiley, C. A., & McCutchan, J. A. (1995). Immune predispositions for cytomegalovirus retinitis in AIDS: The HNRC Group. *Journal of Clinical Investigation, 95*(4), 1741–1746.

Schrier, R. D., Wiley, C. A., Spina, C., McCutchan, J. A., Grant, I., & the HNRC Group. (1996). Pathogenic and protective correlates of T cell proliferation in AIDS. *Journal of Clinical Investigation, 98*(3), 731–740.

Schuckit, M. A. (1994). The treatment of stimulant dependence. *Addiction, 89*(11), 1559–1563.

Schwartzberg, S. S. (1992). AIDS-related bereavement among gay men: The inadequacy of current theories of grief. *Psychotherapy, 29*(3), 422–429.

Schwartzberg, S. S. (1994). Vitality and growth in HIV-infected gay men. *Social Science and Medicine, 38*(4), 593–602.

Sciolla, A. (1995). Sleep disturbance and HIV disease. *Focus: A Guide to AIDS Research and Counseling, 10*(11), 1–4.

Sciolla, A., Brown, S. J., Atkinson, J. H., Summers, J., & Grant, I. (1997, May). *Pilot trial of light treatment for HIV-associated sleep disturbance.* Paper presented at the 150th Annual Meeting of the American Psychiatric Association, San Diego, CA.

Sciolla, A., & Jeste, D. V. (1997). *Use of antipsychotics in the elderly.* Manuscript in preparation.

Sciolla, A., Kripke, D. F., Brown, S. J., Atkinson, J. H., Whitehall, W. W., & Grant, I. (1993, May). *Sleep and light exposure in HIV infected men.* Paper presented at the 146th Annual Meeting of the American Psychiatric Association, San Francisco.

Scott-Algara, D., Vuillier, F., Marasescu, M., de Saint Martin, J., & Dighiero, G. (1991). Serum levels of IL-2, IL-1α, TNF-α, and soluble receptor of IL-2 in HIV-1-infected patients. *AIDS Research and Human Retroviruses, 7*(4), 381–386.

Searight, H. R. (1992). Borderline personality disorder: Diagnosis and management in primary care. *Journal of Family Practice, 34*(5), 605–612.

Seilhean, D., Duyckaerts, C., Vazeux, R., Bolgert, F., Brunet, P., Katlama, C., Gentilini, M., & Hauw, J. J. (1993). HIV-1-associated cognitive/motor complex: Absence of neuronal loss in the cerebral neocortex. *Neurology, 43*(8), 1492–1499.

Selnes, O. A., & Miller, E. N. (1994). Development of a screening battery for HIV-related cognitive impairment: The MACS experience. In I. Grant & A.

Martin (Eds.), *Neuropsychology of HIV infection* (pp.176–187). New York: Oxford University Press.

Selnes, O. A., Galai, N., Bacellar, H., Miller, E. N., Becker, J. T., Wesch, J., van Gorp, W., & McArthur, J. C. (1995). Cognitive performance after progression to AIDS: A longitudinal study from the Multicenter AIDS Cohort Study. *Neurology, 45*(2), 267–275.

Selnes, O. A., Miller, E., McArthur, J., Gordon, B., Munoz, A., Sheridan, K., Fox, R., & Saah, A. J. (1990). HIV-1 infection: No evidence of cognitive decline during the asymptomatic stages. The Multicenter AIDS Cohort Study. *Neurology, 40*(2), 204–208.

Semple, S. J., Patterson, T. L., Straits-Tröster, K., Atkinson, J. H., McCutchan, J. A., Grant, I., & the HNRC Group. (1996). Social and psychological characteristics of HIV-infected women and gay men. *Women and Health 24*(2), 17–41.

Semple, S. J., Patterson, T. L., Temoshok, L. R., McCutchan, J. A., Straits-Tröster, K. A., Chandler, J. L., & Grant, I. (1993). Identification of psychobiological stressors among HIV-positive women: HIV Neurobehavioral Research Center (HNRC) Group. *Women and Health, 20*(4), 15–36.

Sewell, D. D., Jeste, D. V., Atkinson, J. H., Heaton, R. K., Hesselink, J. R., Wiley, C., Thal, L., Chandler, J .L., & Grant, I. (1994a). HIV-associated psychosis: A study of 20 cases. San Diego HIV Neurobehavioral Research Center Group. *American Journal of Psychiatry, 151*(2), 237–242.

Sewell, D. D., Jeste, D. V., McAdams, L. A., Bailey, A., Harris, M. J., Atkinson, J. H., Chandler, J. L., McCutchan, J. A., & Grant, I. (1994b). Neuroleptic treatment of HIV-associated psychosis: HNRC Group. *Neuropsychopharmacology, 10*(4), 223–229.

Shedlack, K. J., Soldato-Couture, C., & Swanson, C. L., Jr. (1994). Rapidly progressive tardive dyskinesia in AIDS [Letter]. *Biological Psychiatry, 35*(2), 147–148.

Shelby, R. D. (1994). Mourning within a culture of mourning. In S. A. Cadwell, R. A. Burnham, & M. Forstein (Eds.), *Therapists on the front line: Psychotherapy with gay men in the age of AIDS* (pp. 53–80). Washington, DC: American Psychiatric Press.

Sherr, L., Hedge, B., Steinhart, K., Davey, T., & Petrack, J. (1992). Unique patterns of bereavement in HIV: Implications for counselling. *Genitourinary Medicine, 68*(6), 378–381.

Siegel, K., & Gorey, E. (1994). Childhood bereavement due to parental death from acquired immunodeficiency syndrome. *Journal of Developmental and Behavioral Pediatrics, 15*(3), S66–S70.

Silberstein, C., Galanter, M., Marmor, M., Lifshutz, H., Krasinski, K., & Franco, H. (1994). HIV-1 among inner city dually diagnosed inpatients. *American Journal of Drug and Alcohol Abuse, 20*(1), 101–113.

Silk, K. R., Lee, S., Hill, E. M., & Lohr, N. E. (1995). Borderline personality disorder symptoms and severity of sexual abuse. *American Journal of Psychiatry, 152*(7), 1059–1064.

Silverstone, P. H. (1996). Prevalence of psychiatric disorders in medical inpatients. *Journal of Nervous and Mental Disease, 184*(1), 43–51.

Snider, W. D., Simpson, D. M., Nielsen, S., Gold, J. W., Metroka, C. E., & Posner, J. B. (1983). Neurological complications of acquired immune deficiency syndrome: Analysis of 50 patients. *Annals of Neurology, 14*(4), 403–418.

Snyder, S., Reyner, A., Schmeidler, J., Bogursky, E., Gomez, H., & Strain, J. J. (1992). Prevalence of mental disorders in newly admitted medical inpatients with AIDS. *Psychosomatics, 33*(2), 166–170.

Sobo, E. J. (1993). Inner-city women and AIDS: The psycho-social benefits of unsafe sex. *Culture, Medicine and Psychiatry, 17*(4), 455–485.

Spector, S. A., Hsia, K., Pratt, D., Lathey, J., McCutchan, J. A., Alcaraz, J. E., Atkinson, J. H., Gulevich, S., Wallace, M., & Grant, I. (1993). Virologic markers of human immunodeficiency virus type 1 in cerebrospinal fluid: The HIV Neurobehavioral Research Center Group. *Journal of Infectious Diseases, 168*(1), 68–74.

Stanley, L. C., Mrak, R. E., Woody, R. C., Perrot, L. J., Zhang, S., Marshak, D. R., Nelson, S. J., & Griffin, W. S. (1994). Glial cytokines as neuropathogenic factors in HIV infection: Pathogenic similarities to Alzheimer's disease. *Journal of Neuropathology and Experimental Neurology, 53*(3), 231–238.

Stern, Y., Liu, X., Marder, K., Todak, G., Sano, M., Ehrhardt, A., & Gorman, J. (1995). Neuropsychological changes in a prospectively followed cohort of homosexual and bisexual men with and without HIV infection. *Neurology, 45*(3, Pt. 1), 467–472.

Stern, Y., Marder, K., Bell, K., Chen, J., Dooneief, G., Goldstein, S., Mindry, D., Richards, M., Sano, M., Williams, J., et al. (1991). Multidisciplinary baseline assessment of homosexual men with and without human immunodeficiency virus infection: III. Neurologic and neuropsychological findings. *Archives of General Psychiatry, 48*(2), 131–138.

Stewart, D. L., Zuckerman, C. J., & Ingle, J. M. (1994). HIV seroprevalence in a chronically mentally ill population. *Journal of the National Medical Association, 86*(7), 519–523.

Stout, J. C., Ellis, R. J., Jernigan, T. L., Archibald, S. L., Abramson, I., Wolfson, T., McCutchan, J. A., Wallace, M. R., Atkinson, J. H., & Grant, I. (in press). Progressive cerebral volume loss in human immunodeficiency virus infection: A longitudinal volumetric MRI study. *Journal of the International Neuropsychological Society.*

Straits-Tröster, K. A., Patterson, T. L., Semple, S. J., Temoshok, L., Roth, P. G., McCutchan, J. A., Chandler, J. L., Grant, I., & the HNRC Group. (1994). The relationship between loneliness, interpersonal competence, and immunologic status in HIV-infected men. *Psychology and Health, 9*, 205–219.

Summers, J., Patterson, T. L., Whitehall, W., Atkinson, J. H., Sciolla, A., Zisook, S., Brown, S. J., Chandler, J. L., Grant, I., & the HNRC Group. (1992, July). *Grief resolution prediction in bereaved men at high risk for human immunodeficiency virus.* Paper presented at the Eighth International Conference on AIDS, Amsterdam.

Summers, J., Robinson, R., Sewell, D., Zisook, S., Atkinson, J. H., Whitehall, W., Chandler, J. L., Grant, I., & the HNRC Group. (1993, June). *The efficacy of short-term group therapy in men with unresolved grief at high risk for HIV.* Paper presented at the Ninth International Conference on AIDS, Berlin.

Summers, J., Zisook, S., Atkinson, J. H., Sciolla, A., Brown, S., Heaton, R., Grant, I., & the HNRC Group. (1995a, October). *Psychiatric and neuropsychological characteristics of AIDS-related elective death.* Paper presented at the conference on Psychopathology, Psychopharmacology, Substance Abuse, and Culture, Los Angeles.

Summers, J., Zisook, S., Atkinson, J. H., Sciolla, A., Whitehall, W., Brown, S., Patterson, T., & Grant, I. (1995b). Psychiatric morbidity associated with acquired immune deficiency syndrome-related grief resolution. *Journal of Nervous and Mental Disease, 183*(6), 384–389.

Susser, E., Miller, M., Valencia, E., Colson, P., Roche, B., & Conover, S. (1996). Injection drug use and risk of HIV transmission among homeless men with mental illness. *American Journal of Psychiatry, 153*(6), 794–798.

Susser, E., Valencia, E., Miller, M., Tsai, W. Y., Meyer-Bahlburg, H., & Conover, S. (1995). Sexual behavior of homeless mentally ill men at risk for HIV. *American Journal of Psychiatry, 152*(4), 583–587.

Swaab, D. F., Fliers, E., & Partiman, T. S. (1985). The suprachiasmatic nucleus of the human brain in relation to sex, age and senile dementia. *Brain Research, 342*(1), 37–44.

Swenson, J. R., Erman, M., Labelle, J., & Dimsdale, J. E. (1989). Extrapyramidal reactions. Neuropsychiatric mimics in patients with AIDS. *General Hospital Psychiatry, 11*(4), 248–253.

Swoyer, J., Rhame, F., Hrushesky, W., Sackett-Lundeen, L., Sothern, R., Gale, H., & Haus, E. (1990). Circadian rhythm alteration in HIV infected subjects. *Progress in Clinical and Biological Research, 341A,* 437–449.

Syndulko, K., Singer, E. J., Nogales-Gaete, J., Conrad, A., Schmid, P., & Tourtellotte, W. W. (1994). Laboratory evaluations in HIV-1-associated cognitive/motor complex. *Psychiatric Clinics of North America, 17*(1), 91–123.

Tozzi, V., Narciso, P., Galgani, S., Sette, P., Balestra, P., Gerace, C., Pau, F. M., Pigorini, F., Volpini, V., Camporiondo, M. P., et al. (1993). Effects of zidovudine in 30 patients with mild to end-stage AIDS dementia complex. *AIDS, 7*(5), 683–692.

Treisman, G. J., Lyketsos, C. G., Fishman, M., Hanson, A. L., Rosenblatt, A., & McHugh, P. R. (1993). Psychiatric care for patients with HIV infection: The varying perspectives. *Psychosomatics, 34*(5), 432–439.

Tunnell, G. (1994). Special issues in group psychotherapy for gay men with AIDS. In S. A. Cadwell, R. A. Burnham, & M. Forstein *Therapists on the front line: Psychotherapy with gay men in the age of AIDS* (pp. 237–254). Washington, DC: American Psychiatric Press.

Vagnucci, A. H., & Winkelstein, A. (1993). Circadian rhythm of lymphocytes and their glucocorticoid receptors in HIV-infected homosexual men. *Journal of Acquired Immune Deficiency Syndromes, 6*(11), 1238–1247.

van Gorp, W. G., Miller, E. N., Marcotte, T. D., Dixon, W., Paz, D., Selnes, O., Wesch, J., Becker, J. T., Hinkin, C. H., Mitrushina, M., et al. (1994). The relationship between age and cognitive impairment in HIV-1 infection: Findings from the Multicenter AIDS Cohort Study and a clinical cohort. *Neurology, 44*(5), 929–935.

Vazeux, R. (1991). AIDS encephalopathy and tropism of HIV for brain mono-cytes/macrophages and microglial cells. *Pathobiology, 59*(4), 214–218.

Verhey, F. R., Jolles, J., Ponds, R. W., Rozendaal, N., Plugge, L. A., de Vet, R. C., Vreeling, F. W., & van der Lugt, P. J. (1993). Diagnosing dementia: A comparison between a monodisciplinary and a multidisciplinary approach. *Journal of Neuropsychiatry and Clinical Neurosciences, 5*(1), 78–85.

Villette, J. M., Bourin, P., Doinel, C., Mansour, I., Fiet, J., Boudou, P., Dreux, C., Roue, R., Debord, M., & Levi, F. (1990). Circadian variations in plasma levels of hypophyseal, adrenocortical and testicular hormones in men infected with human immunodeficiency virus. *Journal of Clinical Endocrinology and Metabolism, 70*(3), 572–577.

Vitkovic, L., Stover, E., & Koslow, S. H. (1995). Animal models recapitulate aspects of HIV/CNS disease. *AIDS Research and Human Retroviruses, 11*(6), 753–759.

Weinrich, J. D., Atkinson, J. H., Jr., McCutchan, J. A., & Grant, I. (1995). Is gender dysphoria dysphoric?: Elevated depression and anxiety in gender dysphoric and nondysphoric homosexual and bisexual men in an HIV sample. HNRC Group. *Archives of Sexual Behavior, 24*(1), 55–72.

Weinrich, J. D., Grant, I., Jacobson, D. L., Robinson, S. R., & McCutchan, J. A. (1992). Effects of recalled childhood gender nonconformity on adult geni-toerotic role and AIDS exposure: HNRC Group. *Archives of Sexual Behavior, 21*(6), 559–585.

Weinrich, J. D., Snyder, P. J., Pillard, R. C., Grant, I., Jacobson, D. L., Robinson, S. R., & McCutchan, J. A. (1993). A factor analysis of the Klein Sexual Orientation Grid in two disparate samples. *Archives of Sexual Behavior, 22*(2), 157–168.

White, D. A., Heaton, R. K., & Monsch, A. U. (1995). Neuropsychological studies of asymptomatic human immunodeficiency virus type-1 infected individu-als. *Journal of the International Neuropsychological Society, 1,* 304–315.

White, J. L., Darko, D. F., Brown, S. J., Miller, J. C., Hayduk, R., Kelly, T., & Mitler, M. M. (1995). Early central nervous system response to HIV infection: Sleep distortion and cognitive–motor decrements. *AIDS, 9*(9), 1043–1050.

Whitfield, J. B., & Martin, N. G. (1985). Individual differences in plasma ALT, AST and GGT: Contributions of genetic and environmental factors, includ-ing alcohol consumption. *Enzyme, 33*(2), 61–69.

Wiener, P. K., Schwartz, M. A., & O'Connell, R. A. (1994). Characteristics of HIV-infected patients in an inpatient psychiatric setting. *Psychosomatics, 35*(1), 59–65.

Wiley, C. A. (1994). Pathology of neurologic disease in AIDS. *Psychiatric Clinics of North America, 17*(1), 1–15.

Wiley, C. A., & Achim, C. (1994). Human immunodeficiency virus encephalitis is the pathological correlate of dementia in acquired immunodeficiency syndrome. *Annals of Neurology, 36*(4), 673–676. (Published erratum appears in same journal, 1995, *37*(1), 140.)

Wiley, C. A., Achim, C. L., Schrier, R. D., Heyes, M. P., McCutchan, J. A., & Grant, I. (1992). Relationship of cerebrospinal fluid immune activation associated factors to HIV encephalitis. *AIDS, 6*(11), 1299–1307.

Wiley, C. A., Masliah, E., & Achim, C. L. (1994). Measurement of CNS HIV burden and its association with neurologic damage. *Advances in Neuroimmunology, 4*(3), 319–325.

Wiley, C. A., Schrier, R. D., Nelson, J. A., Lampert, P. W., & Oldstone, M. B. (1986). Cellular localization of human immunodeficiency virus infection within the brains of acquired immune deficiency syndrome patients. *Proceedings of the National Academy of Sciences USA, 83*(18), 7089–7093.

Williams, J. B., Rabkin, J. G., Remien, R. H., Gorman, J. M., & Ehrhardt, A. A. (1991). Multidisciplinary baseline assessment of homosexual men with and without human immunodeficiency virus infection: II. Standardized clinical assessment of current and lifetime psychopathology. *Archives of General Psychiatry, 48*(2), 124–130.

Zegans, L. S., Gerhard, A. L., & Coates, T. J. (1994). Psychotherapies for the person with HIV disease. *Psychiatric Clinics of North America, 17*(1), 149–162.

Zierler, S., Feingold, L., Laufer, D., Velentgas, P., Kantrowitz-Gordon, I., & Mayer, K. (1991). Adult survivors of childhood sexual abuse and subsequent risk of HIV infection. *American Journal of Public Health, 81*(5), 572–575.

Zimmerman, M. (1994). Diagnosing personality disorders. A review of issues and research methods. *Archives of General Psychiatry, 51*(3), 225–245.

Zisook, S., Shuchter, S. R., & Summers, J. (1995). Bereavement, risk, and preventative intervention. In B. Rafael & B. D. Burrows (Eds.), *Handbook of preventative psychiatry* (pp. 203–222). Amsterdam: Elsevier.

Zorrilla, E. P., McKay, J. R., Luborsky L., & Schmidt, K. (1996). Relation of stressors and depressive symptoms to clinical progression of viral illness. *American Journal of Psychiatry, 153*(5), 626–635.

Zorrilla, E. P., McKay, J. R., Luborsky, L., & Schmidt, K. (1996). Relation of stressors and depressive symptoms to clinical progression of viral illness. *American Journal of Psychiatry, 153*(5), 626–635.

5

Pharmacological Interventions for Neuropsychiatric Symptoms of HIV Disease

MARY M. C. WETHERBY
JOSEPHA A. CHEONG
DWIGHT L. EVANS
FREDERICK A. SCHMITT

INTRODUCTION

Opportunistic infections of the central nervous system (CNS) in human immunodeficiency virus (HIV) infection can result in changes in brain function. However, cognitive deficits commonly present as primary complaints in HIV-seropositive patients, even without evidence of CNS opportunistic infections. It is therefore believed that cognitive impairment in HIV is directly associated with the effects of the retrovirus on the brain, rather than with the secondary complications of immunosuppression (Ho et al., 1985; Poser et al., 1988).

The neuropsychiatric manifestations of HIV infection include both cognitive and affective changes. The Centers for Disease Control 1987 criteria included the presence of cognitive impairment (dementia) in seropositive individuals as sufficient for the diagnosis of AIDS. Given the prevalence of CD4+ T-cell testing, the revised 1993 CDC criteria emphasize CD4+ T-lymphocyte count categories, as well as expanded clinical categories. HIV encephalopathy continues to be listed as one of the diseases indicative of AIDS.

Cognitive changes have been reported in seropositive but otherwise asymptomatic persons (see Chapter 1, this volume). Depressive symptoms, although warranting treatment, have not been found to confound neuropsychological testing results in HIV infection (Grant et al., 1993; Hinkin et al., 1992). As the course of HIV disease progresses, cognitive symptoms usually become more prevalent. Evidence of functional changes found with neuropsychological testing has not been reliably associated with structural brain imaging. Data suggest that memory dysfunction in HIV disease is associated with structural abnormalities in the fornix (Kieburtz et al., 1990), and that slowing of cognitive processing speed is related to atrophy documented by structural imaging (Levin et al., 1990); yet the lack of routinely documented structural imaging abnormalities in early HIV infection (Post et al., 1991) suggests that neurocognitive dysfunction may provide an early indicator of CNS involvement in HIV infection.

For example, studies including those of Saykin et al. (1988) found no statistically significant correlations between neuropsychological test data and magnetic resonance imaging (MRI) abnormalities in seropositive persons with lymphadenopathy. However, the persons studied by Saykin et al. (1988) showed neuropsychological impairments. One might therefore hypothesize that changes in neurocognitive function may provide an early indicator of CNS involvement in HIV infection. An earlier study by Grant et al. (1987), on the other hand, suggested better than chance agreement rates between MRI and neuropsychological test data. The authors suggested that the CNS impact of HIV disease may occur early in the course of the disease and cause mild cognitive deficits in otherwise asymptomatic persons. Furthermore, van Gorp et al. (1992), using positron emission tomography (PET), found significant correlations between cerebral metabolic activity in the basal ganglia, thalamus, and temporal lobe and severity of overall neurological abnormalities. Single-photon emission computerized tomography (SPECT) studies also suggest variations in cortical perfusion for HIV-1-infected mildly demented and cognitively normal subjects, compared with normal controls (Harris, Pearlson, McArthur, Zeger, & LaFrance, 1994). These data suggest the presence of cerebral blood flow and metabolic abnormalities in HIV-1-infected individuals with and without dementia.

Given the prevalence of neuropsychiatric disorders in HIV disease, this chapter is intended to review some of the antiretroviral and neuropsychiatric pharmacotherapies used in efforts to ameliorate symptoms of HIV-associated neuropsychiatric disease.

HIV-1-ASSOCIATED DEMENTIA COMPLEX AND MINOR COGNITIVE/MOTOR DISORDER

In 1991, a working group of the American Academy of Neurology (AAN, 1991) published a classification system for neurological manifestations of HIV Type 1. The AAN's schema of the CNS disorders related to HIV-1 infection includes HIV-1-associated dementia complex, characterized by cognitive and motor impairment, behavioral change, and impairment in activities of daily living detected by history, neurological, and neuropsychological procedures. However, neuropsychological functioning must be assessed during periods of lucidity (no delirium), and neuropsychiatric symptoms must not be attributable to causes other than HIV-1 infection. For those patients whose myelopathy is more severe than their cognitive impairment, the diagnosis of HIV-1-associated myelopathy may be assigned. This acquired myelopathy may include lower-extremity weakness, incoordination, urinary incontinence, paraparesis, lower-extremity spasticity, and other neurological signs.

The AAN's category of HIV-1-associated minor cognitive/motor disorder is reserved for patients with normal or close-to-normal functioning in activities of daily living (social and occupational functioning). These patients do not meet the criteria for HIV-1-associated dementia complex or HIV-1-associated myelopathy. Although the results of mental status examination, brain imaging, and neurological exams may be within the normal range, symptoms often include impaired attention or concentration, mental slowing, impaired memory, slowed movements, and/or incoordination.

The study of neurocognitive symptoms associated with HIV infection has resulted in a number of staging schemes such as the AAN's. Price and Brew (1988) provided an earlier conceptualization for staging severity of the AIDS dementia complex (ADC). Further discussion of the clinical criteria for dementia associated with HIV infection is beyond the scope of this chapter, however (for a review, see Becker, Martin, & Lopez, 1994).

COGNITION IN HIV-1 INFECTION

Several early studies of cognition in HIV-1 infection concentrated on the prevalence of neuropsychological abnormalities. The results of many of these studies questioned the relationship between HIV infection and cognitive abnormalities. An early review by Marotta and Perry (1989) addressed the question of early neuropsychological dysfunction caused by HIV. They concluded that the mixed results reported in previous studies were attributable to methodological problems and/or differences in the sensitivity of the neuropsychological measures that were employed (see also Bornstein, 1994; van Gorp, Lamb, & Schmitt, 1993b). Early reports from the Multicenter AIDS Cohort Study (MACS) did not indicate significant rates of early cerebral impairment in HIV-seropositive patients (McArthur et al., 1989b). The early MACS data suggested that the majority of asymptomatic, seropositive individuals had neither neurological nor neuropsychological deficits, and that confounding factors (e.g., substance use disorders, other preexisting conditions) should be considered when evaluating these individuals' mental abilities (Wilkins et al., 1990).

Later reports from the MACS effort found significant differences on memory, motor, and psychomotor tests between HIV-1-seronegative and symptomatic seropositive subjects. However, neuropsychological abnormalities in the asymptomatic seropositive subjects were not statistically different from those of the seronegative controls (Miller et al., 1990). Furthermore, a longitudinal MACS comparison of neuropsychological tests results obtained semiannually found no evidence of cognitive decline in asymptomatic seropositive subjects over a 1-year period (Selnes et al., 1990). Overall, the MACS data suggested that roughly 13% of asymptomatic seropositive and 28% of symptomatic seropositive subjects showed cognitive deficits, in comparison to 14% of seronegative controls (Miller, Satz, & Visscher, 1991). Y. Stern (1991), however, has proposed one explanation for why the MACS data have not reflected higher rates of cognitive dysfunction in HIV-positive asymptomatic individuals: The use of a screening test battery (intended to detect the need for more extensive testing) may have limited the administration of potentially more sensitive measures. Moreover, 47% of those MACS subjects who were to receive further testing were not assessed, because either time/scheduling constraints or subject refusal.

Early cognitive symptoms in HIV-1 infection have been reported in many studies using tests of processing speed and memory (Law et al., 1994; Martin et al., 1992; Martin, Heyes, Salazar, Law, & Williams, 1993; Rubinow, Berrettini, Brouwers, & Lane, 1988; Wilkie, Eisdorfer, Morgan, Loewenstein, & Szapocznik, 1990). Saykin et al. (1988) and Y. Stern et al. (1991) have posited that neuropsychological and neurological changes are the first detectable signs of HIV-1 infection in the CNS. Cognitive symptoms appear to progress in parallel with the immunological and systemic effects of HIV (e.g., Bornstein et al., 1991), and poorer neuropsychological test performance is associated with a significantly increased risk of mortality (Mayeux et al., 1993). These data therefore suggest a definable syndrome related to cognition in HIV-positive asymptomatic individuals, and an evolving impact of HIV on the brain.

In a recent study, Stern, Silva, Chaisson, and Evans (1996) evaluated the relationship between cognitive reserve and early indicators of cognitive deficits in HIV-1-seropositive subjects. Education, occupation, and premorbid intelligence were used to derive scores of cognitive reserve. Greater deficits were exhibited by the lower cognitive reserve group on neuropsychological measures of attention, information processing speed, verbal learning and verbal memory, and executive and visuospatial functioning. The authors concluded that those with greater cognitive reserve may be less sensitive to the initial CNS effects of HIV, while those with less cognitive reserve may present with neuropsychological impairment earlier.

HIV'S IMPACT ON THE BRAIN

Even though the prevalence of CNS impairment appears to be variable in the early stages of HIV disease, the likelihood of significant cognitive and motor dysfunction increases as HIV disease progresses (van Gorp et al., 1993a). For example, a case study of a man with early HIV dementia (McArthur et al., 1989a) revealed neuropsychological deficits without excessive depressive symptoms. Autopsy findings included astrocytosis of white matter, mild pallor of myelin staining in the absence of inflammation, multinucleated giant cells, and brain atrophy. Several other studies have suggested that basal ganglia atrophy, especially of the caudate nucleus, best correlates with AIDS dementia (Petito, 1993; Wiley et al., 1991). A recent article by the HIV Neurobehavioral Research Center (HNRC) Group (Heaton et al., 1995) found a pattern of cognitive impairment in 389 nondemented HIV-infected males that was most consistent with early involvement of subcortical or frontostriatal systems. Consistent with earlier reports from the HNRC (Jernigan et al., 1993), impairment in HIV-infected subjects was related to measures of brain atrophy on MRI. Increased rates of neuropsychological impairment were found in each successive stage of HIV-1 infection (Heaton et al., 1995).

Cognitive symptomatology often exists in the absence of major systemic opportunistic infections or neoplasms. In an early report, Navia and Price (1987) presented data on 29 patients who developed ADC in the absence of a diagnosis of full-blown AIDS. Six patients were asymptomatic, and the remainder exhibited only mild symptoms of ADC. Most of these patients survived for only a short time (5–16 months) or died without exhibiting systemic manifestations of AIDS. Autopsy of selected subjects revealed white matter and subcortical gray matter changes, with relative preservation of cortical gray matter. However, it is important to note that although neuropsychological deficits have been demonstrated in individuals with HIV infection, there is no justification for discrimination in the workplace (Sidtis & Price, 1990). Clearly, neuropsychological deficits are not precursors or results of every case of HIV-1 infection.

The observation that the frequency of neuropathological changes in HIV disease is not necessarily correlated with clinically observed symptoms has been explained in part by the concept of "cognitive reserve" (Satz, 1993), as well as by methodological concerns (Bornstein, 1994; van Gorp et al., 1993b). It has been suggested (Satz, 1993; Satz, Morgenstern, & Miller, 1993) that cognitive reserve (i.e., the amount of brain reserve a person has available for cognition, as a result of education, occupation, or other factors) influences the vulnerability of the CNS to the early effects of HIV infection, as well as other neurological and dementing disorders (Katzman et al., 1988). Therefore, if cognitive or cerebral reserve actually reflects observable differences in brain structure and function, persons with lower reserve (educational or occupational levels would serve as surrogate markers for this) might be at a greater risk of cognitive impairment in HIV disease if other potentially confounding variables are controlled. This would suggest that measures of cognitive reserve, as partially indexed by education and occupation, could account for a larger proportion of the variance in predicting which individuals could develop cognitive dysfunction and dementia for a wide range of neurological diseases (Y. Stern et al., 1994).

Chronological age has also been examined as a possible risk factor for cognitive impairment in HIV infection. Van Gorp et al. (1994) investigated this problem in relation to the cognitive reserve concept, the basic premise of which in this instance is that younger individuals are less susceptible to dementia than older individuals because of a greater brain reserve. When expected cognitive changes associated with normal aging were considered, however, there was no relationship among age, HIV infection, and neuropsychological impairment.

ETIOLOGY OF NEUROPSYCHOLOGICAL CHANGES IN HIV-1 INFECTION

One of the leading hypotheses to explain brain dysfunction in HIV-infected individuals is microphage or microglial neurotoxicity (Lipton,

1991). Also, HIV or its components can directly affect neurons or astrocytes, eventually leading to the loss of neurons and brain atrophy (Petito, 1993). Berger and Levy (1991) suggested several potential mechanisms of HIV neuropathogenesis, including (1) neurotropism of the virus—namely, a propensity to infect glial cells and perhaps even neurons; (2) direct cell toxicity due to viral proteins of HIV; (3) elaboration of toxic cellular products, such as cytokines, as a consequence of infection; (4) induction of an autoimmune response; (5) infectious cofactors; (6) metabolic and nutritional abnormalities; and (7) an alteration of the blood–brain barrier.

As mentioned previously, evidence suggests that the caudate nucleus and basal ganglia are primary areas of HIV pathogenesis (Aylward et al., 1995; Martin et al., 1993; Rottenberg et al., 1987; van Gorp et al., 1992). In addition to neuroimaging and neurochemical procedures, this line of investigation has used neuropsychological tests that are sensitive to basal ganglia dysfunction. One of these procedures, for example, evaluates motor skill learning through the use of a pursuit-rotor task (Martin et al., 1993). Performance on the pursuit-rotor task is not associated with markers of immune system status, but is linked to cerebrospinal fluid (CSF) levels of the neurotoxin quinolinic acid (Heyes et al., 1991, 1992). Cognitive impairment and symptoms of dementia are also associated with increased p24 antigen levels (viral load) in CSF and blood (Royal, Selnes, Concha, Nance-Sproson, & McArthur, 1994). These results (Martin et al., 1992, 1993; Royal et al., 1994) suggest one important structural region and neurotoxic mechanism, in addition to viral proteins (Berger & Levy, 1991), for the pathogenesis of HIV-related neuronal dysfunction.

Additional clues for the etiology and course of HIV-1 infection can be found in persons who have survived HIV infection for more than 10 years without developing AIDS. Cao, Quin, Zhoang, Safrit, and Ho (1995) and Pantaleo et al. (1995) agree that there are low viral titers in individuals who remain asymptomatic despite HIV infection. Their asymptomatic status appears to be characterized by a combination of strong, virus-specific immune responses and some degree of attenuation of HIV-1 (Cao et al., 1995), with intact lymph node architecture and immune function (Pantaleo et al., 1995).

DESIGN OF THERAPEUTIC STRATEGIES

One manifestation of AIDS in the brain is neuronal loss. Cortical neuron and retinal ganglion cell neuron loss ranging from 18% to 50% has been demonstrated in selected CNS autopsies in AIDS patients

(Everall, Luthbert, & Lantos, 1991; Ketzler, Weis, & Haug, 1990; Tenhula et al., 1992; Wiley et al., 1991). Given this dramatic change in brain structure secondary to the impact of HIV infection, therapies that can reverse or arrest CNS effects of HIV processes are important. In a review of therapeutic strategies to prevent neuronal injury, Lipton (1994) suggested a final common neural pathway related to neurological and neuropsychological dysfunction in HIV involving overstimulation of N-methyl-D-aspartate receptors. Excitatory amino acids such as glutamate and quinolinate are involved in the excessive stimulation of neurons, resulting in neuronal injury or death. Lipton (1994) has suggested that although various cell interactions are likely to lead to neuronal loss in AIDS, this final common pathway is amenable to pharmacotherapy.

In another review, Coffin (1995) has discussed the pathogenesis of HIV, which he feels should be considered in the design of therapeutic strategies. Believing that the latent phase of HIV-1 is actually a period of viral activity, Coffin has proposed a steady-state model in which the high turnover rate of cells characterizes HIV. This steady state eventually results in an accumulation of viral mutations that are resistant to antiretroviral drugs. Coffin (1995) has concluded that the dynamics of this process should be considered by investigators developing pharmacotherapies for HIV.

Results of a study by Larder, Kemp, and Harrigan (1995) demonstrated that *in vitro* mutational data involving suppression of viral resistance may aid in the selection of efficacious drug combinations. One cause of the limited duration of benefit during treatment of HIV-1 infection with single antiretroviral drugs is the likely emergence of drug-resistant strains. These authors found that mutants resistant to zidovudine (ZDV) became phenotypically sensitive *in vitro* through mutation of residue 184 of viral reverse transcriptase to valine. This process induced resistance to 2′-deoxy-3′-thiacytidine (3TC), without coresistance. Although valine-184 mutants rapidly emerged with the combination therapy, the majority of samples assessed from subjects receiving the combination therapy (ZDV plus 3TC) remained ZDV-sensitive at 24 weeks of therapy. The authors claim that the ZDV-3TC combination is the most effective pairing of drugs to date with regard to the magnitude and duration of changes in CD4 counts and viral load.

Mizrachi et al. (1995) explored improved therapy for AIDS dementia through enhanced delivery of effective antiretroviral agents to the CNS, using an animal model. Redox trappings of drugs in the brain were made possible by a novel ZDV chemical delivery system. The authors concluded that this system is capable of achieving improved retroviral activity through the delivery of higher ZDV doses to lympho-cytes and neural cells. Also using an animal model, Limoges, Persidsky, Bock, and Gendelman (1997) evaluated the potential efficacy of anti-inflammatory therapy for HIV dementia. Dexamethasone was adminis-tered to HIV-1 encephalitic mice. Results suggested astrogliosis and increased apoptosis of neurons, indicative of a worsening of neuropa-thology after treatment. Mechanisms for the effects appeared to be increased viability of HIV-infected macrophages and an incomplete suppression of neurotoxic inflammatory secretions suggesting that glucocorticosteroids may not be indicated for the treatment of HIV encephalitis.

ANTIRETROVIRAL PHARMACOLOGY FOR NEUROPSYCHIATRIC AND OTHER SYMPTOMS OF HIV DISEASE

Efficacy of Antiretroviral Agents in Adults

One current pharmacotherapy for the treatment of immunological and cognitive symptoms of HIV/AIDS, based on the evidence from many clinical trials, is ZDV. Toxic side effects of ZDV include nausea, headaches, myalgias, and anemia (Richman et al., 1987). Early studies of ZDV showed both neuropsychological and neurological benefits in HIV-positive adult patients. Schmitt et al. (1988) studied 281 patients with AIDS and advanced AIDS-related complex who were being treated with ZDV. Neuropsychological evaluation revealed gains in cognitive functioning, with the most marked improvement occurring in the AIDS patients, suggesting partial amelioration of neuropsychological dysfunc-tion with ZDV therapy. Yarchoan et al. (1988) had earlier reported that seven seropositive patients benefited from ZDV therapy in terms of neurological and neuropsychological functioning. Three of these pa-tients had dementia; two had peripheral neuropathy; one had dementia and peripheral neuropathy; and one had paraplegia. Three of the patients demonstrated sustained improvements 5–18 months after initial administration of the ZDV. Yarchoan et al. (1988) agreed that the results suggested that certain HIV-associated abnormalities may in part be reversible with the use of ZDV.

Later, Gorman et al. (1993) compared 25 HIV-positive men who were already taking ZDV to 25 seropositive men who claimed they were not taking the drug. ZDV was found to have a statistically significant effect only on clinical ratings of patient functioning. However, the authors noted that since none of the subjects had seriously impaired scores on initial neuropsychiatric measures, the study may have been limited in its ability to show improved scores with ZDV. Rather, they concluded that their findings may be more appropriately interpreted to suggest a lack of deterioration in cognitive functioning with ZDV therapy.

A multicenter study of patients with dementia symptoms (Sidtis et al., 1993) reemphasized previous findings of a therapeutic CNS benefit of ZDV. Forty subjects with mild to moderate ADC were placed on varying schedules of ZDV or placebo. Three treatment arms consisted of 400 mg of ZDV, 200 mg of ZDV, or a placebo, all given five times daily. After 16 weeks of treatment, subjects initially placed in the placebo group were randomly assigned to one of the two active treatment arms. Overall, neuropsychological functioning (average normalized scores for all of the neurocognitive tests) improved with active treatment. Patients receiving the higher dosage of ZDV (a total of 2000 mg daily) seemed to show more improvement.

Gray et al. (1994) examined the benefit of ZDV therapy for HIV encephalitis over a 10-year period. A total of 192 AIDS cases were examined neuropathologically; these included (1) patients who had never received ZDV, (2) patients who received treatment for over 3 months until death, and (3) patients whose treatment terminated more than 1 month before death. Results suggested that ZDV significantly reduced the occurrence of productive HIV encephalopathy, with discontinuation of the drug possibly favoring onset of brain infection. Substitution therapy with dideoxyinosine (ddI) also appeared to have a protective effect.

In a recent case study presentation, Akula, Rege, Dreisbach, Dejase, and Lertora (1997) suggested that valproic acid (an anticonvulsant) was involved in increasing CSF ZDV levels in a patient with AIDS. Increased CSF levels of ZDV, given the interaction with valproic acid, may contribute to higher ZDV levels in the brains of patients with HIV-related encephalopathy and therefore result in improved neurocognitive functioning.

Efficacy of Antiretroviral Agents in Children

HIV/AIDS in children may be manifested through cognitive and neurodevelopmental deficits, behavioral problems, physiological impairment, and other medical complications. Because of the developmental deficits observed in children with HIV infection, including delays in the development of language, neuropsychological evaluations of children with HIV/AIDS are often difficult (Brouwers, Moss, Wolters, & Schmitt, 1994). Nonetheless, the clinical efficacy of certain agents has been evaluated for changes in neuropsychiatric symptoms (Schmitt, Dixon, & Brouwers, 1994).

An early study at the National Cancer Institute (Pizzo et al., 1988) examined 21 children aged 14 months to 12 years who were given ZDV by continuous intravenous infusion. All patients were symptomatic; 13 of them exhibited neurodevelopmental abnormalities and had acquired HIV perinatally or through transfusions. Neuropsychological measures varied according to the patients' age or stage of development. The neuropsychological outcome data indicated that Verbal and Performance intelligence quotient (IQ) scores rose in the 13 patients with neurodevelopmental abnormalities and in 5 additional patients in whom encephalopathy had not previously been diagnosed. Ten of the 13 children with encephalopathy were further followed for 12 months (Brouwers et al., 1990). After 12 months of ZDV therapy, the previously acquired gains in IQ points were maintained. Gains in adaptive behavior were also noted after 6 months of therapy. The data also suggested that antiretroviral treatment of children may be more successful if begun during the asymptomatic stage of HIV.

A recent study by Nozyce et al. (1994) examined the effects of oral ZDV on 54 symptomatic African-American and Hispanic HIV-positive children aged 2 months to 12 years who had acquired HIV through vertical transmission. Neurodevelopmental functioning was evaluated with standard measures of adaptive behavior and intelligence, or with special tests designed for younger children whose impairments were too severe to be tested otherwise. No improvement in neurodevelopmental functioning was noted. The authors suggested that reasons for this finding, compared to other studies demonstrating positive effects of ZDV in children, might have included the use of subjects from varying ethnic, social, and economic strata and the difference in route of administration (steady-state levels of ZDV through continuous infusion vs. intermittent oral administration). Also, since neurodevelopmental status in this study remained stable, it was possible that oral ZDV had a positive effect in inhibiting further decline.

Wolters, Brouwers, Moss, and Pizzo (1994) examined seropositive asymptomatic and symptomatic European-American, African-American, and Hispanic children who were receiving continuous-infusion or intermittent oral ZDV. The children had been infected either through transfusion or vertically. Adaptive behavioral ratings and intelligence measures were obtained. Results indicated that children with or without encephalopathy showed similar improvement in all behavioral domains except for motor skills. Improvements in cognitive ability were accompanied by reductions in aberrant social-emotional behaviors.

Another antiretroviral agent, ddI, has also been used in the treatment of pediatric HIV infection. An early trial involved oral administration of ddI to 43 symptomatic HIV-positive children, 16 of whom had previously received ZDV (Butler et al., 1991). Because of disparities between the groups of children studied, analysis of neuropsychological functioning was conducted individually. An increase in IQ score was found for 2 of the 11 symptomatic patients and for 4 of 14 patients with baseline IQ scores within the normal range. No change occurred for the children with IQs above 110 at baseline. Changes in IQ scores were not found to be influenced by previous pharmacotherapy, method of acquisition of HIV, presence of encephalopathy, or changes in CD4 count or p24 antigen levels. Nor did there appear to be a correlation between ddI dose and cognitive gains. A positive correlation between the plasma concentration of orally administered ddI and increase in IQ score was reported for those children for whom data were available with normal IQ scores at baseline. The authors concluded that optimal results with ddI may be obtained through the use of close monitoring and adjustment in order to obtain ideal plasma concentration levels of this drug.

Pizzo et al. (1990) have examined a third antiretroviral agent, dideoxycytidine (ddC), to ascertain its effectiveness when used in conjunction with ZDV with the goal of suppressing ZDV's side effects (e.g., neuropathy and immunosuppression). Fifteen asymptomatic seropositive children aged 6 months to 13 years were orally administered either ddC alone or ddC with ZDV on an alternating schedule. IQ scores were generally found to decline from baseline levels during the administration of ddC alone, with restoration to baseline during the alternating regimen. Follow-up evaluations showed no significant change in overall score. All four children with initial evidence of encephalopathy improved behaviorally. On the alternating schedule, no neuropathy was observed. The authors concluded that in some children ddC appears to have antiretroviral effects and to be safe when administered for short intervals.

In summary, the data from studies of antiretroviral agents in HIV-infected adults and children suggest that improvement with these agents in the neuropsychiatric manifestations of HIV disease may be related to several factors. These factors seem to involve the route of administration and dose, which in turn affect the agents' penetration into the brain.

NONRETROVIRAL PHARMACOLOGY FOR NEUROPSYCHIATRIC SYMPTOMS IN HIV DISEASE

In addition to the cognitive dysfunction that accompanies the progression of HIV disease, behavioral and affective dysfunction in HIV disease has been widely documented (Evans & Perkins, 1990). These

HIV-associated symptoms may present as apathy and withdrawal, agitated psychosis, and personality change (Sidtis, 1994). Most of the major psychiatric disorders have been reported to occur in the HIV/AIDS patient population, including adjustment disorder, mood and psychotic disorders, anxiety disorders, and personality disorders (R. A. Stern, Perkins, & Evans, 1995; O'Dowd, Natali, Orr, & McKegney, 1991; Evans & Perkins, 1990). Other diagnoses that occur at a high rate are substance use disorders involving both alcohol and other substances (R. A. Stern et al., 1995; O'Dowd et al., 1991). Psychiatric symptoms and syndromes have been reported at various stages in HIV illness. Whether they are directly related to HIV CNS infection or are functional problems of new onset is not yet clear. In some cases, however, the onset of psychiatric symptoms and syndromes in HIV-positive patients has been directly linked to various aspects of AIDS, such as medication side effects, opportunistic infections, metabolic abnormalities, and malignancies (O'Dowd et al., 1991). According to Perry et al. (1990), the predominant current and lifetime Axis I disorders in one HIV-infected sample were major depression, dysthymia, substance dependence, and anxiety disorders.

Grief Reaction and Suicide

Not unexpectedly, individuals who have been newly diagnosed as HIV-positive will experience a process similar to a grief reaction associated with a dysphoric and anxious mood. Affective disorders, such as major depression or an anxiety disorder, must be differentiated from situation-appropriate grief in order to determine whether or not psychopharmacological intervention is indicated. Close monitoring of the grief reaction is recommended to provide early detection for the development of an adjustment disorder, one of the most common psychiatric diagnoses in all stages of HIV infection (O'Dowd et al., 1991).

With the high prevalence of psychiatric disorders and multiple psychosocial stressors associated with HIV infection, the HIV-positive patient, not surprisingly, is at risk for suicidal ideation and suicide. Although one study (McKegney & O'Dowd, 1992) reported a markedly increased risk of suicide in the HIV/AIDS patients (36 times greater than that of age-matched men without AIDS and 66 times greater than that of the general population), other studies have found that asymptomatic HIV-1-infected patients are more likely than AIDS patients to have suicidal ideation. In addition, previous history of suicidal ideation and/or psychiatric treatment correlated more significantly with current suicidal ideation than did HIV/AIDS status (Marzuk et al., 1988; McKegney & O'Dowd, 1992).

As it is in any patient population, suicidality in HIV/AIDS patients is an issue of great concern. Because extensive counseling is a key intervention for suicidality, it may be clinically significant to identify whether suicidal ideation is likely to occur at the early versus later stages of HIV illness. Once this determination has been made, therapy that would address such issues as day-to-day management, living arrangements, and ethical/legal issues as they occur in the various stages of the illness may help to alleviate the overwhelming stress of being HIV-positive. This in turn may decrease the risk of patients' developing suicidal ideation as the illness progresses (R. A. Stern et al., 1995).

Adjustment Disorder

As previously mentioned, one of the most common psychiatric diagnoses in the HIV/AIDS population is adjustment disorder (O'Dowd et al., 1991). This is not surprising, since being diagnosed as HIV-positive and the associated social stigma of the illness are significant stressors. According to several researchers, most individuals with HIV infection exhibit good coping capacity and are able to maintain hope over time; however, the associated psychosocial stressors and subsequent losses may occur more rapidly than an individual can adapt to such events (Leserman, Perkins, & Evans, 1992; Rabkin, Williams, Neugebauer, Riemen, & Goetz, 1990). In addition, the development of cognitive impairment as seen in HIV-1-associated dementia can further impair coping skills and subsequently precipitate the development of an adjustment disorder (R. A. Stern et al., 1995). Coping skills may be greatly facilitated by such interventions as education and community outreach. Although the value of psychotherapy, both individual and group, has been shown to be clinically significant, it has yet to be systematically quantified (Evans & Perkins, 1990; O'Dowd et al., 1991).

Depression

Many depressive symptoms, such as fatigue, weight loss, and anorexia, are also very common symptoms associated with the progression of HIV illness; this complicates the process of diagnosing depression in the HIV/AIDS patient. An added difficulty is that the bradykinesia or psychomotor slowing associated with HIV-1-associated dementia may be mistaken for a symptom of a primary depressive disorder. A recent report, however, suggests that complaints of fatigue and insomnia in asymptomatic HIV-infected patients are suggestive of a mood disorder (Perkins et al., 1995).

The differentiation between major depressive disorder and a

depressive disorder secondary to HIV infection is an important one, because anecdotal evidence suggests that the HIV-related depressive disorder is more likely to respond to antiretroviral treatment than to traditional antidepressant therapy (Evans & Perkins, 1990). The prevalence of major depression across the various stages of HIV illness has not been well defined. Several studies have demonstrated that the prevalence of major depression is higher in asymptomatic HIV-infected gay men than in the general population, but is similar to the prevalence in seronegative, at-risk gay men (Atkinson et al., 1988; Brown et al., 1992; Perkins et al., 1994; Williams, Rabkin, Remien, Gorman, & Ehrhardt, 1991).

Major depression occurring in the asymptomatic stage is not secondary to the effects of HIV-1 on the brain, according to recent data (Evans & Perkins, 1990). Antidepressant therapy of primary depressive disorder may be limited by HIV/AIDS patients' apparently increased sensitivity to the side effects of such medication. This sensitivity is similar to the medication sensitivity noted in elderly and medically frail patients. General principles of medication use similar to those for the elderly and medically frail are recommended for HIV/AIDS patients. These guidelines include lower starting doses (equivalent to one-quarter to one-half of the standard doses) and a slower titration schedule (Hintz, Kuck, Peterkin, Volk, & Zisook, 1990). Both the traditional antidepressants and the newer agents, such as the selective serotonin reuptake inhibitors (SSRIs), have been shown to be effective in the treatment of major depressive disorder. Anecdotally, the SSRIs are well tolerated, particularly when started at lower doses and slowly increased. Electroconvulsive therapy has also been reported as effective, although it may potentiate the development of confusion (Schaerf, Miller, Lipsey, & McPherson, 1989).

Severely ill and depressed AIDS patients may benefit from the use of a quick-acting, quick-mobilizing agent such as methylphenidate and/or dextroamphetamine (Fernández et al., 1988; Fernández & Levy, 1994). Psychostimulants may also be used in patients without depression who have HIV-related cognitive impairment; improvement in cognitive function may be seen within several days (Fernández & Levy, 1994). The usual starting dose is 5–10 mg twice a day, with a gradual increase to a total daily dose of 20–30 mg (Holmes, Fernández, & Levy, 1989). These patients need to be monitored carefully for the development or worsening of insomnia and/or anorexia.

It is also suggested that the use of antidepressant medication may decrease perceived somatic and affective symptoms in medically symptomatic individuals with HIV and AIDS (Ferrando, Goldman, & Charness, 1997). Selective serotonin reuptake inhibitors (SSRIs) utilized over a six-week period included sertraline, paroxetine, and fluoxetine. Fluoxetine appeared to be the most consistently effective and well-tolerated SSRI, although sample size, nonrandom assignment, and the lack of a placebo control prevented a definitive conclusion regarding differential effectiveness and tolerability of the SSRIs in treating HIV disease.

Antidepressant medication may also be utilized in the treatment of pain, often an issue in HIV-related disease (Atkinson & Grant, 1994). Tricyclic antidepressant medication appears to be useful in the treatment of neuropathic pain and chronic headaches, two types of pain conditions often endured by those with symptomatic HIV and AIDS. However, the anticholinergic properties of tricyclics may result in increased memory dysfunction. Anticonvulsant medications and SSRI treatment, as well as other psychotropic treatment, have also been used to treat pain syndromes in HIV disease.

Anxiety

HIV/AIDS patients are not more likely than the general population to develop anxiety disorders per se; however, anxiety is often present as a component of other psychiatric disorders (e.g., adjustment disorder or depression) in this population (Bialer, Wallack, & Snyder, 1991). Anxiety may also be present secondary to an underlying illness, such as hypoxia or HIV-related infection or neoplastic process ("Medical News," 1982). Moreover, individuals with preexisting anxiety disorders are at risk for exacerbations when exposed to the numerous psychosocial stressors of becoming HIV-positive. Situationally appropriate anxiety may be successfully addressed with cognitive-behavioral techniques; however, over extended periods of time, the need for psychopharmacological intervention may become evident (Fernández & Levy, 1994). Benzodiazepines, particularly agents with short and intermediate half-lives (e.g., lorazepam and oxazepam), are commonly initiated. In the hospitalized HIV/AIDS population, benzodiazepines are the most commonly prescribed psychotropic medications because of their sedative/hypnotic and anxiolytic properties (Ochitill, Dilley, & Kohlwes, 1991). To avoid the CNS depressant and neurocognitive impairment potential of benzodiazepines, a decreased dose and increased dosing interval are recommended, as well as time-limited use. An alternative to benzodiazepines is the nonbenzodiazepine anxiolytic buspirone, which has lower potential for oversedation, abuse, and dependence than the traditional anxiolytics. A possible disadvantage of buspirone is the 2 to 3-week delay after initiation of therapy before a consistent anxiolytic effect is obtained. Asymptomatic HIV patients, as well as those in the early stages of HIV illness, are more likely to benefit from buspirone than those in the more advanced stages are (Fernández & Levy, 1994).

Psychosis

Psychosis, in association with neurocognitive impairment, is not uncommon in the more advanced stages of HIV illness. The wide range of presentation varies from paranoid delusions and auditory hallucinations to manic symptoms and catatonia (Evans & Perkins, 1990). These symptoms respond to treatment with neuroleptics in doses equivalent to 40–80 mg of chlorpromazine daily for delirium and approximately 125 mg of chlorpromazine daily for new-onset psychosis (Breitbart, 1993; Sewell, 1993). HIV patients apparently have an increased sensitivity to the dopamine-blocking properties of antipsychotics, and subsequently have an increased susceptibility to the development of severe extrapyramidal symptoms and acute dystonic reactions. These patients also have an increased sensitivity to the anticholinergic side effects of the neuroleptics. Although formal studies have yet to be completed, low doses and a slow titration schedule are recommended for the initiation of antipsychotic agents in this population. High-potency neuroleptics may cause more extrapyramidal side effects, but these may be preferable to the oversedation and confusion associated with the low-potency neuroleptics. Close monitoring for the development of side effects, including neuroleptic malignant syndrome, is necessary for any HIV/AIDS patient on neuroleptic medication (R. A. Stern et al., 1995; Fernández & Levy, 1994).

Mania

Mania in HIV/AIDS patients has not been extensively studied. Much of the current literature on the treatment of mania in HIV/AIDS patients consists of retrospective chart reviews and clinical anecdotes. Although lithium has been shown to be effective in the treatment of mania in this patient population, its efficacy is limited by the associated gastrointestinal and neurotoxic side effects, particularly diarrhea and sedation (Ayuso, 1994; Jernigan et al., 1993). Despite these side effects, lithium's ability to induce leucocytosis and neutrophilia is seen as a potential advantage in the treatment of ZDV-induced neutropenia (Evans & Perkins, 1990). In addition to lithium, such agents as valproic acid, carbamazepine, and clonazepam have been shown to be effective in the treatment of acute mania in HIV-1-infected patients (Keck, McElroy, & Nemeroff, 1992). One retrospective case review of 11 HIV patients with acute mania reported poor tolerance to lithium and neuroleptics, in contrast to 100% therapeutic response to the initiation of various anticonvulsants, including clonazepam, phenytoin, carbamazepine, and valproic acid (Halman, Worth, Sanders, Renshaw, & Murray, 1993).

CONCLUSIONS

HIV's impact on the CNS can be devastating in terms of direct retroviral effects, secondary CNS infections, and general physical debilitation. Given our limited understanding of the effects of HIV infection on the CNS, research is needed to clarify how HIV-associated minor cognitive/motor disorder develops and why there is a progression in some persons to HIV-associated dementia complex. To this end, more studies are necessary that use measures of CNS functioning (e.g., laboratory, imaging, and neuropsychological tests) in order to identify the earliest symptoms of HIV-associated minor cognitive/motor disorder. These approaches might also lend themselves to the efforts to determine which factors might define those persons whose CNS symptoms progress to clinical dementia. Work should continue to focus on current and as yet undefined CSF markers of HIV's impact on the brain and their relationship to neuropsychiatric dysfunction. These markers might also prove to be useful in determining when antiretroviral therapy should be initiated, and which agent(s) should be used, to lessen or reverse HIV's deleterious effects on the CNS. Furthermore, such markers should be useful in determining the impact of current and future antiretroviral agents (Syndulko et al., 1994). Changes in cognitive symptoms in seropositive persons should also be evaluated when psychopharmacological agents are used in conjunction with antiretroviral therapies, especially given the impact of psychopharmacological agents on neurotransmitters.

Although the treatment of HIV-associated neuropsychiatric disease and symptoms has progressed over the past decade, the impact of antiretroviral treatment accompanied by neuroprotective agents needs to be evaluated (particularly those agents that have neuroprotective potential and are commonly used to treat psychiatric symptoms). Since HIV infection can result in both neuropsychiatric and medical illnesses, antiretroviral and other pharmacological agents (antifungal, antimicrobial, psychopharmacological) are often used in tandem. Given HIV's impact on the brain, it is therefore not surprising that the treatment of neuropsychiatric symptoms must be undertaken carefully, and that certain agents (e.g., neuroleptics, tricyclic antidepressants) may exacerbate symptoms of HIV-associated cognitive/motor dysfunction (e.g., Ayuso, 1994; Berman & Kim, 1994).

Finally, CNS penetration of antiretroviral agents appears to be the key factor in many of the studies reviewed in this chapter. As new antiretroviral therapies are developed, they should continue to be evaluated for their ability to penetrate the CNS and to ameliorate or retard the neuropsychiatric sequelae of HIV infection.

REFERENCES

Akula, S. K., Rege, A. B., Dreisbach, A. W., Dejace, P. M., & Lertora, J. J. (1997). Valproic acid increases cerebrospinal fluid zidovudine levels in a patient with AIDS. *American Journal of Medical Sciences, 313*(4), 244–246.

American Academy of Neurology (AAN). (1991). Nomenclature and research case definitions for neurologic manifestations of human immunodeficiency virus-type 1 (HIV-1) infection: Report of a working group of the American Academy of Neurology AIDS Task Force. *Neurology, 41,* 778–785.

Atkinson, J. H., & Grant, I. (1994). Natural history of neuropsychiatric manifestations of HIV disease. *Psychiatric Clinics of North America, 17,* 17–32.

Atkinson, J. H., Grant, I., Kennedy, C. J., Richman, D. D., Spector, S. A., & McCutchan, J. A. (1988). Prevalence of psychiatric disorders among men infected with the human immunodeficiency virus. *Archives of General Psychiatry, 48,* 859–864.

Aylward, E. H., Brettschneider, P. D., McArthur, J. C., Harris, G. J., Schlaepfer, T. E., Henderer, J. D., Barta, P. E., Tien, A. Y., & Pearlson, G. D. (1995). Magnetic resonance imaging measurement of gray matter volume reductions in HIV dementia. *American Journal of Psychiatry, 152,* 987–994.

Ayuso, J. L. (1994). Use of psychotropic drugs in patients with HIV infection. *Drugs, 47*(4), 599–610.

Becker, J. T., Martin, A., & Lopez, O. L. (1994). The dementias and AIDS. In I. Grant & A. Martin (Eds.), *Neuropsychology of HIV infection* (pp. 133–145). New York: Oxford University Press.

Berger, J. R., & Levy, J. A. (1991). The human immunodeficiency virus type 1: The virus and its role in neurologic disease. *Seminars in Neurology, 12,* 1–9.

Berman, S. M., & Kim, R. C. (1994). The development of cytomegalovirus encephalitis in AIDS patients receiving ganciclovir. *American Journal of Medicine, 96,* 415–419.

Bialer, P. A., Wallack, J. J., & Snyder, S. L. (1991). Psychiatric diagnosis in HIV-spectrum disorders. *Psychiatric Medicine, 9*(3), 361–375.

Bornstein, R. A. (1994). Methodological and conceptual issues in the study of cognitive change in HIV infection. In I. Grant & A. Martin (Eds.), *Neuropsychology of HIV infection* (pp. 146–160). New York: Oxford University Press.

Bornstein, R. A., Nasrallah, H. A., Para, M. F., Fass, R. J., Whitacre, C. C., & Rice, R. R. (1991). Rate of CD4 decline and neuropsychological performance in HIV infection. *Archives of Neurology, 48,* 704–707.

Breitbart, W. (1993, April). *HIV-1 and delirium.* Abstract presented at the conference on Psychopharmacology of HIV-1 Infection: Clinical Challenges and Research Directions, Office of AIDS Programs, National Institute of Mental Health, Washington, DC.

Brouwers, P., Moss, H., Wolters, P., Eddy, J., Balis, F., Poplack, D. G., & Pizzo, P. A. (1990). Effect of continuous-infusion zidovudine therapy on neuropsychologic functioning in children with symptomatic human immunodeficiency virus infection. *Journal of Pediatrics, 117,* 982–985.

Brouwers, P., Moss, H., Wolters, P., & Schmitt, F. (1994). Developmental deficits and behavioral change in pediatric AIDS. In I. Grant & A. Martin, (Eds.), *Neuropsychology of HIV infection* (pp. 310–338). New York: Oxford University Press.

Brown, G. R., Rundell, J. R., McManis, S. E., Kendall, S. N., Zachary, R., & Temoshok, L. (1992). Prevalence of psychiatric disorders in early stages of HIV infection. *Psychosomatic Medicine, 54,* 588–601.

Butler, K. M., Husson, R. M., Balis, F. M., Brouwers, P., Eddy, J, El-Amin, D., Gress, J., Hawkins, M., Jaroswski, P., Moss, H., Poplack, D., Santacroce, S. (1991). Dideoxyinosine in children with symptomatic human immunodeficiency virus infection. *New England Journal of Medicine, 324,* 137–144.

Cao, Y., Qin, L., Zhang, L., Safrit, J., & Ho, D. D. (1995). Virologic and immunologic characterization of long-term survivors of human immunodeficiency virus type 1 infection. *New England Journal of Medicine, 332*(4), 201–208.

Centers for Disease Control (CDC). (1987). Revision of the CDC surveillance case definition for acquired immunodeficiency syndrome. *Morbidity and Mortality Weekly Report, 36*(5–7), 1–15.

Centers for Disease Control (CDC). (1992). 1993 revised classification system for HIV infection and expanded surveillance case definition for AIDS among adolescents and adults. *Morbidity and Mortality Weekly Report, 41*(No. RR-17), 1–19.

Coffin, J. M. (1995). HIV population dynamics *in vivo:* Implications for genetic variation, pathogenesis, and therapy. *Science, 267,* 483–489.

Evans, D. L., & Perkins, D. O. (1990). The clinical psychiatry of AIDS. *Current Opinion in Psychiatry, 3,* 96–102.

Everall, I. P., Luthbert, P. J., & Lantos, P. L. (1991). Neuronal loss in the frontal cortex in HIV infection. *Lancet, 337,* 1119–1121.

Fernández, F., Adams, F., Levy, J. K., Holmes, V. F., Neidhart, M., & Mansell, P. W. A. (1988). Cognitive impairment due to AIDS-related complex and its response to psychostimulants. *Psychosomatics, 29,* 38–46.

Fernández, F., & Levy, J. K. (1994). Psychopharmacology in HIV spectrum disorders. *Psychiatric Clinics of North America, 17*(1), 135–148.

Ferrando, S. J., Goldman, J. D., & Charness, W. E. (1997). Selective serotonin reuptake inhibitor treatment of depression in symptomatic HIV infections and AIDS: Improvements in affective and somatic symptoms. *General Hospital Psychiatry, 19,* 89–97.

Gorman, J. M., Mayeux, R., Stern, Y., Williams, J. B. W., Rabkin, J., Goetz, R. R.,

& Ehrhardt, A. A. (1993). The effect of zidovudine on neuropsychiatric measures in HIV-infected men. *American Journal of Psychiatry, 150,* 505–507.

Grant, I., Atkinson, J. H., Hesselink, J. R., Kennedy, C. J., Richman, D. D., Spector, S. A., & McCutchan, J. A. (1987). Evidence for early central nervous system involvement in the acquired immunodeficiency virus (HIV) infections. *Annals of Internal Medicine, 107,* 828–836.

Grant, I., Olshen, R. A., Atkinson, J. H., Heaton, R. K., Nelson, J., McCutchan, J. A., & Weinrich, J. D. (1993). Depressed mood does not explain neuropsychological deficits in HIV-infected persons. *Neuropsychology, 7,* 53–61.

Gray, F., Belec, L., Keohane, C., De Truchis, P., Clair, B., Durigon, M., Sobel, A., & Gherardi, R. (1994). Zidovudine therapy and HIV encephalitis: A 10-year neuropathological survey. *AIDS, 8,* 489–493.

Halman, M. H., Worth, J. L., Sanders, K. M., Renshaw, P. F., & Murray, G. B. (1993). Anticonvulsant use in the treatment of manic syndromes in patients with HIV-1 infection. *Journal of Neuropsychiatry, 5*(4), 430–434.

Harris, G. J., Pearlson, G. D., McArthur, J. C., Zeger, S., & LaFrance, N. D. (1994). Altered cortical blood flow in HIV-seropositive individuals with and without dementia: A single photon emission computed tomography study. *AIDS, 8,* 495–499.

Heaton, R. K., Grant, I., Butters, N., White, D. A., Kirson, D., Atkinson, J. H., McCutchan, J. A., Taylor, M. J., Kelly, M. D., Ellis, R. J., Wolfson, T., Velin, R., Marcotte, T. D., Hesselink, J. R., Jernigan, T. L., Chandler, J., Wallace, M., Abramson, I., & the HNRC Group. (1995). The HNRC 500: Neuropsychology of HIV infection at different disease stages. *Journal of the International Neuropsychological Society, 1,* 231–251.

Heyes, M. P., Brew, B. J., Martin, A., Price, R. W., Salazar, A. M., Sidtis, J. I., Yerdey, J. A., Mouradian, M. M., Sadler, A. E., & Keile, J. (1991). Quinolinic acid in cerebrospinal fluid and serum in HIV infection: Relationship to clinical and neurologic status. *Annals of Neurology, 29,* 202–209.

Heyes, M. P., Jordan, E. K., Lee, K., Saite, K., Frank, J. A., Shoy, P. J., Markey, S. P., & Shevell, M. (1992). Relationship of neurologic status in macaques infected with the simian immunodeficiency virus to cerebrospinal fluid quinolinic acid and kynurenic acid. *Brain Research, 570,* 237–250.

Hinkin, C. H., van Gorp, W. G., Satz, P., Weisman, J. D., Thommes, J., & Buckingham, S. (1992). Depressed mood and its relationship to neuropsychological test performance in HIV-1 seropositive individuals. *Journal of Clinical and Experimental Neuropsychology, 14,* 289–297.

Hintz, S., Kuck, J., Peterkin, J., Volk, D. M., & Zisook, S. (1990). Depression in the context of human immunodeficiency virus infection: Implications for treatment. *Journal of Clinical Psychiatry, 51,* 497–501.

Holmes, V., Fernández, F., & Levy, J. K. (1989). Psychostimulant response in AIDS-related complex (ARC) patients. *Journal of Clinical Psychiatry, 50,* 5–8.

Ho, D. D., Sarngadharan, M. G., Resnick, L., Dimarzo-Veronese, F., Rota, T. R., & Hirsch, M. S. (1985). Primary human T-lymphotrophic virus type III infection. *Annals of Internal Medicine, 103,* 880–883.

Jernigan, T. L., Archibald, S., Hesselink, J. R., Atkinson, J. H., Velin, R. A., McCutchan, J. A., Chandler, J., & Grant, 1. (1993). Magnetic resonance imaging morphometric analysis of cerebral volume loss in human immunodeficiency virus infection. *Archives of Neurology, 50,* 250–255.

Katzman, R., Terry, R., DeTeresa, R., Brown, T., Davies, P., Fuld, P., Renbing, X., & Peck, A. (1988). Clinical, pathological, and neurochemical changes in dementia: A subgroup with preserved mental status and numerous neocortical plaques. *Annals of Neurology, 23,* 138–144.

Keck, P. E., Jr., McElroy, S. L., & Nemeroff, C. B. (1992). Anticonvulsants in the treatment of bipolar disorder. *Journal of Neuropsychiatry and Clinical Neurosciences, 4,* 395–405.

Ketzler, S., Weis, S., & Haug, H. (1990). Loss of neurons in frontal cortex in AIDS brains. *Acta Neuropathologica, 80,* 90–92.

Kieburtz, K. D., Ketonen, L., Zettelmaier, A. E., Kido, D., Caine, E. D., & Simon, J. H. (1990). Magnetic resonance imaging findings in HIV cognitive impairment. *Archives of Neurology, 47,* 643–645.

Larder, B. A., Kemp, S. D., & Harrigan, P. R. (1995). Potential mechanism for sustained antiretroviral efficacy of AZT-3TC combination therapy. *Science, 269,* 696–699.

Law, W. A., Martin, A., Mapou, R. L., Roller, T. L., Salazar, A. M., Temoshok, L. R., & Rundell, J. R. (1994). Working memory in individuals with HIV infection. *Journal of Clinical and Experimental Neuropsychology, 16,* 173–182.

Leserman, J., Perkins, D. O., & Evans, D. L. (1992). Coping with the threat of AIDS: The role of social support. *American Journal of Psychiatry, 149,* 1514–1520.

Levin, H. S., Williams, D. H., Borucki, M. J., Hillman, G. R., Williams, J. B., Guinto, F. L., Amparo, E. G., Crow, W. N., & Pollard, R. B. (1990). Magnetic resonance imaging and neuropsychological findings in human immunodeficiency virus infection. *Journal of Acquired Immune Deficiency Syndromes, 3*(8), 757–762.

Limoges, J., Persidsky, Y., Bock, P., & Gendelman, H. E. (1997). Dexamethasone therapy worsens the neuropathology of human immunodeficiency virus type 1 encephalitis in SCID mice. *Journal of Infectious Diseases, 175*(6), 1368–1381.

Lipton, S. A. (1991). HIV-related neurotoxicity. *Brain Pathology, 1,* 193–199.

Lipton, S. A. (1994). Laboratory basis of novel therapeutic strategies to prevent HIV related neuronal injury. In R. W. Price & S. W. Perry (Eds.), *Research publications of the Association for Research in Nervous and Mental Disease: Vol. 72. HIV, AIDS and the brain* (pp. 183–202). New York: Raven Press.

Marotta, R., & Perry, S. (1989). Early neuropsychological dysfunction caused by human immunodeficiency virus. *Journal of Neuropsychiatry, 1*(3), 225–235.

Martin, A., Heyes, M. P., Salazar, A. M., Kempen, D. L., Williams, J., Law, W. A., Coats, W. E., & Markey, S. P. (1992). Progressive slowing of reaction time and increasing cerebrospinal fluid concentrations of quinolinic acid in HIV-infected individuals. *Journal of Neuropsychiatry and Clinical Neurosciences, 4,* 270–279.

Martin, A., Heyes, M. P., Salazar, A. M., Law, W. A., & Williams, J. (1993). Impaired motor-skill learning, slowed reaction time, and elevated cerebrospinal fluid quinolinic acid in a subgroup of HIV-infected individuals. *Neuropsychology, 7,* 149–157.

Marzuk, P. M., Tierney, H., Tardiff, K., Gross, E. M., Morgan, E. B., Heg, M. A., & Mann, J. J. (1988). Increased risk of suicide in persons with AIDS. *Journal of the American Medical Association, 259,* 1333–1337.

Mayeux, R., Stern, Y., Tang, M.-X., Todak, G., Marder, K., Sano, M., Richards, M., Stein, Z., Ehrhardt, A. A., & Gorman, J. M. (1993). Mortality risks in gay men with human immunodeficiency virus infection and cognitive impairment. *Neurology, 43,* 176–182.

McArthur, J. C., Becker, P. S., Parisi, J. E., Trapp, B., Selnes, O. A., Cornblath, D. R., Balakrishnan, J., Griffin, J. W., & Price, D. (1989a). Neuropathological changes in early HIV-1 dementia. *Annals of Neurology, 26,* 681–684.

McArthur, J. C., Cohen, B. A., Selnes, O. A, Kumar, A. J., Cooper, K., McArthur, J. H., Soucy, G., Cornblath, D. R., Chmiel, J. S., Wang, M.-C., Starkey, D. L., Ginzburg, H., Ostrow, D. G., Johnson, R. T., Phair, J. P., & Polk, B. F. (1989b). Low prevalence of neurological and neuropsychological abnormalities in otherwise healthy HIV-1-infected individuals: Results from the Multicenter AIDS Cohort Study. *Annals of Neurology, 26,* 601–611.

McKegney, F. P., & O'Dowd, M. A. (1992). Suicidality and HIV status. *American Journal of Psychiatry, 149,* 396–398.

Medical News. (1982). Neurological complications now characterizing many AIDS victims. *Journal of the American Medical Association, 248,* 2941–2942.

Miller, E. N., Satz, P., & Visscher, B. (1991). Computerized and conventional neuropsychological assessment of HIV-1-infected homosexual men. *Neurology, 41,* 1608–1616.

Miller, E. N., Selnes, O. A., McArthur, J. C., Satz, P., Becker, J. T., Cohen, B. A., Sheridan, K., Machado, A. M., van Gorp, W. G., & Visscher, B. (1990). Neuropsychological performance in HIV-1-infected homosexual men: The Multicenter AIDS Cohort Study (MACS). *Neurology, 40,* 197–203.

Mizrachi, Y., Rubenstein, A., Harish, Z., Biegon, A., Anserson, W. R., & Brewster, M. E. (1995). Improved brain delivery and *in vitro* activity of zidovudine through the use of a redox chemical delivery system. *AIDS, 9,* 153–158.

Navia, B. A., & Price, R. W. (1987). The acquired immunodeficiency syndrome dementia complex as the presenting or sole manifestation of human immunodeficiency virus infection. *Archives of Neurology, 44,* 65–69.

Nozyce, M., Hoberman, M., Arpadi, S., Wiznia, A., Lambert, G., Dobroszycki, J., Chang, C. J., & St. Louis, Y. (1994). A 12-month study of the effects of oral zidovudine on neurodevelopmental functioning in a cohort of vertically HIV infected inner-city children. *AIDS, 8,* 635–639.

Ochitill, H., Dilley, J., & Kohlwes, J. (1991). Psychotropic drug prescribing for hospitalized patients with AIDS. *American Journal of Medicine, 90,* 601–605.

O'Dowd, M. A., Natali, C., Orr, D., & McKenney, F. P. (1991). Characteristics of patients attending an HIV-related psychiatric clinic. *Hospital and Community Psychiatry, 42,* 615–618.

Pantaleo, G., Menzo, S., Vaccarezza, M., Graziosi, C., Cohen, O. J., Demarset, J. F., Montefiori, D., Orenstein, J. M., Fox, C., Schrager, L. K., Margolick, J. B., Buchbinder, S., Giorgi, J. V., & Fauci, A. S. (1995). Studies in subjects with long-term nonprogressive human immunodeficiency virus infection. *New England Journal of Medicine, 332,* 209–216.

Perkins, D. O., Leserman, J., Stern, R. A., Baum, S. F., Liao, D., Golden, R. N., & Evans, D. L., et al. (1995). Somatic symptoms and HIV infection: Relationship to depressive symptoms and indicators of HIV disease. *American Journal of Psychiatry, 152*(12), 1776–781.

Perkins, D. O., Stern, R. A., Golden, R. N., Murphy, C., Naftolowitz, D., & Evans, D. (1994). Mood disorders in HIV infection: Prevalence and risk factors in a nonepicenter of the AIDS epidemic. *American Journal of Psychiatry, 151,* 233–236.

Perry, S., Jacobsberg, L. B., Fishman, B., Frances, A., Bobo, J., & Jacobsberg, B. K. (1990). Psychiatric diagnosis before serological testing for the human immunodeficiency virus. *American Journal of Psychiatry, 147,* 89–93.

Petito, C. K. (1993). What causes brain atrophy in human immunodeficiency virus infection? *Annals of Neurology, 34,* 128–129.

Pizzo, P. A., Butler, K., Balis, F., Brouwers, P., Hawkins, M., Eddy, J., Einloth, M., Falloon, J., Husson, R., & Jarosinski, P. (1990). Dideoxycytidine alone and in an alternating schedule with zidovudine in children with symptomatic human immunodeficiency virus infection. *Journal of Pediatrics, 117,* 799–808.

Pizzo, P. A., Eddy, J., Falloon, J., Ballis, F., M., Murphy, R. E., Moss, H., Wolters, P., Brouwers, P., Jarosinski, P., & Rubin, M. (1988). Effect of continuous intravenous infusion of zidovudine (AZT) in children with symptomatic HIV infection. *New England Journal of Medicine, 319,* 889–896.

Poser, S., Luer, W., Eichenlaub, D., Pohle, H. D., Weber, T., Jurgens, S., & Felgenhauer, K. (1988). Chronic HIV encephalitis: II. Clinical aspects. *Klinische Wochenschrift, 66,* 26–31.

Post, M. J. D., Berger, J. R., & Quencer, R. M. (1991). Asymptomatic and neurologically symptomatic HIV-seropositive individuals: Prospective evaluation with cranial MR imaging. *Radiology, 178,* 131–139.

Price, R. W., & Brew, B. J. (1988). The AIDS dementia complex. *Journal of Infectious Diseases, 158,* 1079–1083.

Rabkin, J. G., Williams, J. B. W., Neugebauer, R., Remien, R. H., & Goetz, R. (1990). Maintenance of hope in HIV-spectrum homosexual men. *American Journal of Psychiatry, 147,* 1322–1326.

Richman, D. D., Fischl, M. A., Grieco, M. H., Gottlieb, M. S., Volberding, P. A., Laskin, O. L., Lesdom, J. M., Groodman, J. E., Mildvan, D., & Hirsch, M. S. (1988). The toxicity of azidothymidine (AZT) in the treatment of patients with AIDS and AIDS related complex: A double-blind, placebo controlled trial. *New England Journal of Medicine, 317,* 192–197.

Rottenberg, D. A., Moeller, J. R., Strother, S. C., Sidtis, J. J., Navia, B. A., Dhawan, V., Ginos, J. Z., & Price, R. W. (1987). The metabolic pathology of the AIDS dementia complex. *Annals of Neurology, 22,* 700–706.

Royal, W., III, Selnes, O. A., Concha, M., Nance-Sproson, T. E., & McArthur, J. C. (1994). Cerebrospinal fluid human immunodeficiency virus type 1 (HIV-1) p24 antigen levels in HIV-1-related dementia. *Annals of Neurology, 36,* 32–39.

Rubinow, D. R., Berrettini, C. H., Brouwers, P., & Lane, H. C. (1988). Neuropsychiatric consequences of AIDS. *Annals of Neurology, 23*(Suppl.), S24–S26.

Satz, P. (1993). Brain reserve capacity on symptom onset after brain injury: A formulation and review of evidence for threshold theory. *Neuropsychology, 7,* 273–295.

Satz, P., Morgenstern, H., & Miller, E. (1993). Low education as a possible risk factor for cognitive abnormalities in HIV-1: Findings from the Multicenter AIDS Cohort Study. *Journal of Acquired Immune Deficiency Syndromes, 6,* 503–511.

Saykin, A. J., Janssen, R. S., Sprehn, G. C., Kaplan, J. E., Spira, T. J., & Weller, P. (1988). Neuropsychological dysfunction in HIV-infection: Characterization in a lymphadenopathy cohort. *International Journal of Clinical Neuropsychology, 10,* 81–95.

Schaerf, F. W., Miller, R. R., Lipsey, J. R., & McPherson, R. W. (1989). ECT for major depression in four patients infected with human immunodeficiency virus. *American Journal of Psychiatry, 146,* 782–784.

Schmitt, F. A., Bigley, J. W., McKinnis, R., Logue, P. E., Evans, R. W., & Drucker, J. L. (1988). Neuropsychological outcome of zidovudine (AZT) treatment of patients with AIDS and AIDS-related complex. *New England Journal of Medicine, 319,* 1573–1578.

Schmitt, F. A., Dixon, L. R., & Brouwers, P. (1994). Neuropsychological response to antiretroviral therapy in HIV infection. In I. Grant & A. Martin (Eds.), *Neuropsychology of HIV infection* (pp. 276–294). New York: Oxford University Press.

Selnes, O. A., Miller, E., McArthur, J., Gordon, B., Munoz, A., Sheridan, K., Fox, R., Saah, A. J., & the Multicenter AIDS Cohort Study. (1990). HIV-1 infection: No evidence of cognitive decline during the asymptomatic stages. *Neurology, 40,* 204–208.

Sewell, D. (1993, April). *HIV-associated psychosis.* Abstract presented at the conference on Psychopharmacology of HIV-1 Infection: Clinical Challenges and Research Directions. Office of AIDS Programs, National Institute of Mental Health, Washington, DC.

Sidtis, J. J. (1994). Evaluation of the AIDS dementia complex in adults. In R. W. Price & S. W. Perry (Eds.), *Research publications of the Association for Research in Nervous and Mental Disease: Vol. 72. HIV, AIDS and the brain* (pp. 273–287). New York: Raven Press.

Sidtis, J. J., Gatsonis, C., Price, R. W., Singer, E. J., Collier, A. C., Richman, D. D., Hirsch, M. S., Schaerf, F. W., Fischl, M. A., & Kieburtz, K. (1993). Zidovudine treatment of the AIDS dementia complex: Results of a placebo-controlled trial. *Annals of Neurology, 33,* 343–349.

Sidtis, J. J., & Price, R. W. (1990). HIV-1 infection and the AIDS dementia complex. *Neurology, 40,* 323–326.

Stern, R. A., Perkins, D. O., & Evans, D. L. (1995). Neuropsychiatric manifestations of HIV-1 infections and AIDS. In D. J. Kupfer & F. E. Bloom (Eds.), *Psychopharmacology: The fourth generation of progress* (pp. 1545–1558). New York: Raven Press.

Stern, Y. (1991). The impact of human immunodeficiency virus on cognitive function. *Annals of the New York Academy of Sciences, 640,* 219–223.

Stern, Y., Guriand, B., Tatemichi, T. K., Tang, M. X., Wilder, D., & Mayeux, R.

(1994). Influence of education and occupation on the incidence of Alzheimer's disease. *Journal of the American Medical Association, 271,* 1004–1010.

Stern, Y., Liu, X., Marder, K., Todak, G., Sano, M., Ehrhardt, A., & Gorman, J. (1995). Neuropsychological changes in a prospectively followed cohort of homosexual and bisexual men with and without HIV infection. *Neurology, 45*(3, Pt. 1), 467–472.

Stern, Y., Marder, K., Bell, K., Chen, J., Dooneief, G., Goldstein, S., Mindry, D., Richards, M., Sano, M., & Williams, J. (1991). Multidisciplinary baseline assessment of homosexual men with and without human immunodeficiency virus infection. *Archives of General Psychiatry, 48,* 131–138.

Stern, Y., Silva, S. G., Chaisson, N., Evans, D. L. (1996). Influence of cognitive reserve on neuropsychological functioning in asymptomatic human immunodeficiency virus-1 infection. *Archives of Neurology, 53.* 148–153.

Syndulko, K., Singer, E. J., Nogales-Gaete, J., Conrad, A., Schmid, P., & Tourtellotte, W. W. (1994). Laboratory evaluations in HIV-1-associated cognitive/motor complex. *Psychiatric Clinics of North America, 17,* 91–123.

Tenhula, W. N., Xu, S. Z., Madigan, M. C., Heller, K., Freeman, W. R., Sadun, A. A. (1992). Morphometric comparisons of optic nerve axon loss in acquired immunodeficiency syndrome. *American Journal of Ophthalmology, 113,* 14–20.

van Gorp, W. G., Hinkin, C., Satz, P., Miller, E. N., Weisman, J., Holston, S., Drebing, C., Marcotte, T. D., & Dixon, W. (1993a). Subtypes of HIV-related neuropsychological functioning: A cluster analysis approach. *Neuropsychology, 7,* 62–72.

van Gorp, W. G., Lamb, D., & Schmitt, F. A. (1993b). Methodologic issues in neuropsychological research with HIV-spectrum disease. *Archives of Clinical Neuropsychology, 8,* 17–33.

van Gorp, W. G., Mandelkern, M. A., Gee, M., Hinkin, C. H., Stern, C. E., Paz, D. K., Dixon, W., Evans, G., Flynn, F., Frederick, C. J., Ropchan, J. R., & Blahd, W. H. (1992). Cerebral metabolic dysfunction in AIDS: Findings in a sample with and without dementia. *Journal of Neuropsychiatry, 4,* 280–287.

van Gorp, W. G., Miller, E. N., Marcotte, T. D., Dixon, W., Paz, D., Selnes, O., Wesch, J., Becker, J. T., Hinkin, C. H., Mitrushina, M., Satz, P., Weisman, J. D., Buckingham, S. L., & Stenquist, P. K. (1994). The relationship between age and cognitive impairment in HIV-1 infection: Findings from the Multicenter AIDS Cohort Study and clinical cohort. *Neurology, 44,* 929–935.

Wiley, C. A., Masliah, E., Morey, M., Lemere, G., DeTeresa, R., Grafe, M., Hansen, L., & Terry R. (1991). Neocortical damage during HIV infection. *Annals of Neurology, 29,* 651–657.

Wilkie, F. L., Eisdorfer, C., Morgan, R., Loewenstein, D. A., & Szapocznik, J. (1990). Cognition in early human immunodeficiency virus infection. *Archives of Neurology, 47,* 433–440.

Wilkins, J. W., Robertson, K. R., van der Horst, C., Robertson, W. T., Fryer, J. G., & Hall, C. D. (1990). The importance of confounding factors in the evaluation of neuropsychological changes in patients infected with human immunodeficiency virus. *Journal of Acquired Immune Deficiency Syndromes, 3,* 938–942.

Williams, J. B. W., Rabkin, J. G., Remien, R. H., Gorman, J. M., & Ehrhardt, A. A. (1991). Multidisciplinary baseline assessment of homosexual men with and without human immunodeficiency virus infection: Standardized clinical assessment of current and lifetime psychopathology. *Archives of General Psychiatry, 48*, 124–130.

Wolters, P. L., Brouwers, P., Moss, H. A., & Pizzo, P. A. (1994). Adaptive behavior of children with symptomatic HIV infection before and after zidovudine therapy. *Journal of Pediatric Psychology, 19*, 47–61.

Yarchoan, R., Thomas, R. V., Grafman, J., Wichman, A., Dalakas, M., McAtee, N., Berg, G., Fischl, M., Perno, C. F., Klecker, R. W., Buchbinder, A., Tay, S., Larson, S. M., Myers, C. E., & Broder, S. (1988). Long-term administration of 3'-azido-2',3'-dideoxythymidine to patients with AIDS-related neurological disease. *Annals of Neurology, 23*(Suppl.), S82–S87.

6

Psychosocial Interventions in Persons with HIV-Associated Neuropsychiatric Compromise

STEPHAN L. BUCKINGHAM
MICHAEL SHERNOFF

INTRODUCTION

Psychotherapists working with people with HIV/AIDS must be prepared to assess and provide effective psychosocial interventions for individuals who exhibit symptoms of HIV-associated central nervous system involvement. Appropriate psychosocial interventions for these persons often differ from traditional psychotherapy and counseling. For nonmedical clinicians, evaluating the extent to which presenting symptoms are due to HIV-associated neuropsychiatric compromise or represent a reaction to the multiple stresses of living with HIV/AIDS can be a challenging and difficult clinical challenge, and requires skills that most such clinicians do not learn during graduate training. For this reason, it is essential for a nonmedical clinician to have a close working relationship with a client's primary care physician, since referring the client to a neuropsychologist or neurologist for a more complete evaluation when there is suspected organic compromise may need to be done quickly. As Ostrow (1996) notes:

> Both anxiety and depression can be accompanied by mild cognitive deficits such as poor concentration or short term memory difficulty. For the person with HIV-infection these symptoms can themselves be stressful, because they may be experienced as indicators of early HIV brain involvement. If the cognitive symptoms are mild and in keeping with the degree of affective dysfunction, the patient should be counseled that the symptoms will probably disappear when the anxiety or depression is adequately treated. However, if the cognitive symptoms appear to be out of proportion to the degree of affective involvement or they do not respond to adequate antidepressant or anxiolytic treatment, then a neuropsychological evaluation is indicated, even in patients with >500 CD4 cells. (pp. 871–872)

For a clinician engaged in long-term therapy with an HIV-infected individual, it may be easier to notice initial signs of cognitive or mood impairment than it is for a clinician just beginning to work with an HIV-infected individual; in the latter case, the clinician does not have a baseline assessment of mood, affect, or psychological functions antedating the client's becoming symptomatic with HIV. When a clinician has regular weekly sessions with an HIV-infected client, very often he or she will be the first professional to recognize symptoms of physical, mental, or emotional impairment that indeed could be organic in nature. It is also important to note that some patients may be referred for psychotherapy specifically because of the cognitive changes that have been detected. In addition, some patients may present with complaints of cognitive compromise and the resulting emotional distress this perceived deterioration causes as the reasons they are seeking professional assistance.

Once clinicians have the necessary basic understanding of the common mental status changes that are associated with HIV disease, and specifically with HIV-associated cognitive/motor complex as defined by the American Academy of Neurology (1991), they will understand several important implications of these changes for clinical practice. Thus, they will be better able to provide appropriate treatment and assist the persons diagnosed.

CASE EXAMPLE

The following case illustrates the subtle onset of HIV-related symptoms of central nervous system involvement. It also shows how the therapist's own discomfort with the patient's cognitive changes produced an attempt to protect the patient, which delayed their dealing with these changes during the course of treatment, and the need for practical considerations in dealing with HIV-associated cognitive/motor complex.

Tony was a 33-year-old entertainment attorney whose response to the sudden and unexpected breakup of a 7-year relationship was to call in sick to work and spend a week drinking, using drugs, and having anonymous sex several times daily. One morning, Tony called to discuss entering treatment; he was frightened that he was placing his job in jeopardy, and felt that his entire life was falling apart.

By the time Tony and a new partner began to date, both were practicing safer sex, but Tony had spent years engaging in unprotected and risky sex before it was known that HIV was sexually transmitted. Two years after beginning therapy, Tony discovered a lesion on his foot that was diagnosed as Kaposi's sarcoma. His diagnosis was a complete surprise to him because he had been feeling terrific, working out at the gym, and not suffering from symptoms of any kind until he discovered the lesion. His initial reactions to the diagnosis were anger and denial.

Over the 3 years following his diagnosis, Tony lost over 40 pounds and became disfigured by edema and lesions. Tony had always been an extremely articulate and intelligent man, who spoke very quickly and prided himself for thinking quickly on his feet. As time went on, the therapist began to notice that Tony was speaking more slowly and taking longer to respond to questions. There were often long silences during sessions, during which Tony appeared to be staring off into space, forgetting the thread of the conversation. Tony also became defensive when asked to answer questions on a mental status exam. The therapist justified his not confronting Tony with these observations on the grounds that he did not want to increase Tony's discomfort, but he spent increasing amounts of time in his own supervision addressing his avoidance of the unpleasant realities of Tony's diminishing cognitive abilities. It soon became clear to the therapist that he did not want to face and deal with his own discomfort about the mental deterioration of this well-liked patient, and thus irresponsibly neglected to note these instances whenever they occurred.

One day Tony did not appear for his regularly scheduled appointment. When the therapist called Tony at his office to ask why he had missed the session, Tony sounded confused and said that he was certain the appointment was the next day. The therapist assured him that the appointment was that day, Tuesday—the same day and time they had been having sessions for the past 5 years. Tony admitted that this frightened him, and finally acknowledged to the therapist that he had recently noticed other indications of memory loss and a growing disorientation.

The session was rescheduled for the following day, and the therapist asked for and received Tony's permission to telephone him a couple of hours before the session to remind him about it. During the session, Tony was asked his feelings about having to be called to be reminded about the appointment. This prompted him to rage: "AIDS! It's taking over my life, and I'm losing control of my body and mind." Soon he burst into tears, pounded the couch, and said, "Needing you to remind me about our appointment makes me feel the same way that [I feel about] knowing I've known the name for this thing that I am sitting on for the last 30 years, yet for the life of me I can't remember now what it is called. I can't really continue to practice law, since I'm not even aware that I'm missing important details in contracts I read."

> As the therapist listened to Tony, he became teary and overcome with sadness for this man. Inquiring about Tony's fears and feelings regarding his memory loss became a manageable way for Tony to talk about how AIDS was robbing him of the rest of his life. The psychotherapy began to focus on the concrete ways Tony could compensate for his memory loss, as well as on all of the feelings accompanying his need for these accommodations to his neuropsychiatric impairment. It was only at the urging of the therapist that Tony reported his symptoms to his primary care physician, who, because he was seeing Tony only monthly, hadn't noticed the mental deterioration. A neuropsychological evaluation revealed a probable diagnosis of an HIV-related dementia. These results precipitated discussions about the need for him to stop work and go on disability. Tony's memory loss also required him to ask his friends more directly for help. His increased dependence upon other people to help him adjust to losing his memory raised a host of feelings, which were explored continuously until his death a few months later.

As Tony's case illustrates, psychosocial interventions with clients who have HIV-related neuropsychiatric impairment require the use of a variety of skills. Traditional psychotherapy can help an affected individual express his or her feelings about the condition; it may even be the place where mental or emotional disability is first addressed. With such a patient, it is often useful for the mental health professional to take on a counseling role, which includes concrete problem solving in helping the patient make necessary adjustments for coping with disorientation, memory loss, reduced mobility, labile moods, and even psychotic decompensations. In addition to therapy and counseling, a case management approach is beneficial in terms of helping mobilize and prepare the entire group of individuals affected by the client's mental and emotional deterioration.

PRACTICAL CONSIDERATIONS

Many patients complain that the simple things in life now create the most frustration for them. When clinicians hear patients report difficulty in dealing with formerly easily handled activities of daily living, they are often uncertain of how to be most helpful while remaining clinically appropriate. When a patient with HIV infection reports experiencing diminished mental capacity, a more active and at times even directive series of interventions may be appropriate to ensure that treatment remains useful to the patient in his or her new and cognitively limited state. Unfortunately, actively making suggestions or being directive is contrary to traditional psychoanalytic training. Even many nonpsychoanalytic therapists are cautious and reluctant about changing how they work with patients in the midst of an ongoing treatment. These interventions should be conceptualized as counseling techniques, rather than as psychotherapy per se. Counseling differs from psychotherapy in that it focuses on concrete problem solving; it is often exactly what a patient experiencing early or advanced HIV-related dementia most needs from his or her mental health professional.

Table 6.1 (adapted from Buckingham & van Gorp, 1988) lists several practical recommendations that can greatly assist a person who is struggling with cognitive changes and the limitations that these changes represent. In particular, the conspicuous placement of a large calendar near the bedside or in the living space will help the individual remain oriented to the month, date, and year. Frequent notes, reminders, and appointment books serve as important memory aids since research has shown that patients with HIV-associated dementia benefit from cueing and recognition approaches (van Gorp, Hinkin, Satz, Miller, & D'Elia, 1993).

Because many patients with HIV-1-associated cognitive/motor complex also present with motor and gait disturbances, living arrangements should avoid structures with many steps, because the patients may fall or find climbing steps difficult.

Both the cognitive and the motor slowing that these patients experience often make it difficult for them to function in situations requiring quick decisions and actions. For example, working in a busy office setting may frustrate a mildly impaired patient who is in the early stages of the dementia process, and this frustration may promote a sense of failure and lack of coping. When a patient who suffers from

TABLE 6.1. Practical Considerations and Recommendations for Persons with HIV-Associated Dementia

Forgetfulness

1. Use calendars and appointment books.
2. Place Post-It notes in conspicuous places as reminders.
3. Make lists (questions for your physician, groceries needed, people to call, etc.).
4. Develop a list of important things to check when leaving the residence (stove, lights, etc.).
5. Use an alarm clock as a reminder for medications.
6. Keep a list of medications with dosages and times taken.
7. Ask for help if medications must be taken at different times and dosages.
8. Keep a journal detailing complex projects.
9. Use a cassette tape recorder to dictate thoughts and questions.
10. Purchase a noise-activated key chain.
11. Keep a telephone log and important numbers by the phone.

Slowed speech

1. Allow more time for collecting your thoughts and for conversations.
2. Don't hurry; give yourself permission to take your time.
3. Keep talking. Good conversation is good practice.

Visual–spatial problems

1. Don't drive if you are unable to do so.
2. If you are able to drive, plan routes in advance, allow plenty of time, and take a friend along when you can.
3. Use verbal directions instead of maps.
4. Realistically assess whether you are still able to drive at night.
5. Cease driving at night if your vision has become too impaired for you to be able to do so safely.

Depression and social withdrawal

1. Plan recreational activities.
2. Be an active participant.
3. Rekindle old hobbies and interests or create new ones.
4. Directly ask friends and family members to initiate social contacts, and instruct them not to take "no" for an answer unless you are too ill to socialize.

Concentration problems, inattentiveness, or distractibility

1. Try to limit distractions by confining your activities to a single task.
2. Meet with people one at a time.
3. Break large tasks down into more manageable jobs.
4. Turn the TV off when you are conversing or need to concentrate.
5. Don't drive in heavy traffic.

Problems with sequential reasoning or multistep tasks

1. Don't take on new or unfamiliar job responsibilities.
2. Avoid tasks in which speed of performance is important.
3. Simplify such things as meal preparation.
4. Plan activities when you are at your best (e.g., if you are a "morning person," schedule activities for the morning).

Note. Adapted from Buckingham and van Gorp (1988). Copyright 1988 by Family Service America, Inc. Adapted by permission.

any level of HIV-related cognitive impairment reports to the therapist that he or she is feeling increased levels of anxiety and/or depression, it is appropriate for the therapist to reflect back to the patient that the patient's current mental and cognitive limitations may be contributing to his or her emotional distress and to an overall sense of feeling overwhelmed. Having to stop working is often a traumatic loss for a person with AIDS and brings with it a corresponding loss in self-esteem and self-definition. Exploring potential options where the patient may be able to feel useful in a safe environment, such as volunteering at a local AIDS service organization or in a self-help group for people with HIV/AIDS, can be a useful intervention.

Whenever possible, demented patients should be in environments that are familiar and that have sufficient structure and support. Unfamiliar environments with no one to assist in activities of daily living may decrease independence and increase confusion even in a patient with mild dementia. Hospitalizations are often times when a patient in any stage of dementia is easily confused and overwhelmed by being in a new and unfamiliar environment. The therapist should encourage the patient's significant others to bring calendars and familiar photos or mementos to the hospital room to help orient the patient. In addition, placing important phone numbers next to the hospital phone can help reduce anxiety. One man, a former actor who had been able to remember pages of scripts, was no longer able even to remember his home phone number near the end of his illness. During his final hospitalization, his lover taped a note to the telephone that said: "For help call . . . " followed by both his home and office numbers, so that the patient could easily contact him at any time.

Patients with HIV-1-associated cognitive/motor complex may have sufficient *motivation* to undertake activities or tasks, but may lack the initiative needed for actually beginning the activity. This is common in other subcortical disturbances (e.g., Parkinson's disease), and assistance in initiating desired activities and tasks by family members or loved ones may provide the crucial impetus.

If a patient is a single parent, the therapist must do a careful assessment of whether the patient's reduced cognitive and concentration skills may endanger the children, or may contribute to their being neglected or abused. One woman with advanced AIDS was having difficulty finding her way to the office of the therapist she had been seeing for several years. One day this woman reported to the therapist that she had kept her young daughter waiting after school, because she herself was wandering around the neighborhood lost and confused. When she had not claimed her daughter after an hour, the school called the woman's mother, who came right away and brought her

granddaughter to her apartment. The child was understandably frightened by her mother's not keeping to their regular schedule. Once the
therapist learned about this incident, she called a family session with
the patient and the patient's mother and siblings, in order to develop
a plan that would ensure safety and continuity of care for the young
daughter. This practical, creative, and often unconventional management approach is not a traditional psychoanalytic or psychotherapeutic
one, but such an approach is needed in order to provide a comprehensive level of psychosocial support to patients suffering from HIV-related
cognitive impairment.

Another sensitive issue is at what point a referral to an HIV-
related day treatment program is an appropriate intervention by the
therapist. When introducing this or other issues relating to a patient's
need for assistance, the therapist must be sensitive and skillful. A
central difficulty in attempting to enlist family, friends, and other
caregivers in helping the patient who is cognitively impaired is the
treading of a fine line in avoiding having people do things for the
patient that the patient can still do for himself or herself. Developing
ways to ensure that the patient is compliant with an extensive schedule of infusions and oral medications is another example of how the
therapist, together with family and friends, may need to function as a
case manager for the individual experiencing HIV-related memory
loss and disorientation.

As illustrated by the case above in which the woman was too
disoriented to remember the location of her child's school, patients
with advanced HIV-related cognitive impairment may be too disoriented to be able to travel unaccompanied to or from the therapist's
(or any other health care professional's) office. If a patient does not
have a companion, friend, or aide to ensure his or her safe arrival, it
may become necessary for the therapist to consider doing home visits
if the patient still wishes to continue having sessions. Obviously, when
travel time to and from the patient's home is figured in, home sessions
make greater time demands on the therapist. In some cases, the patient
may live too far away from where the therapist either works or lives
for home visits to be practical. However, in cases where home visits are
possible, they serve multiple purposes. They can provide the patient
with a source of support, comfort, and continuity in his or her
life—factors that may be all too rare because of the complications
associated with advanced or terminal-stage AIDS. In addition, a home
visit provides the therapist with the opportunity to assess what level of
care the patient is receiving or in need of, if he or she is still capable
of living independently. In some cases it will be obvious from the
condition of the home or apartment that the individual should no

longer be living alone. A home visit then gives the therapist an opportunity to raise this painful and difficult issue with the patient.

When neuropsychiatric impairment increases to the point at which the patient is no longer able to concentrate long enough to follow the thread of a normal conversation during a psychotherapy session, the therapist can be comforting and helpful in ways that are not traditional forms of psychotherapy. One useful option is for the therapist to read or recite meditations, poetry, or visualizations to the patient, in the hope of calming an agitated state and temporarily reducing fears. One of us is trained in hypnotherapy and finds doing relaxation and pain control work while a patient is in hypnotic trance to be very effective clinical tools. Similarly, guiding a patient in visualizations is very useful if the therapist makes some audiotapes and leaves them with the patient, so the patient can experience this kind of relief between sessions.

EDUCATIONAL CONSIDERATIONS

Not surprisingly, family members or significant others are often frustrated by the physical and mental debilitation their loved one is experiencing. They may have a "need to blame," and they may unconsciously act this out by attributing a patient's forgetfulness to noncompliance, willful stubbornness, or manipulation. This is a common occurrence, and the clinician must be vigilant to educate those close to the demented patient about the actual limitations their loved one is facing. Slowing, confusion, and forgetfulness are all characteristics of HIV-associated dementia; when present, they probably do not reflect intentional manipulation, but actual brain changes resulting in clinical symptomatology.

Providing information and educational resources to patients diagnosed with more or less severe cognitive decline associated with HIV is another important factor in the care of these patients. Many such patients have little or no understanding of neurological functioning or the diseases that affect cognition. Thus, it is often a useful intervention for the therapist to suggest a "family" session for the patient and all of the important caregivers in his or her system. The focus of this session should be psychoeducational: All present should be educated about the nature of HIV dementia, told what new symptoms to be on the lookout for, and given suggestions for managing the cognitive impairment. Most patients, upon hearing the term "dementia," envision the most severe clinical characteristics—usually those associated with Alzheimer's disease, such as complete memory loss and "vegetable"-like mannerisms. Providing patients with a better understanding of neuropsychological functioning and the kind of changes associated with subcortical disease will greatly reduce the fears and worries of those affected.

CLINICAL CONSIDERATIONS

Assessment of clinical depression is important in any patient with HIV, but this is especially true when questions arise regarding the patient's mental functioning. When slowing, forgetfulness, and concentration problems are present, the clinician must attempt to differentiate the effects of depression from early signs of HIV-associated dementia. This is best done by inquiring into the mood state of the individual and being alert to atypical signs of pessimism, feelings of worthlessness, and suicidality. Since most patients diagnosed with HIV-associated dementia are aware of their declining mental capabilities, they may be understandably depressed. This, coupled with the well-established and broad range of psychosocial assaults associated with HIV, creates a high-risk situation for patients who are also experiencing cognitive impairment. If signs of depression are present, the depressive condition should be appropriately treated. Depression can further encroach upon the mental capacities of an already impaired individual.

Assessment of suicide potential is also important in these patients, in light of the increased prevalence of depression in patients with various subcortical diseases (e.g., Parkinson's or Huntington's disease). Crisis resources should be available to the clinician involved with this population, in the event that an impaired patient experiences suicidal intent. The unique mix of psychosocial trauma with a probable biological contribution to depression in this group creates fertile ground for suicidal intent and planning. The clinician must be vigilant and resourceful when signs of suicidality are present. (See Chapter 8, this volume.)

It is important for psychotherapists who work with people with HIV/AIDS to be able to differentiate between an individual who is irrationally suicidal and one who rationally wishes to choose what is known as "self-deliverance" from the ravages of the final stages of a terminal illness. Most patients with end-stage AIDS who discuss wanting to end their own lives often suffer from inadequately treated pain or untreated depression. Once these conditions are successfully treated, some people still feel that "enough is enough" and it is time to die. Self-deliverance is about dying with dignity. It is not always simply about the control of pain in end-stage illness; it is about ending suffering, and suffering can take many forms that compromise quality of life. The medical director of San Francisco General Hospital's AIDS Clinic, Dr. John Stansell, has said, "The simple fact is that there are some patients for whom we cannot make death a tolerable process" (quoted in

Holtby, 1997, p. 40). Many patients we have seen who discuss wanting to have the means available to end their own lives raise this subject long before the onset of dementia. These same individuals express the fear that if they become demented, they may lose their ability to act rationally on their desire to end their lives. This is where serious ethical issues arise for the professional who supports a patient's right to choose the timing of his or her own death. Clearly, once an individual has lost the ability to think clearly, there is a question about how "rational" the person's decision to end his or her life can be.

In one study, 83.3% of people with AIDS said that euthanasia or assisted suicide was a choice they were considering, and reported that the knowledge that they could take their own lives helped them to cope. Many of these respondents stated that they liked to be in control of all aspects of their lives, so it made sense that they be in control of their deaths (Ogden, 1994). Many persons with HIV/AIDS fear that once they become demented they will lose their window for self-deliverance, and discuss with trusted friends concrete plans for being helped to end their own lives. Even for health care professionals who believe in assisted suicide, one foundation of this belief is the ability of the patient to make a rational choice for himself or herself, as noted above. Once a person has become demented, he or she may no longer have the cognitive ability to initiate self-deliverance. Therefore, prior planning and specific instructions are crucial if this has been the planned choice of the neuropsychologically impaired patient prior to the onset of symptoms of dementia. Obviously this places enormous strains upon the patient's partner or other caregiver, who will be responsible for initiating an assisted suicide. (Suicide and HIV disease are discussed further in Chapter 8 of this volume.)

Psychotherapy may also serve as a supportive environment for patients wishing to discuss estate planning, advanced medical directives, medical power of attorney, and living wills. In addition to the legal issues inherent in these topics, concretely planning for the end of one's life has significant emotional ramifications, which become complicated as cognitive impairment sets in. Because wills and other legal documents are sometimes contested after death on the grounds of alleged mental incompetence, referral for neuropsychiatric evaluation by a second mental health professional is one way of possibly establishing the patient's level of competence prior to his or her death. It should be noted that compromised neuropsychological performance alone does not necessarily render a patient legally incompetent. (See Chapter 10 of this volume for further discussion of this issue.)

In many cases, countertransference issues arise for therapists who work with patients diagnosed with HIV-associated dementia. Professionals who work with cognitively impaired patients frequently experience countertransference problems because of their own inability to reverse the course of the mental deterioration. As the case of Tony described earlier in this chapter illustrates, it is not helpful to treatment when both the therapist and patient avoid bringing up indications of the onset of AIDS dementia complex during the course of psychotherapy. Presentation of symptoms of HIV-associated dementia gives both the patient and therapist concrete evidence of the fact that HIV disease is progressing; this raises a host of understandable feelings (most often powerlessness and anger), which the clinician must be prepared to recognize in order for them not to interfere with effective treatment. These dynamics are particularly important for clinicians, because HIV is still a relatively new, lethal, and predominantly sexually transmitted disease that was first identified in socially stigmatized groups. Identification and acknowledgment of countertransference issues are crucial and require that the clinician have adequate self-awareness to respond effectively.

CONCLUSIONS

Much of this chapter has discussed how the cognitive changes associated with HIV infection can create a clinical situation that stretches the boundaries of traditional psychotherapy and the role of the clinician. Given the current changes in health and mental health care delivery, such as managed care, clinicians who work with people with HIV/AIDS must be able to deal with a wide range of clinical problems and disorders. HIV-1-associated cognitive/motor complex is a good example of how clinicians must respond to a greater range of clinical phenomena while at the same time being specialists. The interventions we have described here can make a critical difference in the care and management of patients who have HIV-associated dementia. Through early detection, accurate differential diagnosis, and sound clinical intervention, practitioners can increase the quality of care available to all those affected by such dementia.

REFERENCES

American Academy of Neurology. (1991). Nomenclature and research case definitions for neurologic manifestations of human immunodeficiency virus—type 1 (HIV-1) infection: Report of a working group of the American Academy of Neurology AIDS Task Force. *Neurology, 41,* 778–785.
Buckingham, S. L., & van Gorp, W. (1988). AIDS-dementia complex: Implications

for practice. *Social Casework: The Journal of Contemporary Social Work, 69,* 371–375.

Holtby, M. (1997). HIV, suicide and hastened death. *National Social Work AIDS Network Readings and Writings, 2*(1), 36–49.

Ogden, R. (1994). *Euthanasia, assisted suicide and AIDS.* New Westminster, British Columbia: Peroglyphics.

Ostrow, D. (1996). Mental health issues across the HIV-1 spectrum for gay and bisexual men. In R. Cabaj & T. Stein (Eds.), *Textbook of homosexuality and mental health* (pp. 859–880). Washington, DC: American Psychiatric Press.

van Gorp, W., Hinkin, C., Satz, P., Miller, E., & D'Elia, L. F. (1993). Neuropsychological findings in HIV infection, encephalopathy, and dementia. In Parks, Zec, & Wilson (Eds.), *Neuropsychology of Alzheimer's disease and other dementias* (pp. 153–185). New York: Oxford University Press.

7

Issues for Caregivers, Families, and Significant Others

IAN STULBERG

JILL SHAPIRA

INTRODUCTION

From virtually every perspective, the HIV epidemic is unique and challenges our more traditional notions—of disease and the disease process; of the delivery of medical care; of the relationship between the provider and the consumer of medical care; of human developmental stages and human sexuality; and of our attitudes toward those who are ill and of the provision of services to them. Just as the disease process of HIV is exacerbated by the fact that it is caused by immune suppression, which leaves its victims vulnerable to an incredible array of infections and medical complications, the psychosocial environment of HIV/AIDS is made more complex and problematic by an atmosphere of fear, prejudice, and moral righteousness. And the complexity of issues in both the medical and environmental spheres results in the unique and overwhelming psychosocial issues with which both people with HIV/AIDS and their caregivers must contend (Stulberg & Buckingham, 1988). As we examine the psychosocial issues specific to both personal and professional caregivers of people suffering from neuropsychiatric complications of HIV/AIDS, we will see not only that they encompass many of the issues typical for caregivers of people with other, non-HIV-related neuropsychiatric illnesses (specifically Alzheimer's disease), but that they are further complicated by the medical and environmental factors unique to HIV (Boccellari & Zeifert, 1994).

This chapter examines issues relevant to all those who provide care to a person with AIDS (PWA). "Personal caregivers" are lovers, family members, and friends who have a primary emotional bond with the individual who is ill. "Professional caregivers" are health care providers who enter into contracts with patients and their significant others to contribute physical care and emotional support when the need arises. As the mental status of a PWA declines, professional caregivers work together with personal caregivers to ensure an optimal quality of life for the PWA. This chapter begins with a discussion of general psychosocial issues related to HIV/AIDS and to the concomitant neuropsychiatric complications (our primary emphasis here is on dementia). Specific intervention strategies for caregivers are then reviewed. And, finally, recommendations for caregivers are offered.

PSYCHOSOCIAL ISSUES OF PERSONAL CAREGIVERS

The caregivers of PWAs may differ from more traditional caregivers in many significant ways. For example, caregivers of people with Alzheimer's disease have traditionally been female family members. Caregivers of PWAs, however, may *include* family members, but are much more likely to be partners (most often male), as well as members of an extended network of friends (frequently *previous* partners), neighbors, and community volunteers (Wardlaw, 1994). This phenomenon is one aspect of the unique environment of the AIDS epidemic: Because most PWAs in the United States are also members of previously stigmatized groups, they may have a greater likelihood than other people of being alienated from families of origin, and thus relying more heavily on "families of choice."

Although the phenomenon of PWAs being cared for by their "chosen families" is one of the more positive and uplifting consequences of the epidemic, the downside is that families of choice do not automatically come with the same legal rights and guarantees as families of origin. Family-of-choice members may face challenges to their roles as caregivers, as well as to their rights of inheritance, by family-of-origin members who have difficulty accepting the lifestyle of a PWA.

Moreover, whereas Alzheimer's disease strikes individuals in the latter stages of life, AIDS primarily affects individuals who are in the prime productive periods of their lives (over 80% are between the ages of 20 and 50), which means that their caregivers also tend to be much younger than "traditional" caregivers. Increased stress may be a consequence of assuming a caregiving role at a young age, as well as of preparing for the death of a partner or friend some 30–50 years prematurely. Caregiving responsibilities at a younger age may also mean a lack of financial resources and hampered career development (Folkman, Chesney, & Christopher-Richards, 1994). The parental caregiver of an adult child with AIDS may experience stress unique to the untimely loss of a child, which undermines the parent's sense of developmental life stages.

The pervasiveness of AIDS, particularly in the gay community, adds a further complication to the role of caregiver. One study found that almost 54% of urban gay and bisexual men had provided informal care to a loved one with AIDS (Folkman et al., 1994). A study of AIDS caregivers conducted at the University of California at San Francisco (UCSF) found that 96% of caregivers had lost at least one close friend to AIDS, and, furthermore, that 76% of traditional family member caregivers knew at least one person who had died of AIDS (Wardlaw, 1994). Consequences of providing care for someone with AIDS in the midst of a community that has been devastated by the disease may include difficulty in obtaining help and support from others, and/or a reluctance to ask for support from others already burdened with loss and caretaking responsibilities (Levin, Buckingham, & Hart, 1996); the inability to "get a break" from the illness, which pervades all aspects of one's life and thus provides constant reminders of illness and death (Boccellari & Zeifert, 1994); and, ultimately, an impaired ability to process one's grief appropriately because of the experience of "providing care under the burden of chronic, unresolved grief" (Wardlaw, 1994, p. 376).

The stigmatized nature of the AIDS epidemic may also complicate caregivers' access to support: They may be reluctant to acknowledge the true nature of their loved ones' illness to others, or they may be forbidden to do so *by* their loved ones (Stulberg & Buckingham, 1988). The burden of caregiving can become immense for such individuals, who may become PWAs' sole source of both practical and emotional support.

Perhaps the issue for HIV/AIDS caregivers that sets them furthest apart from more traditional caregivers is the fact that because HIV is a communicable disease and is most often spread via sexual activity, a caregiver is also susceptible to the illness of his or her loved one. Indeed, the UCSF caregiver study found that 35% of "nontraditional" caregivers were themselves HIV-positive (Wardlaw, 1994). It is difficult to imagine the emotional implications of caring for someone whose inevitable decline foretells the experience that probably awaits the caregiver, who may also have to go through this experience *without* similar involvement from a loved one (Kain, 1996). For a caregiver who is not HIV-infected, sex and intimacy issues may become major sources of conflict and concern: What does it mean when the primary means of expressing closeness and caring to a loved one has also become a potential means of exposing oneself to death?

What is more, noninfected caregivers must assume a level of precaution in the provision of practical support to their loved ones, which is not the case for caregivers in other settings. Fear of contagion may be a particularly salient issue for family caregivers, who may be confronting AIDS for the first time while providing care to their loved ones and may not have the level of sophistication about the disease and its transmission that is common within affected communities.

As noted in the introduction to this chapter, AIDS caregiving is further complicated by the fact that caregivers are not simply responding to a single medical entity, but to a myriad of infections and medical complications. In addition to neuropsychological problems PWAs are susceptible to gastrointestinal disturbances, including unrelenting diarrhea; eye infections, which may lead to blindness; peripheral neuropathy, which causes pain in the extremities and makes ambulation difficult; chronic fevers and drenching night sweats; and profound fatigue—among others. Clearly, caregiving responsibilities may increase exponentially as a PWA's medical picture becomes more complicated and extensive. Such responsibilities may include assistance with activities of daily living, including bathing, feeding, cooking, cleaning, shopping, and providing transportation; management of the loved one's legal and financial concerns; coordination of outside services and resources; and provision of in-home medical care, including injections and intravenous therapies. All these responsibilities must be assumed in addition to being the primary source of emotional support to the PWA (Kain, 1996). The UCSF study indicated that caregivers spent an average of 100 hours per week with their loved ones (L. Wardlaw, personal communication, 1995).

Because it is rare for a PWA to demonstrate symptoms of cognitive impairment prior to the experience of other physical manifestations of HIV (Buckingham & van Gorp, 1994), it is possible that a caregiver will be confronted with neuropsychological complications in his or her loved one after already having reached a level of physical and emotional exhaustion from months or years of caretaking responsibilities (Levin et al., 1996; Monahan & Hooker, 1995). A sibling of a PWA told one of us that he knew nothing about HIV-associated dementia when his brother began demonstrating symptoms, but he acknowledged being too overwhelmed with other-responsibilities to have the energy to find out more about it: "It was just another thing he had."

The statement above may be typical for many caregivers, who may be so overwhelmed by their situation that they are unable or unwilling to cognitively process what is happening to them and their loved ones. Such individuals may adopt a "just put one foot in front of the other" approach to getting through each day. Consequently, it is not surprising that these caregivers either may be oblivious to early symptoms of cognitive impairment or may assume that they are attributable to other interpersonal factors.

However, it is easy for *any* individual who has not been educated in the often subtle manifestations of HIV-associated dementia to misinterpret or misunderstand such symptoms when they arise—regardless of whether or not he or she has *also* had to contend with emotional and physical exhaustion! Many of the early symptoms of dementia (flat affect, memory problems, distractibility, etc.) are often attributed to other causes, such as depression, stubbornness, or anxiety, by both personal and professional caregivers (Buckingham & van Gorp, 1994; Boccellari & Zeifert, 1994). The fact that people with dementia may have difficulty recalling new information, but may be able to recognize it when prompted, may cause a caretaker to assume that a PWA is simply being willful or manipulative: "He remembers what he *wants* to remember!" (Buckingham & van Gorp, 1994). This picture is further complicated by the fact that the actual occurrence of depression in PWAs may be particularly high (up to 76% may experience depressed mood); moreover, individuals suffering from subcortical brain impairment are susceptible to mood disorders that are attributable in part to their central nervous system complications (Buckingham & van Gorp, 1994).

Although simple ignorance regarding dementia, and/or the experience of being overwhelmed by caretaking responsibilities, may be the primary explanation(s) for such misunderstandings, the role that denial may play in these situations should not be underestimated. It is probably safe to say that most caregivers would prefer to think that their loved ones are "just being stubborn" than that the PWAs are starting to lose their mental faculties. Many caregivers will tell themselves, "This is just a phase she's going through. Things will get back to normal again soon." One complication for such caregivers is that they develop such an *external* point of focus—in order to get through each day—that they may fail to process what is happening to them emotionally, thereby leaving their *inner* resources undeveloped. These individuals are much less likely to be able to acknowledge and, ideally, to grieve for the losses as they occur, and may therefore be particularly unprepared at the end for their loved ones' death.

Cognitive changes resulting from early stages of such neuropsychological disorders as dementia or progressive multifocal leukoencephalopathy (PML) may result in a degree of paranoia and distrustfulness on the part of PWAs, which—along with other symptoms mentioned above (e.g., apathy, mental inflexibility)—may be misunderstood by their caregivers. Without an awareness of organicity as a factor in such personality changes, the caregivers are likely to personalize exchanges with their loved one: They may feel hurt, abused, or at fault, or assume that something has changed in their relationship (Wardlaw, personal communication, 1995). Such experiences can contribute to an overall feeling on the caregivers' part of "rudderlessness" or confusion about what exactly is going on.

Of course, even though being made aware of the presence of neuropsychological complications may provide some alleviation of the above-noted stresses by clarifying the situation, it still leaves the caregivers with the devastating reality that their loved ones' mental faculties are deteriorating—and, furthermore, that there is very little medical science can do to treat the situation. Neuropsychological impairment is often identified by both PWAs and their caregivers as their worst HIV-related nightmare (Kain, 1996). No matter how overwhelming other medical manifestations of HIV/AIDS may be, PWAs are still left with the possibility of communicating effectively with their loved ones about their experience. And although personality changes may occur in PWAs in *reaction* to the various stresses of their illness, these changes generally are not perceived to be as global, irreversible, or devastating as the changes that may result from neuropsychological impairment. One lover of a PWA with PML told one of us, "It was one of the major shocks of my life to see someone I knew so well change in front of my eyes." Others providing care to loved ones with dementia have stated that they felt as if they were caring for "a stranger" (Wardlaw, personal communication, 1995).

As a PWA's mental faculties begin to deteriorate, the practical issue of providing for his or her needs and safety becomes more of a priority. The need for the caregiver to assume many of the responsibilities previously managed by the PWA may create numerous emotional conflicts with the PWA, as well as psychological obstacles with which the caregiver must contend.

Addressing the issue of shifting responsibilities from the PWA to the caregiver is a delicate psychological task, as it may symbolize the acknowledgment of the PWA's real or eventual deterioration—a reality that both the PWA and his or her caregiver may be reluctant to confront (Livingston, 1996; Wardlaw, 1994; Folkman et al., 1994). A common coping defense of many PWAs is a reluctance to acknowledge a decline in physical capabilities to others; however, as difficult as it may be to admit the limitations of their *physical* abilities, the acknowledgment that they may no longer be capable of making their own decisions is likely to be an even greater psychological hurdle to cross. It is very often the case that PWAs will demonstrate enough impairment in mental faculties to cause their caregivers concern, but will retain sufficient cognitive abilities to resist suggestions and offers of assistance from others.

Whether and when to assume responsibilities for PWAs may be extremely difficult decisions for caregivers to make, as they may raise concerns about invading the PWAs' privacy, undermining their autonomy, and contributing to feelings of powerlessness and loss of control. The caregivers, in turn, may struggle with their own feelings of guilt and resentment over this issue (Folkman et al., 1994; Boccellari & Zeifert, 1994).

When a PWA's cognitive impairment has progressed to the point that he or she is unable to be safely left alone, the caregiver may be faced with the issue of placement in an outside facility. In the UCSF caregivers study, dementia was among the most frequently mentioned reasons for placing a PWA in a hospice or skilled nursing facility (Wardlaw, personal communication, 1995). Even when placement options are readily available to PWAs (generally only in large metropolitan areas), their caregivers may struggle with feelings of guilt at having failed or abandoned the loved ones. Often the caregivers will have promised the loved ones early in the disease process to care for them at home until the end. When the reality of the PWAs' caretaking needs subsequently exceeds the caregivers' ability to provide adequate and safe care, the decision to place the PWAs can be an agonizing one.

Many times, however, placement options are extremely limited or nonexistent—particularly for PWAs whose medical status is stable, but whose cognitive impairment is so severe that it necessitates 24-hour care. Many existing facilities may refuse admission because of concerns about their ability to manage the PWAs' medical needs. Others may require a "rehabilitative" psychiatric diagnosis (Lee & McGill, 1991). Access to some facilities may be denied because of inadequate financial or insurance resources. Such situations severely test the practical, as well as psychological and emotional, resources of caregivers.

Among the myriad of difficult emotions common to caregivers of PWAs suffering from cognitive impairment, anger may be among the most prevalent (Livingston, 1996; Monahan & Hooker, 1995). Given that one of caregivers' primary motivations is to obtain proper medical care for the PWAs (Powell-Cope, 1994), when no adequate or truly effective medical care exists for conditions like dementia or PML, the caregivers may be left with feelings of great frustration and rage—feelings that they may be at a loss to express and direct effectively (Stulberg & Buckingham, 1988).

Guilt is perhaps the other feeling most common to caregivers (Levin et al., 1996). Guilt may be associated both with what a caregiver failed to do (provide "better" care, protect the loved one from harm, or even *cure* the loved one of illness) and with what he or she *did* do or wanted to do (take personal time away from caretaking responsibilities, experience pleasure outside the relationship). Guilt is also potentially one of the most harmful of emotions for caregivers, as their defense against it may be to extend their caretaking responsibilities even further and to deny themselves pleasure or respite of any kind. Clearly, the psychological health of caregivers in this situation is severely at risk.

PSYCHOSOCIAL RESPONSES
OF PROFESSIONAL CAREGIVERS

Many different professionals provide health care to PWAs: social workers, nurses, physicians, psychologists, and home health aides. Caring for any sick person creates demands upon health care providers, but the special circumstances of AIDS cause many professional caregivers to experience exceptional stress. The fact that many health care workers face contagion is documented in several studies (Blumenfield, Smith, Milazzo, Seropian, & Wormser, 1987; Link, Feingold, Charap, Freeman, & Shelov, 1988; Pleck, O'Donnell, O'Donnell, & Snarey 1988; Richardson & Lochner 1987), even though very few cases of health care workers' contracting HIV are documented (Brewington, 1994).

The incurable nature of AIDS means that professional caregivers experience multiple losses as patients eventually die (Lovejoy, 1988). Macks and Abrams (1992, p. 291) conclude that this can result in "bereavement overload," in which "people cannot complete grieving [for] one loss before confronting the next one." In addition, feelings of helplessness and futility may result from the knowledge that as yet no cure exists (Van Servellen & Leake, 1994).

Because professional health care providers bring their own cultural beliefs, values, and attitudes into the work setting, at least some of them may have difficulty in providing care to persons with a different sexual orientation. Homophobia is frequently named as a psychological stressor in clinical observations, anecdotal reports, and questionnaire surveys (Silverman, 1993). Some providers are comfortable with homosexual clients, but resent working with patients who contracted HIV through injection drug use or prostitution.

When a PWA develops dementia, additional stressors emerge. It is often difficult to "connect" personally with a demented patient; thus a provider gives care in a vacuum, without the benefit of a mutual patient–provider relationship. Also, the usual age for dementia to occur is much older than that seen in AIDS, as noted earlier. It is emotionally difficult for a professional to accept severe cognitive impairment in a person close to his or her own age, and this causes an uncomfortable sense of vulnerability.

Hospital staff members are often constrained by institutional policies that stimulate grievances and psychosocial concerns of patients. Foley and Fahs (1994) interviewed 50 hospitalized PWAs. Themes related to depersonalizing behaviors by staff members and communication deficits emerged. These patients interpreted the required hospital routine as uncaring and depersonalized attitudes on the part of the nursing staff. The patients also experienced communication deficits when they were not given enough information. The competing demands of compassionate patient care and institutional requirements compound the stress upon hospital personnel. Staff members may not know the answers to the difficult questions of patients and caregivers, such as the possibility of cognitive recovery or the speed of mental decline.

Because demented patients are unable to meet their own self-care needs, health care workers depend upon personal caregivers to provide necessary care for the patients at home. Yet friends and family members are quickly overwhelmed, and must themselves be supported by the professional caregivers. Thus, the circle of people needing care enlarges. Community resources vary, depending upon population size and prevalence of HIV infection (Boccellari & Zeifert, 1994). Unfortunately, resources are more difficult to find for patients with cognitive and behavioral problems. Their need for constant supervision is often unmet within the existing structure of health care, and this situation provokes feelings of frustration and helplessness among both personal and professional caregivers.

SPECIFIC CAREGIVER INTERVENTIONS

Although many of the following recommended interventions are specific to a professional caregiving situation, a number of interventions are also applicable to personal caregivers as well.

Interventions for Patients with Mild Impairment

Once the features of cognitive dysfunction are apparent, a complete medical, neurological, and neuropsychological assessment is performed to assess for other, treatable conditions, such as concurrent physical illness, nutritional deficiency, side effects of medications, anxiety, or depression. Providing the patient with complete information about the reason for and conduct of each scheduled examination helps alleviate undue anxiety about the assessment process. The professional team reviews the information and then formulates suggestions to reinforce strengths and compensate for cognitive deficits. The plan of care is individualized and designed in collaboration with the PWA and personal caregiver(s).

When patients have a mild degree of cognitive impairment, the role of the professional team is to help the PWAs and caregivers establish realistic goals that are within the PWAs' present capabilities. Cognitive strengths are identified and reinforced. Personal caregivers are encouraged to allow the PWAs as much independence and control as possible. The following interventions (Boccellari & Zeifert, 1994; Ungvarski & Staats, 1995) should be established as soon as cognitive impairment is identified. Personal caregivers also find these coping strategies helpful.

Since forgetfulness is a predominant problem, methods that help PWAs attend to the environment and retrieve previously learned information are useful. Talking aloud while performing a task focuses attention. Similarly, the use of memory aids, such as writing down all appointments and chores to do, supplements impaired memory function. Personal caregivers can also provide written reminders of scheduled activities. When telephoning, health professionals should first make sure that PWAs have paper and pencil handy before providing the PWAs with any information. It is recommended that both personal and professional caregivers make reminder calls before scheduled appointments.

PWAs and their caregivers are encouraged to examine daily tasks and identify which ones have become too difficult or stressful. Perhaps tasks can be redistributed; paying bills could be traded for doing the dishes every night, for example. In addition, nonstressful mental stimulation is important. Board games, crossword puzzles, and video games can be enjoyed by both PWAs and their caregivers.

Clients are asked to identify what times of the day are best for them. By scheduling appointments during these times, and by encouraging clients to avoid doing too many tasks at one time, professional caregivers can help reduce fatigue for the PWAs. Adequate rest is important for both PWAs and caregivers, and discussion about which activities are essential and which ones can be delayed is encouraged by members of the health care team.

Stress reduction is important for both PWAs and their caregivers. Many relaxing activities can be done together, such as walking, massage, listening to music, attending movies, and visiting with friends and family members. Incorporating routine into daily activities, while cognitive strengths exist fosters better retention of skills.

Finally, beneficial coping strategies that PWAs and caregivers are already employing may be identified by asking them to relate positive or meaningful experiences that occur. Learning to "seize the moment" and enjoy ordinary events (Folkman et al., 1994) early in the course of the disease helps buffer dysphoria and maintain positive morale during later and more difficult stages.

Interventions for Patients with HIV-Associated Dementia Complex

Although the course of HIV-associated dementia is variable, this syndrome is progressive and incurable. In the early stages, the strategies discussed above are helpful in maintaining autonomy and independence in clients and their personal caregivers. However, in later stages of dementia, PWAs are no longer able to monitor their own self-care activities, and the roles and responsibilities of both personal and professional caregivers expand. Caregivers learn to structure the environment of the demented individuals, and generally accept more of a directive function (Boccellari & Zeifert, 1994). Health professionals, especially nursing staff members in hospital settings, provide more direct care, and are thus able to compare and share strategies with personal caregivers to ensure high-quality patient care. Spending time with hospitalized patients' friends and family members also allows the professional team to assess these individuals' specific physical and emotional needs related to the caregiving role.

Because patients with dementia present with differing degrees of impairment, professional caregivers should conduct ongoing assessments of cognitive and behavioral function. This is especially important when patients are hospitalized in an unfamiliar environment and removed from a regular routine. It is also helpful to note whether patients are more alert during specific times of the day; perhaps diagnostic tests or teaching sessions can be scheduled to maximize patient participation.

Since thinking and communication problems are features of HIV-associated dementia, caregivers need to allow enough time for working with these individuals. It is best to reduce background noise, make eye contact, and speak slowly to get and maintain the PWAs' attention.

Caregivers should present information slowly, giving only one command at a time. Written instructions and nonverbal communication strategies can be used to supplement the spoken word. For example, a caregiver can pantomime the gesture of drinking when asking whether a PWA would like some juice. Dementia patients have difficulty monitoring their own feelings and are sensitive to the emotional states of others; the rushed behavior of a nurse may be misinterpreted as anger and may precipitate an agitated reaction. A well-timed calming breath before beginning a counseling session or entering a patient's room helps dissipate some of the normal hassles of the day for busy staff members.

Demented individuals often have severe memory problems that worsen considerably when they are presented with a new situation, such as hospitalization. Staff members should always introduce themselves each time they meet with patients and orient them to their surroundings and the time of day; they should also explain carefully what is going to happen before initiating an activity. A blackboard listing the day's activities facilitates orientation. A patient should be kept in the same room whenever possible, and family and friends should be encouraged to bring personal items from home. Rearranging of items should be avoided. Placing written and pictorial labels on the closet and bathroom is helpful to some. Caregivers can maintain as much structure in patient's daily routine as possible by following the patients' usual patterns in bathing and eating. Flexibility on the,part of professional caregivers is clearly beneficial to these patients.

Problems with motor weakness, balance, and coordination also occur in people with HIV dementia. Caregivers and staff members may notice a change in handwriting, or difficulty tying shoelaces, zipping clothes, or using buttons (Boccellari & Zeifert, 1994). Adaptive devices may prove helpful, and consultation with a physical or occupational therapist is suggested. These individuals are at risk for falls, particularly when hospitalized or in new environments. Supervision of all ambulatory activities is desirable. Nursing staff can learn from personal caregivers how patients manage at home; information shared between personal and professional caregivers helps patients maintain as much independent functioning as possible, and also alerts the staff to acute changes in the patients' behavior. A sudden worsening of mental status may indicate the presence of a delirium due to the effects of a physical condition or medication.

Interventions for Patients with Delirium and Dementia

Delirium is often seen in patients with dementia, as individuals with compromised brain function are at risk of developing this acute confusional state (Cummings, Benson, & LoVerme, 1980). If delirium is misdiagnosed as the dementia related to HIV/AIDS, treatable conditions may remain unrecognized. Even if a patient has an underlying cognitive impairment, any sudden change in behavior should be carefully evaluated, and reversible illnesses (e.g., pneumonia, urinary tract infection) can then be promptly treated. Personal caregivers are often the first to identify acute alterations in mental status or behavior; professional caregivers depend on these observations as well as their own baseline evaluations. Patients with delirium should be hospitalized while the cause of the problem is identified and appropriate treatment ordered.

When delirium is present, the goal of professional caregivers is to provide all necessary care, as delirious patients are unable to meet their own physical and emotional needs. Confused patients must be protected from environmental or self-imposed harm.

Patients in this confusional state are intermittently disoriented to their surroundings; this may precipitate agitated behaviors. Each time a caregiver enters a delirious patient's room, the caregiver should remind the patient where he or she is. In addition, a large poster can be placed on the wall with a message such as this: "Jim Smith, you are in Community Hospital." Some individuals benefit from having the television or radio on, whereas others only become more confused with additional stimuli. A caregiver should provide identification each time the room is entered and explain what will be done in direct statements—for example, "Mr. Smith, I am your nurse, Carol. I will take your temperature now." The caregiver should also make sure that the patient can perceive the environment correctly; if glasses are normally worn, the personal caregiver should be asked to bring them to the hospital. The patient's life experiences or special interests can be used as an "internal orientation"; the caregiver can ask about previous occupations, hobbies, or pets. The effectiveness of each strategy should be evaluated with ongoing assessment, and the ones that are helpful in decreasing each patient's behavioral disturbances should be documented (Shapira, Roper, & Schulzinger, 1993; Swanson, Cronin-Stubbs, & Colletti, 1990).

Confused patients become agitated because they feel a threat to their safety. Caregivers can validate their feelings by calmly stating, "I understand you feel afraid. I will not harm you. I am here to help you." If a patient is at risk for self-harm through pulling out intravenous tubings or falling from bed, chemical or physical restraint may be necessary. A low dose of a major tranquilizer, such as haloperidol (0.5 mg) or thioridazine (10 mg), may be prescribed. However, some patients become even more confused and agitated with these medications; careful observation helps determine the effectiveness of the medication.

It is important to offer emotional support to the personal caregivers of confused and agitated patients. It can be quite disturbing for them to see their loved ones out of control and unable to communicate. They may also be embarrassed about unusual behaviors. Family members and friends should be allowed to express their fears and dismay. If they wish to participate in a patient's care, staff members can suggest ways to be helpful; for example, a personal caregiver can sit by the bedside and talk to the patient, or assist with meals. Staff members should also explain that a medical condition is responsible for a patient's actions, and that the patient should return to a previous level of functioning when the acute illness abates. Personal caregivers should be kept informed about patients' progress, and anticipatory planning for discharge should be encouraged.

Support for Personal Caregivers of Hospitalized Patients

As patients become progressively more impaired, demands upon their personal caregivers increase. Loved ones often suffer more than patients, who may not realize the extent of their difficulties. When a patient is hospitalized, the treatment team has the opportunity to explore how the caregiver is adjusting to these increased responsibilities, and to discover what assistance is needed. Both the emotional and physical needs of the caregiver are considered. It is essential to identify what the caregiver believes to be the most problematic issues, and to make sure that these are adequately addressed. Support of the caregiver who provides daily care is a prime objective.

When a patient is hospitalized, many of the physical tasks usually done at home are performed by members of the nursing staff. Personal caregivers differ in their response to hospitalization. Some are able to accept the extra time as a form of respite from total responsibility, and to catch up on chores or sleep. Other caregivers are concerned about the quality of care provided in a new environment, and feel uneasy leaving patients alone. Professional staff members can explore with such caregivers what they can do to gain trust, and thus allow the caregivers time for personal activities. It is important to provide caregivers with clear information about what can and cannot be expected during the hospitalization; this helps them make informed decisions in how to use their time while their loved ones are hospitalized.

Planning for a patient's eventual discharge begins early in the course of hospitalization, and often depends upon the ability or inability of the personal caregiver to provide constant care to the impaired individual. It is important to determine first whether the caregiver wishes to provide this high-demand care, and then how the professional team can support the decision. If there is a lack of knowledge about specific aspects of physical care, staff members should allow enough time to teach the caregiver the necessary skills, so that a measure of confidence is obtained. Staff members should also stress the need for help, because no one person can do everything; friends and family members may be mobilized to assist, and formal support services should be explored. The treatment team members serve as patient advocates by making certain that the home environment is as safe as possible and that patients are protected from wandering and getting lost outside of the home.

Home care may not be appropriate in all cases, depending upon the physical and emotional resources of the primary caregiver. There may be situations when it is not in a patient's best interest to return home, if the level of care required is more than the personal caregiver can provide. Honest communication between the treatment team and the personal caregiver helps obtain optimal care for the patient, while supporting the personal caregiver's need to make a difficult placement decision.

RECOMMENDATIONS FOR PERSONAL CAREGIVERS

The process of educating patients and caregivers is more successful if health professionals first gain an understanding of the clients' belief systems about changes in cognitive status and dementia. For example, dementia is commonly associated with the elderly, or may be considered a mental illness with concomitant bizarre and violent behaviors.

Clarifying misperceptions before offering specific recommendations enhances the learning potential. In addition, numerous studies demonstrate that ethnocultural attitudes and values about HIV/AIDS provide the framework for current knowledge and behavioral practices of diverse populations (Bowser, 1992; Diaz, Buehler, & Castro, 1993; Elder-Tabrizy, Wolitski, & Rhodes, 1991; Eversley, Newstetter, & Avins, 1993; Flaskerud & Uman, 1993; Wyatt, 1991). Awareness and support of a client's cultural background help establish a sensitive and trusting professional relationship.

As it does in so many other areas, identified earlier, HIV/AIDS also challenges our more traditional notions of the appropriate role of mental health professionals. The complexity of the psychosocial issues faced by PWAs and their caregivers may mean developing more flexible professional boundaries; this may include seeing clients in their homes, as well as in hospital and other health care settings, and interacting more significantly with the caregivers, family members, and friends of clients. This work may also demand of mental health professionals that they also become strong client advocates and educators as a means of lessening the potential psychosocial consequences inherent in the environment of HIV/AIDS.

On the practical level, in order to prevent or to lessen the severity of such consequences, it becomes important for both PWAs *and* their caregivers to plan for the future—in effect, to plan for the worst-case scenario. Clearly, taking such initiatives may be extremely difficult psychologically for many individuals, whose primary coping style may be to remain focused on the positive (Livingston, 1996). However, by framing such activities in terms of empowerment and of providing PWAs and their caregivers with more control over their lives, the mental health professional may be able to overcome psychological defenses against taking such action. The same reframing intervention may be effective in alleviating the guilt of many caregivers, who feel that by assuming practical responsibilities for their loved ones with cognitive impairment, they are undermining the loved ones' autonomy and control.

Planning for the future involves getting various legal and financial matters in order—making a will, establishing a legal/financial power of attorney, and establishing a durable power of attorney for health care. (For a full discussion of these and other legal matters, see Chapter 10, this volume.) To avoid successful challenges of wills, especially in cases where dementia or other cognitive impairments are factors, it is recommended that individuals videotape themselves reciting the stipulations of wills. It is also highly recommended that PWAs add trusted loved ones as signatories on their bank accounts, to facilitate the assumption of financial responsibility by the loved ones, should the need arise. One of us had personal experience with an individual who became so demented that he stopped paying his bills. Having made no provision for anyone else to manage his affairs, he ultimately lost his health insurance because he failed to pay his premiums.

By designating an agent for durable power of attorney for health care, individuals can be assured that their wishes regarding health care decisions will be followed in the event that they are not able to make them themselves. Establishing such a power of attorney is especially important for PWAs who are alienated from their families of origin, because, in the absence of such a document, next of kin are generally consulted about health care decisions.

Planning may also include researching patients' health and disability insurance benefits, as well as any benefits that may be available from public assistance programs. All too often PWAs wait until a medical crisis occurs or until they decide to go on disability before investigating such resources, only to discover that the benefits available to them are severely deficient or inadequate to cover their needs. Knowing in advance what may be available from community HIV/AIDS organizations in the way of practical support (transportation, in-home assistance, shopping, etc.) will also help PWAs and their caregivers plan more effectively for their futures.

Early detection and diagnosis of cognitive impairment are extremely important on a number of levels. They can provide caregivers with a sense of grounding—a context within which to understand what they are going through. Detection and diagnosis also allow caregivers to plan more effectively for the future, to pace themselves, and to develop their inner resources. A caregiver who is aware that his or her loved one's behavior is related to medical rather than interpersonal factors may also be more willing to accept outside sources of support for caretaking responsibilities. Finally, an awareness of the existence of cognitive impairment can assist caregivers in not personalizing—and thereby possibly deescalating—conflicts that they may be experiencing with their loved ones. It may be devastating to realize that the interpersonal difficulties one is experiencing with a loved one are the result of organic factors related to HIV/AIDS; however, such a realization is apt to be less upsetting than the assumption that such difficulties indicate a failure of the relationship itself.

In contrast to the scenarios discussed above, there are PWAs and caregivers who automatically assume that *any* mental difficulties are signs of dementia. In such situations, a neuropsychological assessment can also assist in the identification of other, non-HIV-related sources of cognitive impairment; this may serve to relieve the anxiety of these individuals, who may have automatically assumed "the worst." Neuropsychological assessments are also recommended even for PWAs who have not yet exhibited any symptoms of brain involvement. Such assessments can provide baselines for future comparison, should difficulties arise subsequently.

It is recommended that mental health professionals explore options for obtaining neuropsychological testing for those clients (probably the majority) without adequate insurance resources to cover it. Free assessments may be available through local HIV/AIDS support organizations or through clinical trials or studies being conducted at academic research sites around the United States.

The term "dementia" is often used in a fairly casual—and inaccurate—manner within the HIV/AIDS community, by PWAs, personal caregivers, *and* health care professionals (Kain, 1996). It is therefore extremely important that PWAs and caregivers receive accurate, appropriate education about the conditions they may be dealing with. Boccellari and Zeifert (1994) suggest that when PWAs and caregivers are encouraged to discuss their own conceptions of and concerns about dementia, health care professionals will be able to intervene with accurate information, clarifying any misunderstandings the clients may have.

Obtaining emotional and psychological support for what they are going through is perhaps the most obvious, as well as the most important, recommendation for caregivers. Individual therapy and caregiver support groups are effective alternatives or adjuncts for caregivers reluctant to burden friends and families or depend on them for their support. This is especially true for those individuals who, because of the stigma associated with HIV, do not have access to the personal support resources normally available in similar, non-HIV-related situations. For some individuals, therapy may be the only "break" they receive from the continuous bombardment of HIV/AIDS in their personal lives.

Support groups can be particularly effective in providing caregivers with a perspective on their experience, through the feedback they are able to receive from others in a similar situation. By way of the examples of others who have gone through it before, groups can provide reassurance that a caregiver's experience is not unique and that he or she *will* survive it. Support groups are also good sources of information on resources that may be available, as well as on effective interventions caregivers may utilize with their loved ones. Unfortunately, studies have shown that most caregivers do not participate in either individual therapy or support groups (Wardlaw, 1994). Whether this is a consequence of ignorance about their availability or value, or of a reluctance to make time for themselves, remains unclear.

It is imperative that mental health professionals assist caregivers in processing feelings of guilt and other dysfunctional thoughts and emotions that may prevent them from accessing external sources of support and attending to their own needs. Individuals whose personal resources have been severely depleted are less likely to be able to provide high-quality care to others.

RECOMMENDATIONS FOR PROFESSIONAL CAREGIVERS

As stated in a previous section of this chapter, there are many reasons for health care providers to experience stress when caring for patients with HIV-related dementia. Investigators characterize the effects of these stressors as "burnout" (Bennett, Michie, & Kippax, 1991; Lovejoy, 1988; Macks & Abrams, 1993; Van Servellen & Leake, 1994). Maslach and Jackson (1981) identify three components of burnout: emotional exhaustion, with feelings of being overextended by one's work; depersonalization, as one becomes unfeeling and impersonal with clients; and a lack of personal accomplishment, with a tendency to evaluate oneself negatively in relation to work duties. The impact of stressors and the potential for burnout can be reduced by institutional support and personal management skills.

Administrators of facilities can encourage all professional caregivers to participate in the decision-making process as much as possible. In addition to sharing unified goals at the organizational level, individual providers must have influence over their own assignments and caseloads (Van Servellen & Leake, 1994). Effective policies should be clearly stated, yet flexible enough to allow off-duty time when needed. Peer support and mentoring systems may prove helpful, as they allow sharing of both expertise and common emotional responses to patients. Lego (1994) describes the success of a formal support group for nursing personnel in reducing anxiety and increasing methods of coping. Individual practitioners can encourage appropriate communication systems, as poor communication among workers is frequently a key stressor. Formal information about patients must be shared, both to allow members to function as a team and to enable members to provide patients with consistent facts. In addition, opportunities for informal communication can be encouraged through relaxed time spent together outside of work (Macks & Abrams, 1992).

By recognizing and attending to feelings perceived as stressful, professional caregivers can then participate in activities that help them cope with the realities of their work. Such activities include relaxation strategies, as well as positive behavioral patterns of diet, exercise, and sleep. The ability to separate work from the rest of one's life is necessary; taking scheduled vacations, and lunch breaks while at work, reinforces this strategy. Perhaps by listening to the suggestions they make to patients and their loved ones, professionals can learn how to help themselves.

CONCLUSIONS

The unique psychosocial issues encountered by both PWAs and their caregivers require an enhanced level of sensitivity and flexibility on the part of mental health professionals working with this client population.

It is important for professionals not only to be informed regarding neuropsychiatric manifestations of HIV, but also to be aware of the biopsychosocial implications of the disease process as a whole, as well as of the environment in which the disease process is played out.

Like pebbles tossed into a pond, those *infected* with HIV are surrounded by expanding waves of *affected* caregivers, both personal and professional. HIV "happens" to all of these individuals, and it is important that those in the mental health profession consider all *affected* parties when developing treatment plans. The creation of "caregiving teams," which include both personal and professional caregivers, allows for the establishment and maintenance of optimal support systems for PWAs. By being sensitive to the issues faced by personal caregivers, mental health professionals are better able to enlist their participation in such a "team"; in turn, this enhances the effectiveness of the professionals' own participation as team members.

REFERENCES

Bennett, L., Michie, P., & Kippax, S. (1991). *AIDS Care, 3,* 181–192.

Blumenfield, M., Smith, P. J., Milazzo, J. C., Seropian, S., & Wormser, G. P. (1987). Survey of nurses working with AIDS patients. *General Hospital Psychiatry, 9,* 58–63.

Boccellari, A., & Zeifert, P. (1994). Management of neurobehavioral impairment in HIV-1 infection. *Psychiatric Clinics of North America, 17*(1), 183–203.

Bowser, B. P. (1992). Cross-cultural medicine a decade later: African-American culture and AIDS prevention—from barrier to ally. *Western Journal of Medicine, 157*(3), 286–289.

Brewington, J. G. (1994). The AIDS epidemic: Caring for caregivers. *Nursing Administration Quarterly, 18*(2), 22–29.

Buckingham, S., & van Gorp, W. (1994). HIV-associated dementia: A clinician's guide to early detection, diagnosis, and intervention. *Families in Society: The Journal of Contemporary Human Services, 75*(6), 333–345.

Cummings, J. L., Benson, D. F., & LoVerme, J. R. (1980). Reversible dementia. *Journal of the American Medical Association, 243,* 2434–2439.

Diaz, T., Buehler, J. W., & Castro, K. G. (1993). AIDS trends among Hispanics in the United States. *American Journal of Public Health, 83*(4), 504–509.

Elder-Tabrizy, K. A., Wolitski, R. J., & Rhodes, F. (1991). AIDS and competing health concerns of blacks, hispanics, and whites. *Journal of Community Health, 16*(1), 11–21.

Eversley, R. B., Newstetter, A., & Avins, A. (1993). Sexual risk and perception of risk for HIV infection among multiethnic family-planning clients. *American Journal of Preventive Medicine, 9*(2), 92–95.

Flaskerud, J. H., & Uman, G. (1993). Directions for AIDS education for Hispanic women based on analyses of survey findings. *Public Health Reports, 108*(3), 298–304.

Foley, M. E., & Fahs, M. C. (1994). Hospital care grievances and psychosocial needs expressed by PWAs: An analysis of qualitative data. *Journal of Nurses in AIDS Care,* 5(5), 21–29.

Folkman, S., Chesney, M., & Christopher-Richards, A. (1994). Stress and coping in caregiving partners of men with AIDS. *Psychiatric Clinics of North America,* 17(1), 35–53.

Kain, C. (1996). *Positive HIV affirmative counseling.* Alexandria, VA: American Counseling Association.

Lee, K., & McGill, C. (1991). Confronting the lack of resources for patients with AIDS dementia complex. *Social Work,* 36(6), 473–475.

Lego, S. (1994). AIDS-related anxiety and coping methods in a support group for caregivers. *Archives of Psychiatric Nursing,* 8(3), 200–207.

Levin, R., Buckingham, S., & Hart, C. (1995). Gay men as caregivers. In V. Lynch & P. A. Wilson (Eds.), *Caring for the HIV/AIDS caregiver* (pp. 73–90). Westport, CT: Auburn House.

Link, R. N., Feingold, A. R., Charap, M. H., Freeman, K., & Shelov, S.P. (1988). Concerns of medical and pediatric house officers about acquiring AIDS from their patients. *American Journal of Public Health,* 78, 455–459.

Livingston, D. (1996). A systems approach to AIDS counseling for gay couples. In M. Shernoff (Ed.), *Human services for gay people* (pp. 83–93). New York: Haworth Press.

Lovejoy, N. (1988). Family and caregiver responses to HIV infection. In G. Gee & T. A. Moran (Eds.), *AIDS: Concepts in nursing practice* (pp. 379–401). Baltimore: Williams & Wilkins.

Macks, J., & Abrams, D. (1992). Burnout among HIV/AIDS health care providers: Helping the people on the frontlines. *AIDS Clinical Review,* 281–299.

Maslach, C., & Jackson, S. E. (1981). The measurement of experienced burnout. *Journal of Occupational Behavior,* 2, 99–113.

Monahan, D., & Hooker, K. (1995). Health of spouse caregivers of dementia patients: The role of personality and social support. *Social Work* 40(3), 305–311.

Pleck, J. H., O'Donnell, L., O'Donnell, C., & Snarey, J. (1988). AIDS phobia, contact with AIDS, and AIDS-related job stress in hospital workers. *Journal of Homosexuality,* 15, 41–54.

Powell-Cope, G. (1994). Family caregivers of people with AIDS: Negotiating partnerships with professional health care providers. *Nursing Research,* 43(6), 324–330.

Richardson, J. L., & Lochner, T. (1987). Physician attitudes and experience regarding the care of patients with acquired immunodeficiency syndrome and related disorders. *Medical Care,* 25, 675–685.

Shapira, J., Roper, J. M., & Schulzinger, J. (1993). Managing delirious patients. *Nursing,* 23, 80–83.

Silverman, D. C. (1993). Psychosocial impact of HIV-related caregiving on health providers: A review and recommendations for the role of psychiatry. *American Journal of Psychiatry,* 150, 705–712.

Stulberg, I., & Buckingham, S. (1988). Parallel issues for AIDS patients, families and others. *Social Casework,* 69(6), 355–359.

Swanson, B., Cronin-Stubbs, D., & Colletti, M. A. (1990). Dementia and depression in persons with AIDS: Causes and care. *Journal of Psychosocial Nursing,* *28*(10), 33–39.

Ungvarski, P. J., & Staats, J. A. (1995). Clinical manifestations of AIDS in adults. In J. H. Flaskerud & P. J. Ungvarski (Eds.), *HIV/AIDS: A guide to nursing care* (pp. 81–133). Philadelphia: W.B. Saunders.

Van Servellen, G., & Leake, B. (1994). Burn-out in hospital nurses: A comparison of acquired immunodeficiency syndrome, oncology, general medical, and intensive care unit nurse samples. *Journal of Professional Nursing, 9*(3), 169–177.

Wardlaw, L. (1994). Sustaining informal caregivers for persons with AIDS. *Families in Society: The Journal of Contemporary Human Services, 75*(6), 373–384.

Wyatt, G. E. (1991). Examining ethnicity versus race in AIDS related sex research. *Social Science and Medicine, 33*(1), 37–45.

8

Suicide and HIV Disease

SHARON M. VALENTE
JUDITH M. SAUNDERS

INTRODUCTION

Statistically, people with HIV infection or neurological diseases such as Huntington's disease have higher rates of suicidal behaviors and suicide than either the general population or people with other life-threatening illnesses (National Center for Health Statistics, 1994). According to Breitbart (1993), AIDS and persistent pain are associated with the highest rates of suicide, euthanasia, and requests for assisted death among people who are HIV-infected. Fatigue, symptom distress, depression, dementia, and other factors also increase suicide risk among patients with HIV/AIDS (Flavin, Franklin, & Frances, 1986; Perry, Jacobsberg, & Fishman, 1990; Perry, Fishman, Jacobsberg, & Frances, 1991; Schneider, Taylor, Hammen, Kemeny, & Dudley, 1991) (see Table 8.1). In a study of 2,793 people who were registered with the National Huntington's Disease Research Roster, suicide was also the reported cause of death among 205 people (7.3%). Suicide was more frequent in all categories of risk (e.g., from possible risk to 50% risk) of Huntington's disease than among the general U.S. population (DiMaio et al., 1993; Lipe, Schultz, & Bird, 1993).

People with HIV disease need routine evaluation of suicide potential (Copeland, 1993; Cote, Biggar, & Dannenberg, 1992). Clinicians who treat patients with HIV-related pain or symptoms, or terminally ill AIDS patients, will need to examine their attitudes toward suicide, to evaluate

TABLE 8.1. Risk Factors for Suicidal Behavior among People with HIV/AIDS

Risk factor	Citations
Organic mental disorder, delirium, dementia	Alfonso & Cohen (1994)
Current AIDS-related death and illness events	Schneider, Taylor, Hammen, Kemeny, & Dudley (1991)
Perceived AIDS risk	Schneider et al. (1991)
Past depression, social isolation	Perry, Jacobsberg, & Fishman (1990); Perry (1990); Schneider et al. (1991)
Alcoholism, other substance abuse	Flavin, Franklin, & Frances (1986)
Hopelessness	Breitbart (1993)
Untreated pain, fatigue, other symptom distress	Breitbart (1993)
Bereavement	Rundell, Kyle, Brown, & Thomason (1992); Schneider et al. (1991)

rationality and suicide risk, and to respond therapeutically to patients who pose serious ethical dilemmas. One prerequisite for this work is a knowledge of the distinctions among various types and degrees of self-destructive thoughts and behaviors. For example, "suicide" itself is defined as an intentional self-inflicted death; "parasuicide" includes all nonfatal suicidal thoughts, acts, or wishes (see Table 8.2 for definitions of these and other terms in suicidology).

Several factors complicate the recognition and treatment of suicidal HIV/AIDS patients. Clinicians may need more in-depth knowledge of research, skill in managing suicidal patients in general, or methods of examining bioethical dilemmas. Patients with terminal illnesses of all types raise complex issues about the right to die with dignity (Battin, 1991; Quill, 1993; Stone, 1997). High-quality management of suicidal HIV/AIDS patients rests on sound scientific knowledge that guides effective evaluation and treatment.

In this chapter, we first take a brief look at traditional and controversial views of suicide in general and in the context of life-threatening illness, and consider the various presentations of suicidal HIV/AIDS patients. We then provide a critical review of the research on HIV and suicide, with an emphasis on risk factors; an overview of assessment and management of suicidal HIV/AIDS patients, together with guidelines for clinical practice; and a discussion of ethical issues related to suicide in the context of HIV/AIDS. The literature suggests that it is dangerous to assume prematurely that ideas of suicide among persons with HIV/AIDS are rational ideas, because suicidal impulses may be cries for help and may be related to physical symptom distress

TABLE 8.2. Definitions of Commonly Used Terms in Suicidology

Term	Definition and examples
Suicide or completed suicide	Taking one's own life intentionally and voluntarily; a mode of death. Example: A woman believed she had AIDS but was never tested. As planned, she took a large quantity of barbiturates at 4:30 P.M., turned on the gas, fell asleep, and died.
Parasuicide or attempted suicide	Nonlethal, deliberate, self-inflicted behaviors that are not intended to cause death. Also called "deliberate self-injury."
Suicidal ideas	All thoughts that may be inferred or observed via behaviors that threaten the person's life.
Suicide gesture	A misleading term, because it implies that some suicidal behaviors are innocuous. Typically used to indicate an act that is not lethal, is not intended to cause death, and is tentative. This term should be avoided.
Indirect self-destructive behavior	A subtle, covert, indirect, and perhaps unconscious method of attempting to end one's life. Examples: Refusing medications, food, or fluids necessary to sustain life; using street drugs; driving recklessly.
Lethality of method/plan	The degree of potential to cause death. Examples: jumping from tall buildings, hanging, and using guns have high lethality.
Survivor-victims	Bereaved individuals who have had a loved one die by suicide.
Psychological autopsy	Investigation of details, deceased's motives, and mode of death via interviewing family, friends, and significant others.

or psychiatric comorbidity (e.g., depression, substance abuse, or anxiety) (Breitbart, 1993).

TRADITIONAL AND CONTROVERSIAL VIEWS OF SUICIDE

The traditional view of suicide as an irrational behavior and a cry for help, which has emerged from studies of psychiatric patients, has provided important standards. These standards indicate a need for understanding a patient's psychodynamics, motives, suicide risk, rationality, and options for improving quality of life. At times when a patient's thinking is impaired by dementia, depression, pain, or drug intoxication, the patient cannot make a rational choice. These standards and the law also hold clinicians accountable for preventing suicide if it is foreseeable and for evaluating and treating pain, depression, and suicidal ideas and attempts (Bongar, 1992). However, people with HIV/AIDS have questioned these traditional views and asserted that they are rational and deserve the right to die. The bioethical dilemmas involved in assisted death, rational suicide, and euthanasia are challenging and may elicit conflicts among a clinician's values and duties.

The clinician's duty to a rational, suicidal person with a life-threatening illness is controversial. Clinicians can have a meaningful role in prevention when suicidal behaviors are impulsive and a cry for help. Alternatively, clinicians can act as advocates for people who are terminally ill, who demonstrate rational thinking, and who seek assistance in dying (Valente & Saunders, 1996a). Although some states have drafted legislation to legalize the health care clinician's role in assisted dying, many people still believe that assisted suicide is unethical and unacceptable, and it remains illegal in most states. Advocacy for rational patients may include encouraging open and candid discussions with significant others about dying, and ensuring that loved ones understand that suicide is not a solution for temporary problems. Advocacy may also include referrals to legal advocates and education about options for refusing food or fluids or for preparing advance directives. Interventions differ for rational and irrational choices. For patients making irrational choices, protection against suicide and precautions to prevent it are warranted (Valente & Saunders, 1996). Formerly rational patients may also develop episodes of dementia, in which their thought processes are impaired.

In considering the rationality of a patient's decision to commit suicide, the clinician must determine that the patient has the capacity to choose suicide freely. Capacity to choose can fluctuate among people with HIV/AIDS, especially among patients with dementia. However, the diagnosis of dementia does not automatically disqualify patients from participating in end-of-life decisions, including suicide. In determining a patient's capacity to choose, the clinician should attend to the side effects of medication, treatable illnesses, and other factors that might influence the patient's capacity. Providing the patient with the best possible circumstances for participating in decisions is the clinician's responsibility, even when such decisions involve refusing treatments or considering rational suicide.

PRESENTATIONS OF SUICIDAL HIV/AIDS PATIENTS

Different pathways lead to suicide. Suicidal people with HIV disease often present themselves for treatment in one of five contexts: (1) covertly suicidal patients complaining of symptom distress; (2) overtly suicidal patients who report their suicidal thoughts or who are brought by their loved ones; (3) patients who have already attempted suicide; (4) suicidal patients whose risk is identified by other staff members; and (5) terminally ill patients whose requests for assisted dying may be labeled as wishes for suicide. A patient's loved ones, friends, and other staff members can provide important observations that can help a clinician determine the motives and precipitants of the patient's suicidal behavior.

Patients will consider suicide for diverse psychological, social, biological, and existential reasons (Armandariz, Saunders, Poston, & Valente, 1997). Many suicidal patients do not want to die, but are desperate for relief of suffering. For others, suicidal thoughts may help control anticipated yet intolerable suffering (e.g., "I can kill myself if my lover dies and I'm a burden to my friends," " . . . if my vision goes and I can't see my garden," or " . . . if fatigue or intolerable pain prevents me from working").

Physiological precipitants may include HIV-related central nervous system abnormalities, such as subcortical disease or dementia; depressive side effects of medication; and alterations in neurotransmitter function. Other physiological causes include blindness, pain (multifactorial), debilitation, diarrhea, and other neurological problems. Feelings of alienation, hopelessness, or isolation may also precipitate suicide. In addition, people may consider suicide because they do not want to be a burden to loved ones. Or suicide may remain an abstract idea until various circumstances, which are personally defined, become intolerable. The rationality of a patient's suicide plans requires examination, and the patient needs a therapeutic environment in which to explore options (Battin, 1991; Saunders & Valente, 1993; Valente & Saunders, 1996a, 1996b).

OVERVIEW OF RESEARCH ON SUICIDE AND SUICIDALITY AMONG PEOPLE WITH HIV DISEASE

Table 8.3 provides a summary of selected research on suicide and suicidality among people with HIV disease.

Rates of Suicide and Suicidal Behaviors

Several researchers have found high rates of suicide and suicidal behaviors among people at different stages of HIV disease. Marzuk et

TABLE 8.3. Summary of Selected Research

Author	Design	Methods	Findings	Notes
Schneiderman et al. (1994)	AIDS (n = 89) and cancer (n = 61) patients with 5 years' life expectancy were offered California durable power of attorney.	Convenience sample accrued through cancer and AIDS clinics.	Most seriously ill patients pondered costs, burdens on others in considering their decisions about advance directives.	
Alfonso & Cohen (1994)	Retrospective analysis of psychiatric consultations— individual case studies.	Case reports.	Essential for caregivers to recognize dementia and be alert to suicide.	Substance abuse increased risks.
McKegney & O'Dowd (1993)	Retrospective study; adult and elderly patients, 1988–1990.	Psychiatric consults, using structured clinical interviews.	322 patients with AIDS were less suicidal than 82 HIV-positive patients and comparable in suicidality to 1,086 HIV-negative or HIV-unknown patients.	Organicity, denial, acceptance, and/or preoccupation with fatal illness may reduce suicidality in AIDS patients.
Copeland (1993)	Retrospective review of 25 cases of suicide among individuals who had AIDS or thought they had AIDS, 1985–1989.	Autopsy of all suicides and data from medical examiner, Dade County, Florida.	Many different of suicide methods were used. Annual suicide rate (166.7/100,000) was 9-fold higher than that for general population (18.6/100,000).	High suicide rates.
Rabkin, Remien, Katloff, & Williams (1993)	53 gay men with opportunistic infections in past 3 years prior, from Gay Men's Health Crisis Center in New York City.	Convenience sample in 1990.	High level of positive emotional health, independent of HIV illness stage.	Before 1990, few met sample criteria.

(continued)

TABLE 8.3. *(cont.)*

Author	Design	Methods	Findings	Notes
Cote, Biggar, & Dannenberg (1992)	165 male and female suicides among persons with AIDS in United States; retrospective study of mortality data, 1987–1989.	Surveillance data and death certificates.	Self-poisoning with drugs was most common method (35%). Rate of suicide (165/100,000) was 7.4-fold higher than that of general population ($p < .05$).	High suicide rates. Both males and females were studied.
Valente, Saunders, & Uman (1993)	A comparative, correlational study of a convenience sample of 223 subjects (91% males; 9% females) at prevention clinics) for AIDS or sexually transmitted diseases. Subjects were either HIV-positive, or seronegative but concerned about risk.	Impact of Events Scale, Beck Depression Inventory (BDI), Beck Hopelessness Scale symptom survey and interview, clinical record review.	People with two or more HIV symptoms had higher risk of depression and more unhealthy or negative self-care behaviors.	BDI and symptom survey and interview identified people with risk of suicide.
Schneider, Taylor, Hammen, Kemeny, & Dudley (1991)	In a convenience sample of 778 gay men with AIDS, 212 reported suicidal ideas over past 6 months. Approx. half were HIV-positive.	Questionnaire.	Current stressors and past levels of adaptive functioning were more powerful predictors of suicide intent among HIV-positive than HIV-negative ideators.	

(continued)

TABLE 8.3. *(cont.)*

Author	Design	Methods	Findings	Notes
Perry, Fishman, Jacobsberg, & Frances (1991)	Comparative study. Random sample of 307 asymptomatic adults (*n* = 204 HIV-negative; 103 HIV-positive).	Psychoeduca-tion was compared with counseling alone, with video, or with stress reduc-tion.	Significant decrease in mean distress after stress reduction training.	Stress reduction training helped.
Breitbart (1990)	Comparison of HIV-positive patients with pain patients and controls in an ambulatory medical clinic.	Current suicidal ideas (BDI item 9).	20–40% of patients had current suicidal ideas; HIV-positive, 26%; HIV-positive with pain, 40%.	Higher rate of suicidal ideas in HIV-positive subjects with pain.
Perry, Jacobsberg, & Fishman (1990)	Subjects (*n* = 301) completed BDI and had counseling for physically asymptomatic HIV-positive and -negative informants who were at risk for HIV infection.	Convenience sample; case reports; interviews about depression; BDI scores on item 9.	HIV-positive subjects reported at suicidal ideas at 2 months; HIV-negative, decreased suicide ideas.	
Rabkin, Williams, Neugebauer, Remien, & Goetz (1990)	208 HIV-positive homosexual patients with good education.	5-year ongoing study.	Despite discrimination and vulnerability, subjects kept a sense of faith.	

Note. Phyllis Oreck assisted with the literature review and summary.

al. (1988), who conducted a retrospective study, reported that the relative suicide risk of New Yorkers aged 29–59 with AIDS was 36 times higher than that of a comparison cohort without AIDS and 66 times higher than that of the general population. Kizer, Green, Perkins, Doebbert, and Hughes (1988) examined California death certificates for 1986 and found that men with AIDS aged 20–39 had a suicide rate 21 times that of men without AIDS. Suicide attempt rates among HIV-infected Air Force personnel (*n* = 15) were reported to be 16–24 times higher than those of their noninfected counterparts (Rundell, Kyle, Brown, & Thomason, 1992). In a study of people at various stages of HIV infection (n = 183), O'Dowd, Biderman, and McKegney (1993) found that patients with either AIDS-related complex or asymptomatic HIV-positive status had significantly more suicidal ideas than those with AIDS.

Areas Studied and Methodological Problems

Some areas remain poorly understood: variations in suicide risk over the course of HIV disease; the motives, precipitants, and psychological profiles of suicide among people with HIV disease as opposed to other neuropsychiatric disorders; patterns among different ethnic, gender, and age groups; and patterns among neurologically impaired patients. HIV testing and suicidal ideas, correlates of suicidal intent, and suicide among psychiatric patients have been studied. Anecdotal data and case studies illustrate suicidal behavior among alcohol-dependent, homosexual men with AIDS; people with HIV-associated dementia or substance abuse; and people responding to a diagnosis of AIDS or the fear of having AIDS (Alfonso & Cohen, 1994; Armandarez et al., 1997; Flavin et al., 1986).

However, different methodologies, definitions, and instruments make it difficult to compare results across studies. Also, most samples have consisted of white, well-educated men. In addition, neither suicides nor HIV-related deaths are accurately recorded in mortality statistics, and most postmortem studies lack an appropriate reference population. These problems pose important methodological challenges in this area of research (Starace, 1993).

Although lists of risk factors grow, no comprehensive theory explains which people with HIV disease versus other neuropsychiatric disorders will be vulnerable to suicide. Some researchers have reported that HIV-positive asymptomatic individuals experience high levels of psychosocial stress, depression, anxiety, and hopelessness (Joe, Knezek, Watson, & Simpson, 1991; Joseph et al., 1990). Others cite contradictory findings, which suggest that the association of psychosocial stress and depression with HIV disease is unclear or unstable (Roth & Breitbart, 1996; Rundell et al., 1992). The relationships among HIV, sexual orientation, and suicide are also unclear (Saunders & Valente, 1988).

Risk Factors for Suicide

Detecting persons with HIV disease who are at risk for suicide is the first step in evaluation, treatment, and suicide prevention. Factors that have been associated with suicide risk in this population are listed in Table 8.1 and discussed below.

Psychopathology

Most researchers confirm that psychiatric symptoms or disorders, particularly depression, occur in 80% of suicidal people. Although low rates of mood disorders were found in one small study of HIV-positive long-term survivors (Rabkin, Remien, Katloff, & Williams, 1993), major depression, substance abuse, and dementia/delirium are critical factors in suicide for many HIV-positive individuals. Whereas suicide attempts, substance dependence, posttraumatic stress disorder, phobias, and schizophrenia are correlates of suicide in general populations, how these factors influence suicide risk across the HIV disease spectrum or in HIV disease versus other neuropsychiatric disorders is unclear.

Case studies illustrate that a few suicidal individuals may actually desire to become HIV-infected. Flavin et al. (1986) described three cases of alcohol-dependent men with suicidal ideation who consciously attempted to contract HIV as a method of committing suicide. In studies of non-HIV-infected populations, suicide rarely occurs in the absence of a psychiatric disorder (Bongar, 1992).

Substance Abuse. Substance abuse or dependence on alcohol or drugs often accompanies or predates suicidal ideas and attempts, and complicates the treatment of suicide. Suicidal individuals often also have a dual diagnosis (e.g., depression and substance abuse). Substance abuse increases impulsivity and may increase risk for HIV infection and reinfection and risk of suicide. The issue of addiction or craving and suicide risk must be addressed in evaluation and treatment, and clinicians need to evaluate whether the addiction is an attempt to self-medicate a psychiatric disorder such as depression. These individuals are a challenge for clinicians and may pose a high risk for poor treatment outcomes.

Dementia and Delirium. The prevalence of organic mental disorders, particularly delirium and dementia, increases as HIV disease progresses, and suicide is a dangerous potential complication of HIV-associated dementia (Alfonso & Cohen, 1994). In contrast with earlier reports of AIDS-related neurological conditions among 40–60% of people with AIDS, brain changes in as many as 90% of people have been reported on autopsy. Dementia affects 7–16% of people with AIDS, but in autopsies brain tissue damage associated with AIDS dementia occurs in up to 66%. The prevalence of depression is increased among people with subcortical dementia. During a psychiatric evaluation, Breitbart (1993) found that most suicidal patients with AIDS or Kaposi's sarcoma had prominent signs of delirium, often in addition to AIDS-associated dementia. However, treatment of delirium often resolved the suicidal ideas or behavior.

Many people with AIDS typically become mildly, or moderately cognitively impaired at some point (Buckingham & van Gorp, 1988; Selnes et al., 1995). AIDS-related dementia begins insidiously, with difficulty in concentrating, impaired recent memory, and slowing of mentation and movement; it progresses steadily or rapidly in many patients to severe global dementia. Symptoms of dementia (e.g., impulsivity, poor judgment, lability, and disinhibition) can increase suicide risk. In their retrospective study, Alfonso and Cohen (1994) reported that one in five persons with HIV seropositivity or AIDS had suicidal behavior. Among patients with subcortical dementia and its associated behavioral disinhibition, substance abuse intensified the risk of suicide. Subcortical dementia and depression are discussed elsewhere in this volume (see Chapters 2 and 4).

Major Depression. Depression is one of the most common psychiatric disorders of HIV-infected people (Markowitz, Rabkin, & Perry, 1994). Because the somatic symptoms of HIV disease mimic those of depression, diagnosis may be difficult. Depression may be related to medication side effects, treatments, or other HIV-related stress issues, and/or to a personal or family history of depression, substance use, multiple losses and loss of social supports or confidants, and advanced HIV infection itself (Markowitz et al., 1994). Marzuk (1991) reported that 50% of people with AIDS who committed suicide were significantly depressed and that 40% had seen a psychiatrist within 4 days before their suicide.

Schneider et al. (1991) examined factors influencing suicide intent among a convenience sample of 778 gay and bisexual men with and without HIV (none with AIDS). The sample was white, well-educated, urban, and well integrated into the white gay community. Using the 27% who reported suicidal ideas, the researchers compared predictors of suicide intent among relatively asymptomatic seropositive and seronegative groups. Among other factors, previous social isolation and depression were significant and powerful predictors of suicide intent among HIV-positive ideators. Some subjects' suicidal ideas may have reflected deficient coping strategies more than psychological distress per se. Schneider et al. also argued that suicide risk is psychologically rather than biologically mediated in the seropositive but asymptomatic population, although this pattern may change as disease progresses. We (Valente & Saunders, 1994) reported that depression and suicidal impulses increased as symptoms increased in our comparative study of relatively healthy seropositive and seronegative men.

Perry (1990) found frequent low-grade depressive symptoms among HIV-positive, at-risk, and seronegative individuals, but depressive disorders occurred most often among those with a history of past depressions, limited social support, and personality disorders. Perry (1990) advised further evaluation and treatment for depressive symptoms accompanied by suicidal ideas. Often, major depression intensifies as HIV disease progresses. Typically, initial episodes of acute depression respond well to treatment with antidepressants and psychotherapy; as depression lifts, suicide risk often increases. Without treatment, major depression tends to heighten suicidal thoughts and risk (U.S. Department of Health and Human Services [DHHS], 1993; Bongar, 1992; Saunders & Valente, 1993)

In non-HIV-infected populations, impaired thinking, impaired problem solving, and stress typically accompany suicidal risk. Suicidal thoughts arise impulsively with overwhelming distress. This pattern may be similar in HIV disease, because clinicians report that many suicidal people with HIV disease have difficulty in noting improvement, progress, or pleasure, or in planning realistic goals (Saunders & Buckingham, 1988). Thus, if they are making progress, they may discount it and thus act out suicidal impulses, despite their clinical improvement.

HIV-Related Stressors and Perceived Risk

Schneider et al. (1991) reported that AIDS-related stressors (AIDS-related deaths and illnesses, as well as perceived AIDS risk), in addition to past levels of poor adaptive functioning (social isolation and depression), were significantly more powerful predictors of suicide intent among HIV-positive than among HIV-negative suicide ideators. Although it has received relatively little investigation, bereavement increases suicide risk among HIV-positive individuals (Schneider et al., 1991; Rundell et al., 1992).

Hope involves confidence in future events and circumstances; hopelessness raises suicide risk, and hopelessness may well increase as HIV/AIDS-related stressors increase. Clinicians can anticipate that suicide risk typically increases at HIV and AIDS diagnosis, at initiation of therapy, at the first opportunistic infection, at each AIDS-related loss, and at exacerbation of symptoms. Often, also, suicide risk may increase at onset of a new illness or treatment that the patient associates with serious disease progression.

Pain is a significant but often neglected stressor in HIV disease, and it too is linked with psychological and functional morbidity (Breitbart, 1993). Common pain syndromes in AIDS patients are listed in Table 8.4. In retrospective studies, approximately 50% of hospitalized

HIV-infected patients required treatment for pain (Breitbart, Rosen-feld, & Passik, 1996; Schofferman & Brody, 1990), but pain is usually undertreated. Breitbart (1993) has asserted that clinicians have not effectively evaluated or treated pain among their HIV-infected clients. Pain profoundly influences emotional distress and has been correlated with depression, functional impairment, and suicidal ideas. In a study of ambulatory HIV-infected patients, Breitbart (1993) reported that 40% of patients with pain reported suicidal ideas; these were more related to concomitant depression than to the intensity of the pain.

PRINCIPLES OF RISK ASSESSMENT

An effective and typical approach to evaluating risk of suicide is to use both clinical and empirical methods of assessment and to interview significant others as well as the patient. A clinician needs to establish rapport with the patient; to detect suicide clues; to ask direct, nonjudgmental questions about suicide; and to determine the circumstances that compromise the patient's desire to live. Flavin et al. (1986) advise clinicians to be alert to subtle indicators of suicide risk. Any suicidal warnings, despair, or hopelessness should be examined.

Although a sensitive topic such as suicide should be broached in a gentle manner, a clinician must ask clear and direct questions about it. When a patient says, "I would rather be dead," the clinician might respond, "You sound sad and discouraged. I wonder—are you feeling so discouraged that you might do something to harm yourself?" If the patient responds affirmatively, the clinician should investigate whether the patient has a plan and a method. The clinician should also explain that no one feels discouraged without reason, but that treatment can

TABLE 8.4. Pain Syndromes in AIDS Patients

Pain related to AIDS	Pain related to AIDS therapy
HIV neuropathy	Antiretroviral agents (zidovudine,
HIV myelopathy	dideoxynosine, dideoxycytidine,
Kaposi's sarcoma	stavudine)
Secondary infections	Biological modifiers (GM-CSF
Organomegaly	[granulocyte macrophage-colony
Myositis	stimulating factors], interferon)
Diarrhea/enteropathy	Chemotherapy (vincristine and others)
Lymphoma	Radiation
Postherpetic neuralgia	Surgery
Arthritis/arthralgias	Medical procedures

Note. Adapted from Breitbart (1993). Copyright 1993 by Lippincott–Raven Publishers. Adapted by permission.

often effectively reduce many symptoms such as depression or pain. Astute clinicians often explore what HIV disease means to patients now, and discuss options for managing distress that may inspire hope and a sense of control. Hope is often encouraged when clinicians emphasize that the members of the clinical staff are committed to supporting their patients throughout this disease. This approach may help covertly suicidal patients to voice their suicidal thoughts. Communicating a genuine interest in patients' feelings is also very important. Principles of therapeutic communication indicate that patients need time to talk about their distressing feelings, and clinicians should avoid the temptation to change the subject, to cheer their patients, or to emphasize only positive options. Such empty reassurance often discounts the patients' distress and increases their despair.

When patients display impulsivity, impaired judgment, or defective memory associated with dementia, close observation and interviews with significant others may be needed to evaluate suicide risk. Clinicians need to attend to increased agitation or a behavior change, and to examine whether these behaviors may indicate an increase in risk of suicide.

The immediate goal of assessment is to detect any planned attempt, the degree of short-term risk, precipitants of suicidal thoughts, and to discover what might reduce suicide potential (e.g., control of pain, treatment of depression, a change in medications). Asking the patient what has prompted consideration of suicide *now* is an effective way to begin evaluation. The next goal is to differentiate a depressive mood resulting from a medical illness (e.g., side effects of medication or HIV-induced dementia) from a more chronic psychiatric disorder such as an anxiety disorder or depression. Finally, the clinician should examine the purpose behind the suicidal impulses and determine whether the patient intends to die, hopes to be rescued, or expects to survive the attempt. Talking with the patient's significant others can help the clinician explore whether the patient has expressed wishes for death or suicide, or has given other clues to suicide.

Assessment includes a review of suicide clues and risk factors, as well as a thorough psychiatric evaluation (see the top portion of Table 8.5). The psychiatric evaluation should include a neurobehavioral mental status evaluation; an assessment of depressive side effects from medications or treatments; and an evaluation for the presence of physical symptom distress, dementia, and depression or other psychiatric symptoms/disorders. A thorough exploration of current and past substance abuse is critical, because depression and suicide risk may increase with detoxification or withdrawal of abused substances, and also with increased use of substances. Exploring the patient's fantasies

TABLE 8.5. Clinical Practice Guidelines

Assessment

Interview patient and significant others about suicide clues/risk factors:
Despair/hopelessness.
Lethality of method/specificity of plans.
Strength of intent (does patient actually wish to die?).
History of past suicide attempts.
Evidence of recent attempts or other indications of imminence.
Both overt verbalizations and covert communications of suicidal ideas.
Sudden increase/recurrence of significant suicidal ideas.
Low impulse control.
Absence of deterrents.
Absence of environmental support or presence of pressure/antagonism
from others.
New, pronounced life stressors.
Appearance of increasing depression (or elation) or substance abuse in
response to new/unusual stressors.
Administer one or more screening instruments:
Scale for Suicide Ideation.
Beck Hopelessness Scale.
Beck Depression Inventory.
Conduct a thorough psychiatric evaluation:
Neurobehavioral mental status evaluation.
Assessment of depressive side effects of medications/treatments.
Assessment of substance abuse.
Evaluation for physical symptom distress, dementia, depression, other
psychiatric symptoms/disorders.

Management

Talk directly and fully about suicidal issues—conduct ongoing evaluation.
Evaluate rationality of choices.
Discuss the situation with consultant.
Treat and reduce pain/other physical symptom distress, dementia, depression,
other psychiatric symptoms/disorders.
Challenge sense of powerlessness/hopelessness and improve resources.
Expand social network and reduce isolation; involve significant others.
Serve as an advocate for patient.
Consider no-suicide contract.
Help patient deal with grief.

For imminent suicidal emergency

Focus on the immediate, pressing problem; understand dimensions of
problem and the dynamics and goal of the suicidal behavior.
Institute suicide precautions and improve safety—consider hospitalization for
acute crisis when choice is not rational, or provide supervision at home and
reduce access to suicide methods (e.g., have medications supervised, remove
other methods).
Seek consultation regarding management and bioethical dilemmas.
Document thorough psychiatric evaluation and suicide assessment (see above),
as well as rationale for treatment decisions.

Note. This table incorporates ideas from Bongar (1992) and Valente (1994).

about suicide and death is also useful. Based upon routine and ongoing assessment of suicide risk, the clinician estimates the lethality of the patient's chosen method and the strength of his or her suicidal intent (see below).

Clinicians need to detect not only direct communications of suicide, but indirect or subtle cries for help. Direct clues to suicide include comments such as "I'm going to kill myself; I'm a burden to my family and I'd be better off dead." Subtle clues include the patient's suggesting that life just isn't worth it, giving away a prized possession, or simply wishing for death. Subtle or disguised references to suicide are more common in some cultures or age groups, such as Hispanic, Asian, and elderly patients (Flaskerud, 1986; Nyamathi, Flaskerud & Leake, 1997). Statistically, the highest suicide rates for black or Hispanic men occur during their young adult years. In addition, they often commit suicide with no prior attempt, although a prior attempt indicates high risk among whites (Hatton & Valente, 1984). Screening instruments (see below) can help identify depression or suicide potential.

Screening

Several checklists help identify patients at risk who need further assessment, but these scales do not diagnose or predict suicide accurately. Commonly used scales include the Scale for Suicide Ideation (SSI), the Beck Hopelessness Scale, and the Beck Depression Inventory (BDI).

The 19-item SSI, developed by Beck (1979) and his colleagues, is a clinically administered scale that measures and evaluates suicidal ideas. Questions ask about reasons for living and dying, desire for suicide, duration or frequency of suicidal ideas, and attitudes toward suicide. It has good reliability and validity among general populations and diverse ethnic groups (α = .89 and interrater reliability α = .83; estimates of concurrent validity, discriminant validity and construct validity, have been favorable).

Another useful scale is the Beck Hopelessness Scale (Wright, Thase, Beck, & Ludgate, 1993), which also has confirmed reliability and validity and has been tested on diverse ethnic populations. In a large study of 1,958 psychiatric patients, 17 who scored 9 or more on the Hopelessness Scale had committed suicide by follow-up 43 months later (Beck, Brown, Berchick, Stewart, & Steer, 1990). People with HIV disease do not like this scale and complain about its items (e.g., the belief in a positive future). We have found this scale useful for symptomatic patients with HIV disease, but not for asymptomatic patients (Valente & Saunders, 1994)

The BDI (Beck & Steer, 1987) has 20 questions and can be completed in 5–10 minutes. Patients rate the frequency over the past 7 days of such behaviors as crying, fatigue, anorexia, and suicidal ideas. Because items on the BDI tap physical illness, symptomatic HIV-positive patients will often have artificially high BDI scores. Because the physical symptoms may arise from HIV disease, depression, or both, some clinicians suggest that the psychological items offer a more reliable index of depression and suicide risk. Possible responses range from 0 ("rarely") to 3 ("very often"). Scores over 11 suggest mild to severe depression, but an interview is needed to evaluate suicide risk. On item 2 (pessimism) and item 9 (suicidal ideas), scores of 2 or higher specifically suggest suicide risk (Berchick & Wright, 1992).

Most screening instruments have not been tested on people with HIV disease, but have been tested on people with cancer (Valente & Saunders, 1994). When people have mild dementia, repeated use of a screening tool over time helps provide a baseline measure. However, dementia may interfere with recall of symptoms over the past 7 days and thus may threaten the reliability of retrospective screening tools.

Determining Risk: Lethality of Method, Strength of Intent, Imminence of Plan

Traditionally, the degree of suicide risk among cognitively unimpaired patients is assessed from data about their suicide plan, method, and intended outcome (i.e., death or rescue). As noted in Table 8.2, "lethality" refers to the degree of deadliness and immediacy that a patient's suicide plan and method entail. Precautions for rescue, a low-lethality method (e.g., a nonlethal dose of medication), and available social support decrease a degree of risk (Bongar, 1992). It should be kept in mind that even critically ill patients have committed suicide. Clinical impressions also provide a barometer of risk.

Among cognitively intact patients, a precise plan for committing suicide in the next 24–48 hours via a lethal method constitutes immediate high risk. Cognitively impaired patients may be impulsive and lack a plan for suicide, so clinicians must look behind increases in general anxiety, distress, impulsivity, and agitation for clues that such patients genuinely want to die. For example, one cognitively impaired patient became increasingly anxious and walked off the nursing unit, saying, "Nobody loves me any more, and I don't like this hotel either." He then climbed the stairs to the top of the building and jumped off. Because he did not talk about suicide or give the usual suicide clues associated with depression, staff members did not suspect that suicide risk lurked behind his dementia and anxiety. Cognitively impaired persons such as this patient may actually not intend to kill themselves, but may accidentally do so in a cry for help or without recognizing the fatal consequences of their behavior.

Although lethal suicide methods can include use of guns or knives, jumping from heights, drowning, asphyxiation via carbon monoxide, and others, medically ill patients typically use an overdose of medications or alcohol, and/or suffocation. Several studies (Marzuk, 1991; DMello, Finkbeiner, & Kocher, 1995; Pugh, Odonnell, & Catalan, 1993) have reported that jumping from a high place is a commonly chosen method of suicide among people with AIDS. Hanging and jumping are also common methods of suicide in hospital settings. Tricyclic antidepressants have frequently been used in lethal suicide attempts (Kapur, Mieczkowski, & Mann, 1992). Generally, combinations of medication and alcohol are potentially lethal. However, doses of opiates that would be lethal for most people are not necessarily lethal for people with a high tolerance. Such patients who overdose on morphine to attempt suicide may awaken without ill effects. Strict safety precautions to prevent suicide are recommended for HIV-positive patients with high risk factors (i.e., males with depression, dementia, persistent pain, substance abuse, prior attempts, social isolation, poor resources, and/or inadequate social support). Psychiatric consultation is useful to confirm the degree of risk and to plan therapeutic interventions.

A short-term risk rating is based upon the individual's intent to die, specific plan for suicide, current distress, and isolation. After risk is estimated, several strategies (e.g., a safe environment, a no-suicide contract, and monitored medications) can reduce suicide potential (Valente, 1993).

Suicidal patients require careful ongoing assessment and monitoring. The astute clinician who suspects suicide risk treats a comment such as "I'll commit suicide if . . . " like a bomb that may explode, and evaluates suicidal plans and their precipitants.

MANAGING SUICIDAL PATIENTS

Clinicians need to review their agency policies and professional standards for managing suicidal patients (Bongar, Maris, Berman, Litman, & Silverman, 1993). Guidelines for reducing suicide risk in the hospital are useful in many clinical settings (Farberow, 1981; Silverman, Berman, Bongar, Litman, & Maris, 1994; Litman, 1995).

Effective interventions include removing methods of suicide, making no-suicide contracts, identifying options, improving problem solving, involving significant others, enhancing the patient's available resources (e.g., pastoral counselors, pain consultant, other health professionals), reducing pain or other physical symptoms, and providing education about treatment. Ongoing risk assessment, psychiatric evaluation, and treatment for dementia, depression, anxiety, and other psychiatric symptoms/disorders are also important. (See the "Management" portion of Table 8.5.)

Establishing Safety and Reevaluating Diagnoses

The first priority is to establish an environment to provide safety by using hospitalization, close supervision, psychiatric consultation, symptom management, and medications. The most common legal action involving suicidal patients is the failure to reasonably protect patients from harming themselves (Bongar et al., 1993). For inpatients, bathrooms are commonly selected locations for suicide attempts, so evaluation of potential hazards in bathrooms (e.g., door hinges or places that would support a strap and a patient's weight) is necessary. Consultation is useful in general, and particularly in cases when poorly controlled pain, anxiety, depression, dementia, substance abuse, or other symptoms or disorders precipitate suicidal impulses. As noted earlier, clinicians cannot afford to be lulled into a false sense of security and must recognize that even critically ill patients have found the stamina to plan and commit suicide.

Patients with delirium, dementia, substance abuse, or other mental disorders who may impulsively attempt suicide require careful supervision and one-to-one observation. Their denials of suicide intent must be considered unreliable and changeable. Complex psychiatric diagnoses often accompany suicidal potential, so psychiatric evaluation and consultation are advisable (Targ et al., 1994). If patients' suicide risk relates to their unrealistic perceptions of disease, education is needed. Risk of suicide also often increases as major depression lifts.

Clinicians must use caution to ensure that diagnoses of depression and dementia are accurate. A common problem occurs when the early apathy of dementia is mislabeled as depression, and the anticholinergic side effects of the antidepressants may include memory loss and other early symptoms of dementia. When depression and dementia coexist, smaller doses of antidepressants are needed to minimize side effects. Patients require constant reassessment for onset and changes in dementia. Patients with subcortical dementia experience forgetfulness, so if they decide to commit suicide at 9 A.M., they may promptly forget this plan. Hence, a patient can report intense suicidal feelings at several different times, and then forget these conversations and deny feeling suicidal. Impaired memory makes denial of suicidal impulses unreliable and makes the clinician's surveillance necessary.

Making No-Suicide Contracts

Asking patients to promise not to harm themselves accidentally or intentionally has been used both to evaluate and to reduce risk among clients who reliably recognize and report their suicide risk and who have a good relationship with their clinicians. A no-suicide contract can often remind a patient that a caregiver is concerned; indeed, it can serve as the patient's lifeline to the clinician. A cognitively impaired patient can carry a written memory aid that says: "I, _____, will *not* forget my bargain with my nurse/doctor, _____. I will not hurt myself. I will call _____ if I feel like hurting myself." This brief note can enhance a patient's memory and reduce a sense of isolation. However, no-suicide contracts are not a guarantee of safety, and they may have limited reliability when manipulation, impulsivity or impaired memory reduces a patient's capacity to keep a bargain (Hatton & Valente, 1984). Some patients have killed themselves even after making a no-suicide contract.

Reducing Physical Symptom Distress

Adequate management of pain, fatigue, and other physical symptoms must be a priority in treating HIV-infected patients with suicidal ideas. Guidelines for effective pain control need to be followed (U.S. DHHS, 1993).

Reducing Social Isolation

Not only is social isolation an important risk factor for direct suicidal behavior, but HIV-infected adolescents and young adults may respond to isolation or ostracism by engaging in direct self-destructive behavior, such as unprotected sex, alcohol/drug use, and antisocial acting out. Various interventions including counseling, can help patients reduce isolation by helping them to become involved in community activities with others, to develop close relationships, and to overcome barriers to socialization. When patients have a deficit in social skills, these interventions can build or strengthen these important skills. The goal of such interventions is to help patients maintain satisfying social relationships, cope with losses, and keep symptoms from interfering with social activities. Use of support groups, home visitors, and consultation can help patients identify their strengths or social skills and improve social interactions. Patients may welcome referrals to community groups where they can be involved as members or volunteers; this can increase their sense of belonging to the community. Telephone contacts, written correspondence, and ham radio and computer communications can provide alternative ways to maintain relationships.

Modifications in the physical environment may also help patients maintain or restore meaningful involvements with others and with social activities. Such modifications may include using memory aids to reduce forgetfulness, as well as altering style of dressing to distract attention from skin rashes or physical problems that cause discomfort in public.

Referral to chaplains or clergy may help patients meet spiritual needs. Although satisfaction with such relationships is subjective, it can often reduce suicide risk. Relationships with health care providers also provide important social support.

Dealing with Grief

HIV-infected patients are likely to experience multiple losses and deaths of friends and significant others, and another goal in such cases is to help patients resolve the tasks of grief. Grief is one of the most universal human responses, and few people find it easy to talk about bereavement or death. Clinicians should encourage patients to express grief, to consider participating in grief support groups or counseling, to manage the feelings of grief, to make sense of the loss of a loved one, and to reestablish social relationships and an interest in others. Cultural traditions will often determine many aspects of grief and establish guidelines for private and public expressions of grief.

Treating Specific Psychiatric Symptoms/Disorders

When specific psychiatric symptoms/disorders (e.g., depression, dementia, anxiety, and substance abuse) are diagnosed, these require specific treatment. Some comments on depression in particular are in order. Although many HIV-infected depressed patients respond to antidepressants and psychotherapy, treatments for patients with HIV disease and chronic depression or depression with dementia are more challenging and less effective. Cognitive therapy or other brief psychotherapy is often effective for managing cognitively intact patients with depression. If loss or conflict trigger suicidal impulses, then psychotherapy can help patients alter perceptions of these problems, plan more constructive responses, and seek significant others who offer resources and support. However, many people with HIV disease become depressed because they have limited resources, live alone in dreary circumstances, and have few people in their lives. Depression is more difficult to treat when few options exist to improve resources, social support, and living conditions. Clinicians can also help facilitate therapeutic interactions or recommend family or network therapy to help patients and loved ones negotiate conflicts.

When this chapter was first written, few drug interactions were reported when depressed HIV-positive persons took antidepressants or other psychiatric medications. However, Rose and Romeyn (1997) highlight new recommendations regarding medication interactions with protease inhibitors. Due to the mechanisms of absorption, distribution, metabolism, and elimination, several psychiatric drugs interact with protease inhibitors. For example, problems (e.g., flushing and abdominal pain) occur when antialcohol drugs (e.g., disulfiram or Antabuse) are taken with agents containing alcohol such as ritonavir. Because protease inhibitors inhibit metabolism of most benzodiazepine antianxiety agents, oversedation and risk of respiratory depression may result from combining drugs. Hence ritonavir should be avoided due to interactions with most benzodiazepines. Instead, lorazepam (Ativan), oxazepam (Serax), and temazepam (Restoril) should be used with ritonavir.

Rose and Romeyn also indicate that "tricyclic antidepressants such as amitriptyline (Elavil), desipramine (Norpramin), and nortriptyline (Pamelor) can build dangerous levels when used with ritonavir and should be taken at reduced levels" (p. 30). Ritonavir may also increase blood levels of some SSRIs. Close monitoring is needed when TCA or when SSRI and TCA combinations are used to treat depression. Avoid prescribing bupropion (Wellbutrin) with ritonavir because hyperconcentrations of this drug can provoke seizures. Combining "ritonavir with trazodone (Desyrel), venlafaxine (Effexor), or nefazodone (Serzone) can possibly trigger dangerous cardiac side effects" (Rose & Romeyn, p. 30).

Dose reduction may be required when common antipsychotics such as holoperidol (Haldol) are prescribed with ritonavir. Close monitoring and dose adjustments may be required when risperidone (Risperdal) is used with ritonavir. Avoid prescribing clozapine (Clozaril) with ritonavir because increased blood concentrations and severe neutropenia may result. No drug interactions have been reported so far with olanzapine (Zyprexa). Pimozide (Orap) should be avoided with ritonavir due to risk of sudden death.

ETHICAL ISSUES

The current controversy regarding euthanasia, assisted dying, and AIDS is based not on facts but on opposing ethical views. Although patients have the right to explore their treatment choices fully and to refuse some or all treatments, some clinicians consider refusal of treatments as tantamount to suicide. The fact remains, however, that until a cure is found, for a person with AIDS, the choice may not be between living and dying, but between dying now and dying later (Yarnell & Battin, 1988).

Debates on this topic are prominent in the mass media, with reports of physician-assisted deaths and publication of how-to-commit-suicide books (Breitbart et al., 1996; Saunders, 1994). Organizations such as the Hemlock Society, Choice in Dying, and Americans Against Human Suffering have sponsored legislative initiatives supporting assisted suicide in California, Oregon, and Washington. Although surveys of health care professionals indicate acceptance of assisted suicide, the American Medical Association Council on Ethical and Judicial Affairs and the California Nurses Association oppose active euthanasia (Lipman & Battin, 1996). Many individuals who support assisted suicide in principle have voiced concern about inadequate safeguards legalizing assisted suicide (Stone, 1997) proposed prior to 1997.

Clinicians may experience conflicts as they consider their duty to prevent suicide and their responsibility to respect patients' autonomy. Some argue that their duty is to respect patients' right and free will to choose suicide instead of a life-threatening disease (i.e., AIDS) that involves pain, fatigue, and unrelieved suffering. Slome, Moulton, Huttine, Gorter, and Abrams (1992) examined physicians' attitudes toward assisted suicide in the context of AIDS; twenty-three percent of the total sample in San Francisco said that they would be likely to grant a patient's initial request for help to commit suicide. However, many HIV/AIDS patients who request suicide may be unable to exercise autonomy because a severe psychiatric disorder such as depression undermines their ability to think clearly (Saunders, 1994). In addition, when clinicians consider granting an initial request for suicide, their approach may overlook the need to improve pain management, reduce other physical symptoms, or improve quality of life. In short, they may fail to evaluate whether the request for suicide is a cry for help or a rational consideration of alternatives.

Still other factors that must be considered in evaluating an HIV/AIDS patient's request for suicide are the effects on this particular patient of HIV disease itself. Some neurocognitive impairment is common in advanced HIV disease, but the rate of progression of HIV dementia is highly variable. Early symptoms may not affect a patient's capacity to make decisions. The patient with HIV-related dementia should continue to make personal decisions autonomously in as many situations as possible. Capacity for decision making may vary from day to day and from one situation to another. The clinician must assess capacity and must not assume that impaired capacity is constant rather than fluctuating.

Rational suicide is a particularly relevant issue in HIV/AIDS. People with terminal illnesses such as AIDS are often the groups used to illustrate arguments for rational suicide. Controversy exists over whether a person of sound mind can plan suicide (Maris, 1983). People who are contemplating suicide because of terminal illness, permanent disability, or advanced old age deserve serious consideration, however, and their requests for suicide should not be automatically disregarded or discounted (Saunders, 1994).

One proponent of rational suicide recommends evaluation of the following criteria for terminally ill adults who plan suicide: (1) a mental status examination showing clear mental processes without depression; (2) motives for suicide that society in general would understand; and (3) evidence that all options have been thoroughly explored before suicide is selected (Siegel, 1986). These criteria, however, may not guide clinicians through more complex situations. For example, one patient with AIDS planned to commit suicide when her pain was overwhelming, her quality of life unacceptable, and her life meaningless. She was receiving psychotherapy and pharmacological treatment for her depression, and she demonstrated clear thought processes about the nature, meaning, and consequences of her suicide plan and all other options. However, it was not clear whether she met the first of Siegel's (1986) criteria. She had mild to moderate depression, but she also had thought clearly about options and the meaning and consequences of her suicide. Moreover, these criteria address the individual but do not consider loved ones, family, or friends.

Clinicians will find Battin's (1991) guidelines a more effective approach to evaluating rational suicide. Battin (1991) advocates discussion of a client's request for help in suicide, and recommends that a mental health professional evaluate various factors in assessing the rationality or irrationality of suicide with the client (see Table 8.6). Although it is still illegal in most states for clinicians actually to *assist* patients in committing suicide (as Battin notes), clients who demonstrate rational decision making about suicide may benefit from legal advocates, education about their options, and palliative care.

When the pain of living is greater than the idea of dying, people may consider suicide as a response to persistent pain, depression,

TABLE 8.6. Questions for Assessment of the Rationality of Suicide

1. What are the purposes and motives of the person considering suicide?
   Is the person making a request for help?
   Why is the person consulting a health professional?
   Is the request for help in suicide a request for someone else to decide?
   Is the suicide plan financially motivated?
   What has kept the person from committing suicide so far?
   Does the person fear becoming a burden?
2. How stable is the request? Has suicide been planned for a long time, or is it a response to a recent event.
3. Is the request consistent with the person's basic values?
4. Are the medical and nonmedical facts cited in the request accurate?
5. Has the person considered the effects of his or her suicide on others?
6. What are the person's suicide plans and options?
   How far in the future would the suicide take place?
   Has the person picked a method of suicide?
   Would the person be willing to tell others about his or her suicide plan?
   Does the person see suicide as the only way out?
7. What cultural influences are shaping a person's choices?
8. Are the person's affairs in order? Have arrangements been made for a funeral, or durable power or attorney in case the suicide attempt is not fatal? *Comment*: In most states a health professional's relationship with a patient implies a legal and professional duty to refrain from assisting suicide; clinicians may not knowingly administer a lethal dose of medication or help clients plan a lethal dose. However, terminally ill patients with suicide plans deserve thoughtful evaluation of their rational and irrational requests, and appropriate treatment options for their depression, pain, or symptom distress. Clinicians need to understand the legal and ethical issues and criteria for evaluating the rationality of suicide.

Note. Adapted from Battin (1991). Copyright 1991 by Hogrefe and Huber Publishers. Adapted by permission.

dementia, or unacceptable quality of life. Sometimes, when a patient says, "I would be better off dead," a clinician may believe that the patient is right. Only a thorough assessment of suicidal intent will identify distressing symptoms that require treatment, such as persistent pain, depression, or dementia. Clinicians cannot assume that suicide risk is absent when suicide is not mentioned, because many patients will not spontaneously mention suicide unless asked. In patients with HIV, suicide risk should be routinely monitored and evaluated.

If a moral conflict about suicide impairs a clinician's ability to care for a suicidal client, a referral should be considered. A clinician is not obligated to meet a patient's demands for specific interventions or advice when, in the clinician's best judgment, doing so is not indicated or appropriate. Regardless of their position on this issue, however, clinicians who treat HIV-infected people have an ethical duty to influence politics and legislation to improve research, clinical services, and access to treatment for this population, as budget cuts continue to reduce funds and services.

SUMMARY AND RECOMMENDATIONS

Because people with HIV disease have high suicide rates, clinicians must evaluate suicide clues and risk factors (see Table 8.1). Early in the course of HIV disease, clinicians need to evaluate suicide risk and concomitant psychiatric syndromes (Marzuk et al., 1988). Clinicians need not only to establish baseline assessments, but to conduct ongoing evaluations of suicide potential. Many people with AIDS develop symptoms of dementia (e.g., impulsivity, poor judgment, lability, and disinhibition), which can increase suicide risk. A thorough diagnostic evaluation, including history, physical examination, and neurobehavioral/psychiatric evaluation, should be conducted to assess suicidality and to rule out organic, mood, and cognitive disorders secondary to or coexisting with HIV infection. In particular, depressive disorders are never "normal" and deserve treatment. It is important to maintain hope and support in those who may see HIV as a reason for having none. A patient's rationality and decision-making capacity regarding suicide require monitoring.

Clinicians need to establish rapport with patients and to ask direct, nonjudgmental questions about suicide. Screening questionnaires can detect or monitor people at risk for depression or suicide. Interviews with significant others are also useful. A clinician's initial goals are to detect a patient's suicide plans, estimate short-term risk, and reduce suicide potential (e.g., control pain, treat depression, change medications). The patient's degree of suicide risk should be estimated; a patient with a precise and lethal suicide plan to be carried out in the next 24–48 hours is at high risk and requires safety precautions. Clinicians must look for more subtle clues such as agitation and death wishes among cognitively impaired patients, who may be impulsive and lack a plan for suicide. Many medically ill people use an overdose of medications or alcohol, and/or suffocation, as methods of suicide. Tricyclic antidepressants have been commonly used in lethal suicide attempts.

The first priority in managing suicidal patients is to establish a safe environment by using hospitalization, close supervision, psychiatric consultation, symptom management, and medications. Clinicians need to establish trusting relationships with patients and to establish safe opportunities for talking about sensitive and troubling topics. Clinicians must recognize that even critically ill patients have found the stamina to plan and commit suicide. Patients with delirium, dementia, substance abuse, or other mental disorders who may impulsively attempt suicide require careful supervision and one-to-one observation. Their denials of suicide must be considered unreliable and changeable. Accurate diagnosis of depression and dementia are critical to effective treatment.

Other effective interventions include reducing pain or other physical symptoms, identifying options, improving problem solving, enhancing resources, involving significant others, and providing education about treatment. Ongoing risk assessment, psychiatric evaluation, and treatment are important. Regardless of treatment chosen, clinicians should consider the stage of HIV disease progression and set realistic goals for therapy. Referrals for individual and group therapy are useful for patients who are depressed or suicidal, and medications (e.g., antidepressants or antianxiety drugs) are often effective for the respective psychiatric disorders.

Ethical conflicts often arise when HIV/AIDS patients refuse treatment or request suicide: Clinicians' duty to prevent suicide conflicts with their responsibility to respect their patients. Many HIV/AIDS patients who request suicide may be unable to exercise autonomy, because depression or another psychiatric disorder, pain or other HIV-related stressors, or HIV disease itself may undermine their ability to think clearly. However, some patients with HIV/AIDS may plan suicide rationally as a way to manage the end of their lives or to avoid disease progression and distress. Dementia itself is not incompatible with a patient's choosing rational suicide, but capacity to participate in personal, health care, or end-of-life decisions will fluctuate or diminish as cognitive impairment progresses. The goal in all cases is to help patients explore their ideas about rational suicide without locking themselves into positions of action. Battin (1991) suggests questions to evaluate a suicidal patient's rationality (see Table 8.6).

REFERENCES

Alfonso, C., & Cohen, M. A. (1994). HIV dementia and suicide. *General Hospital Psychiatry, 16,* 45–46.

Armendariz, A., Saunders, J. M., Poston, S. L., & Valente, S. M. (1997). Exploring a life history of HIV disease and self caring: Alfredo's story. *Journal of Association of Nurses in AIDS Care, 8*(2), 72–82.

Battin, M. (1991). Rational suicide: How can we respond to a request for help? *Crisis, 12,* 73–80.

Beck, A. T. (1979). *Cognitive therapy and the emotional disorders.* New York: New American Library.

Beck, A. T., Brown, G., Berchick, R. J., Stewart, B. L., & Steer, R. A. (1990).

Relationship between hopelessness and ultimate suicide. *American Journal of Psychiatry 147*(2), 190–195.

Beck, A. T., & Steer, R. A. (1987). *Beck Depression Inventory: Manual.* San Antonio, TX: Psychological Corporation.

Berchick, R. J., & Wright, F. D. (1992). Guidelines for handling the suicidal patient. In B. Bongar (Ed.), *Suicide: Guidelines for assessment, management and treatment* (pp. 179–186). New York: Oxford.

Bongar, B. (Ed.). (1992). *Suicide: Guidelines for assessment, management and treatment.* New York: Oxford University Press.

Bongar, B., Maris, R. W., Berman, A. L., Litman, R. E., & Silverman, M. M. (1993). Inpatient standards of care and the suicidal patient: Part I. General clinical formulation and legal considerations. *Suicide and Life-Threatening Behavior, 23*(3), 245–262.

Breitbart, W. (1990). Cancer pain and suicide. In K. Foley, J. J. Barica, & V. Ventafridda (Eds.), *Advances in pain research and therapy* (Vol. 16, pp. 399–412). New York: Raven Press.

Breitbart, W. (1993). Suicide risk and pain in cancer and AIDS patients. In C. R. Chapman & K. M. Foley (Eds.), *Current and emerging issues in cancer pain: Research and practice* (pp. 49–65). New York: Raven Press.

Breitbart, W., Rosenfeld, B. D., & Passik, S. D. (1996). Interest in physician-assisted suicide among ambulatory HIV-infected patients. *American Journal of Psychiatry, 153*(2), 238–242.

Buckingham, S., & van Gorp, W. (1988). Essential knowledge about AIDS dementia. *Social Work, 2,* 112–115.

Copeland, A. R. (1993). Suicide among AIDS patients. *Medicine, Science, Law,. 33*(1), 21–28.

Cote, T., Biggar, R., & Dannenberg, A. (1992). Risk of suicide among persons with AIDS: A national assessment. *Journal of the American Medical Association, 268*(15), 2066–2068.

DMello, D. A., Finkbeiner, D. S., & Kocher, K. N. (1995). The cost of antidepressant overdose. *General Hospital Psychiatry, 17*(6), 454–455.

DiMaio, L., Squitieri, F., Napolitano, G., Campanella, G., Trofatter, J. A., & Conneally, P. M. (1993). Suicide risk in Huntington's disease. *Journal of Medical Genetics, 30*(4), 293–295.

Farberow, N. (1981). Suicide prevention in the hospital. *Hospital and Community Psychiatry, 32*(2), 99–104.

Flavin, D., Franklin, J., & Frances, R. (1986). The acquired immune deficiency syndrome (AIDS) and suicidal behavior in alcohol-dependent homosexual men. *American Journal of Psychiatry, 143*(11), 1440–1442.

Flaskerud, J. (1986). Diagnostic and treatment differences among five ethnic groups. *Psychological Reports, 58*(1), 219–235.

Glick, M. E. (1994, December). HIV damage of nervous system increases. *Being Alive,* p. 15.

Hatton, C. L., & Valente, S. M. (1984). *Suicide: Assessment and intervention.* New York: Appleton-Century-Crofts.

Joe, G. W., Knezek, L., Watson, D., & Simpson, D. D. (1991). Depression and decision-making among intravenous drug users. *Psychological Reports, 68*(1), 339–347.

Joseph, J. G., Caumartin, S. M., Tal, M., Kirshi, J. P., Kessler, R. C., Ostrow, D. G., & Wortman, C. B. (1990). Psychological functioning in a cohort of gay men at risk for AIDS: A three year descriptive study. *Journal of Nervous and Mental Disease, 178*(10), 607–615.

Kapur, S., Mieczkowski, T., Mann, J. J. (1992). Antidepressant medications and the relative risk of suicide attempt and suicide. *Journal of the American Medical Association, 268,* 3441–3445.

Kizer, K. W., Green, M. A., Perkins, C. I., Doebbert, G., & Hughes, M. S. (1988). AIDS and suicide in California. *Journal of the American Medical Association, 260*(13), 1581.

Lipe, H., Schultz, A., & Bird, T. D. (1993). Risk factors for suicide in Huntington's disease: Retrospective case controlled study. *American Journal of Medical Genetics, 48*(4), 231–233.

Lipman, A., & Battin, M. P. (1996). (Eds.). Position papers on euthanasia and assisted suicide [Special issue]. *Journal of Pharmaceutical Care in Pain and Symptom Control 3*(3–4).

Litman, R. E. (1995). Suicide prevention in a treatment setting. *Suicide and Life-Threatening Behavior 25*(1), 134–142.

Maris, R. (1983). Rational suicide: An impoverished self transformation. *Suicide and Life-Threatening Behavior, 12*(1), 4–16.

Markowitz, J. C., Rabkin, J. G., & Perry, S. W. (1994). Treating depression in HIV-positive patients. *AIDS 8*(4), 403–412.

Marzuk, P. M. (1991). Suicidal behaviour and HIV illnesses. *International Review of Psychiatry, 3,* 367.

Marzuk, P. M., Tierney, H., Tardiff, K., Gross, E., Morgan, E., Hsu, M., & Mann, J. (1988). Increased risk of suicide in persons with AIDS. *Journal of the American Medical Association, 259*(9), 1333–1337.

McKegney, P., & O'Dowd, M. (1992). Suicidality and HIV status. *American Journal of Psychiatry, 149*(3), 396–398.

National Center for Health Statistics. (1994). *Vital statistics of the United States.* Washington, DC: U.S. Government Printing Office.

Nyamathi, A., Flaskerud, J., & Leake, B. (1997). HIV-risk behaviors and mental health characteristics among homeless or drug-recovering women and their closest sources of support. *Nursing Research, 46*(3), 133–137.

O'Dowd, M., Biderman, D., & McKegney, F. (1993). Incidence of suicidality in AIDS and HIV+ patients attending a psychiatry outpatient program. *Psychosomatics, 34*(1), 33–40.

Perry, S. (1990). Organic mental disorders caused by HIV: Update on early diagnosis and treatment. *American Journal of Psychiatry, 147*(6), 696–710.

Perry, S., Fishman, B., Jacobsberg, L., & Frances, A. (1991). Effectiveness of psychoeducational interventions in reducing emotional distress after human immunodeficiency virus antibody testing. *Archives of General Psychiatry, 48,* 143–147.

Perry, S., Jacobsberg, L., & Fishman, B. (1990). Suicidal ideation and HIV testing. *Journal of the American Medical Association, 263*(5), 679–682.

Pugh, K., O'Donnell, I., & Catalan, J. (1993). Suicide and HIV disease. *AIDS Care,* 5, 391–400.

Quill, T. (1993). "Doctor, I want to die. Will you help me?" *Journal of the American Medical Association, 270*(8), 870–876.

Rabkin, J. G., Remien, R., Katloff, L., & Williams, J. B. W. (1993). Suicidality in AIDS long-term survivors: What is the evidence? *AIDS Care, 5*(4), 401–411.

Rabkin, J. G., Williams, J. B. W., Neugebauer, R., Remien, R., & Goetz, R. (1990). Maintenance of hope in HIV-spectrum homosexual men. *American Journal of Psychiatry, 147*(10), 1322–1326.

Rose, E., & Romeyn, M. (1997, September). Protease inhibitor drug interactions. *Beta: Bulletin of experimental treatment for AIDS,* pp. 29–38.

Roth, A. J., & Breitbart, W. (1996). Psychiatric emergencies in terminally ill cancer patients. *Hematology/Oncology Clinics of North America, 10*(1), 235–239.

Rundell, J., Kyle, K., Brown, G., & Thomason, J. (1992). Risk factors for suicide attempts in a human immunodeficiency virus screening program. *Psychosomatics, 33*(1), 24–27.

Saunders, J. M. (1994). Ethical issues. In J. Flaskerud & P. Ungvarsky (Eds.), *HIV/AIDS: A guide to nursing care* (3rd ed., pp. 364–388). Philadelphia: Saunders.

Saunders, J. M., & Buckingham, S. L. (1988). Suicidal AIDS patient: When the depression turns deadly. *Nursing, 18,* 60–64.

Saunders, J. M., & Valente, S. M. (1988). Suicide risk among gay men and lesbians. *Death Studies, 11,* 1–23.

Saunders, J. M., & Valente, S. M. (1993). Terminal illness and suicide: A case study. *Suicide and Life-Threatening Behavior, 23*(1), 76–82.

Saunders, J. M., & Valente, S. M. (1996). Hopelessness, intimacy, isolation. In K. M. Casey, F. Cohen, & A. Hughes (Eds.), *Core curriculum for HIV/AIDS nursing care* (pp. 258–272). Philadelphia: Nursecom.

Schneider, S. G., Taylor, S. E., Hammen, C., Kemeny, M. E., & Dudley, J. (1991). Factors influencing suicide intent in gay and bisexual suicide ideators: Differing models for men with and without human immunodeficiency virus. *Journal of Personality and Social Psychology, 61*(5), 776–788.

Schneiderman, L. J., Kronick, R., Kaplan, R. M., Anderson, J. P., & Sanger, R. D. (1994). Attitudes of seriously ill patients toward treatment that involves high cost and burden on others. *Journal of Clinical Ethics, 5*(2), 109–112.

Schofferman, J., & Brody, R. (1990). Pain in far advanced AIDS. In K. M. Foley, J. J. Bonica, & V. Ventafridda (Eds.), *Advances in pain research and therapy* (Vol. 16, pp. 379–386). New York: Raven Press.

Selnes, O. A., Galai, N., Bacellar, H., Miller, E. N., Becker, J. T., Wesch, J., van Gorp, W., & McArthur, J. C. (1995). Cognitive performance after progression to AIDS: A longitudinal study from the Multicenter AIDS Cohort study. *Neurology, 45*(2), 267–275.

Siegel, K. (1986). Psychological aspects of rational suicide. *American Journal of Psychotherapy, 40*(3), 405–418.

Silverman, M. M., Berman, A. L., Bongar, B., Litman, R. E., & Maris, R. W. (1994). Inpatient standards of care and the suicidal patient: Part II. An integration with clinical risk management. *Suicide and Life-Threatening Behavior, 24*(2), 152–169.

Slome, L., Moulton, J., Huffine, C., Gorter, R., & Abrams, D. (1992). Physicians' attitudes toward assisted suicide in AIDS. *Journal of Acquired Immune Deficiency Syndromes 5*(7), 712–718.

Starace, F. (1993). Suicidal behavior in people infected with human immunodeficiency virus: A literature review. *International Journal of Social Psychiatry, 39*(1), 164–170.

Stone, A. A. (1997). Physician assisted suicide and the psychiatric profession. *Harvard Mental Health Letter, 1*, 4–7.

Targ, E. F., Karasic, D. H., Diefenbach, P. N., Anderson, D. A., Bystritsky, A., & Fawsy, F. I. (1994). Structured group therapy and fluoxetine to treat depression in HIV-positive persons. *Psychosomatics, 35*(2), 132–137.

U.S. Department of Health and Human Services (DHHS). (1993). AHCPR Clinical practice guidelines: Depression. In *Depression in primary care* (DHHS Publication No. AHCPR 93-0551, Vol. 1, pp. 1–99.). Washington, DC: U.S. Government Printing Office.

Valente, S. M. (1993). Evaluating suicide in the medically ill patient. *Nurse Practitioner, 18*(9), 41–50.

Valente, S. M., & Saunders, J. M. (1994). Management of suicidal patients with HIV disease. *Journal of Nurses in AIDS Care, 5*(6), 19–29.

Valente, S. M., & Saunders, J. M. (1996a). Case commentaries on assisted suicide and euthanasia. *Journal of Pharmaceutical Care in Pain and Symptom Control, 4*(1–2), 291–344.

Valente, S. M., & Saunders, J. M. (1996b). Powerlessness and guilt. In K. M. Casey, F. Cohen, & A. Hughes (Eds.), *Core curriculum for HIV/AIDS nursing care* (pp. 255–258; 267–269). Philadelphia: Nursecom.

Valente, S. M., Saunders, J. M., & Uman, G. (1993). Self care, psychological distress and HIV disease. *Journal of Nurses in AIDS Care, 4*(4), 15–25.

Wright, J. G., Thase, M. E., Beck, A. T., & Ludgate, J. W. (Eds.). (1993). *Cognitive therapy with inpatients.* New York: Guilford Press.

Yarnell, S. K., & Battin, M. P. (1988). AIDS, psychiatry and euthanasia. *Psychiatric Annals, 18*(10), 598–603.

9

Enhancing Adaptive Function in HIV-Associated Dementia

RAE LYNN BENSON-DUFFY

INTRODUCTION

Clinical occupational therapists work with other clinicians and with many types of patients to promote and enhance the patients' functional abilities. For this to be done in an efficient manner, a patient must first be evaluated in order to determine his or her abilities and deficits. This chapter deals with enhancing function in patients with HIV-associated dementia. To assist such a patient, an occupational therapist must first know what to expect—that is, what cognitive and physical symptoms are associated with HIV-associated dementia. Once an occupational therapist knows what the symptoms are, he or she must then determine how these symptoms affect function in the affected individual. Finally, based on this knowledge, the occupational therapist can make recommendations for environmental, equipment, or other changes to help the person function better in his or her chosen living situation.

CHANGES IN HIV-ASSOCIATED DEMENTIA

The number of patients with HIV who will develop HIV-associated dementia has been shown to range from 15% to 30% (Pulliam, Gascon, Stubblebine, McGuire, & McGrath, 1997). Early symptoms of HIV-associated dementia are often broken down into three categories: cognitive, behavioral, and motor (Maj, 1990). As in any type of dementing illness, reversible causes for such changes need to be carefully evaluated and treated first.

Cognitive problems in this group of patients include forgetfulness; difficulty in organizing thoughts to complete daily tasks; losing track of a conversation; problems with memory and concentration; and overall mental slowing. Often these problems first become apparent to an HIV-infected person and his or her caregiver(s) in the performance of daily tasks. The person may have difficulty in remembering to take medications, going to appointments, returning phone calls, making meals, or answering questions. Often difficulties can arise when the person tries to follow a conversation; the plot of a book, movie, or television show; or even the news. Instrumental activities of daily living can also be greatly affected, as they are generally more complicated and require more planning to accomplish. These include shopping, paying bills, balancing the checkbook, and driving a car, to name a few.

These cognitive changes can lead to needing more time to complete daily tasks. Ideas for helping keep affected individuals able to do more for themselves for a longer period of time are discussed later in this chapter. However, it is important for a therapist to be aware when evaluating a patient that at least some cognitive symptoms can be linked to affective syndromes, such as depression, anxiety, obsessions, compulsions or mania (Fernandez, 1989; Maj, 1990; see also Chapter 4, this volume). In these cases it is important to treat the underlying psychiatric symptoms with psychotherapy and medication, in order to improve functional abilities.

Altered behaviors that may be found in patients with HIV-associated dementia are also often related to psychiatric symptoms, including depression, apathy, reduced spontaneity, psychotic symptoms, and social withdrawal (Fernandez, 1989; Maj, 1990). These symptoms can lead to a decrease in the patients' ability to work productively. Patients may also avoid socializing with friends, family members, or other acquaintances.

It should be noted that in some patients with HIV-associated dementia psychotic symptoms may develop. These symptoms and/or delirium need to be evaluated and treated quickly to prevent any type of permanent brain damage (Fernandez, 1990). Behaviors to observe for include restlessness, irritability, anxiety, difficulty thinking, insomnia, and vivid nightmares. These symptoms often become worse at night because of diurnal variations. Further, with delirium as with HIV-associated dementia, there are often abnormal movement patterns noted. These can include tremor, multifocal myoclonus, asterixis, and floccillation.

Motor changes in the person with HIV-associated dementia resemble a subcortical dementia movement pattern (see Chapters 2 and 4, this volume). They can include changes in muscle tone and coordination, dysgraphia, dysarthria, mild to moderate cerebellar dysfunction, hyperreflexia, and motor weakness (Buckingham & van Gorp, 1994; Fernandez, 1989; Maj, 1990).

These changes can result in problems with daily activities that require good hand skills, such as eating, shaving, and writing. Cerebellar dysfunction can also cause a person to trip or fall more often, or to have difficulty walking up and down stairs or traversing uneven surfaces. In work situations where a person has a job requiring writing, typing, or other clerical skills, motor problems can lead to a decrease in job performance. Because of this, these problems should be addressed early through modifications of a person's work station and/or modification of the job description.

In the later stages of HIV-associated dementia, there is a global deterioration of cognitive and motor abilities (Maj, 1990; Fernandez, 1989). The person may have severe psychomotor slowing, may be confined to a wheelchair or bed most of the time, may have dual incontinence, and may exhibit myoclonus or seizures. Speech is generally slow, with word-finding difficulties apparent. Some patients may progress to mutism and appear to be catatonic. Others may exhibit more socially inappropriate behaviors, such as sexual acting out, biting, poor impulse control, and fecal or urinary smearing (Maj, 1990). Some of these inappropriate behaviors may be related to a concurrent delirium. In these cases, the level of consciousness and apparent cognitive impairment can change from day to day and should be observed to help the person do what he or she is capable of doing.

Although HIV-associated dementia affects adults, there is a related problem in children with HIV known as HIV-1-associated progressive encephalopathy that pediatric therapists should be aware of for treatment purposes (Mintz, 1996). Both of these syndromes can result in severe clinical and pathological deterioration of the central nervous system. Further, opportunistic infections are more likely in these patients, which can cause symptoms of HIV-associated dementia in adults or HIV-1-associated progressive encephalopathy in children (Mintz, 1996).

In children the clinical features of progressive encephalopathy fall into three main categories that are similar to those in adult HIV-associated dementia: impaired brain growth, progressive motor dysfunction, and problems with neurodevelopmental milestones.

Impaired brain-growth is measured by atrophy on neuroimaging and head circumference growth rates in the first two years. Progressive motor dysfunction is similar to that of adults with HIV-associated dementia and can include decreased find motor movement and eventually gross motor skills (Mintz, 1996). The children may also have a "Parkinsonian-like" appearance with rigidity, dystonia, and tremors. In some cases, L-dopa therapy helps improve movements in these children (Mintz, 1996). In younger children there can be problems with neurodevelopmental milestones. These children generally need assistance with activities of daily living (Mintz, 1996) like their adult counterparts. In infants, formal testing has shown that motor skills and prelinguistic abilities are most affected (Mintz, 1996) while school-age children are more likely to have noted cognitive problems, generally noted as attention deficit or attention-deficit/hyperactivity disorders. Attention disorders are often found in adults with HIV-associated dementia as well (Mintz, 1996). In addition, while adults with HIV-associated dementia often have psychiatric syndromes, it is rare in children with progressive encephalopathy, except in the late stages of the disease, and most can be attributed to opportunistic infections (Mintz, 1996).

Although primary depression and psychosis are rare in children, they are increasing in frequency as children are beginning to live longer with HIV infection. As with adults they must be carefully evaluated for other causes of the depression or psychosis. Metabolic or endocrine dysfunction can often be factors (Mintz, 1996).

Finally, children and adults can both benefit from evaluation and treatment by rehabilitation professionals. Occupational, physical, and speech therapists are trained to help remediate and train patients to improve motor and cognitive functioning.

DETERMINING HOW CHANGES TRANSLATE INTO FUNCTIONAL PROBLEMS

In general, occupational therapists attempt to look at what patients can and cannot do, based on what they learn about the patients through observation and testing. This process is the same for patients with HIV-associated dementia as it is for patients with any other syndrome or disorder. By knowing generally what problems to expect in a person with HIV-associated dementia, the occupational therapist has a reference point to begin testing for functional problems. This knowledge will, in turn, lead to the implementation of standard therapeutic measures or the design of new ones to help improve or maintain the patient's function.

Again, cognitive changes in these patients include memory loss, decreased concentration, difficulty in comprehending, psychomotor slowing, and difficulty in processing information. Many of these changes are difficult to test for reliably in the early stages of the HIV-associated dementia, but they can be assessed subjectively through interviewing the person and/or his or her caregiver(s). Subjectively, patients who are depressed report more forgetfulness and problems with other everyday cognitive activities, which are seen on their performance in formal neuropsychological testing (Buckingham & van Gorp, 1994).

For early formal testing, there is one area that is relatively easy to test and has good reliability: psychomotor slowing. Commonly, patients or caregivers will report that the patients have difficulty driving or finding their way, or have had recent auto accidents (Buckingham & van Gorp, 1994). If a person is an office worker or cashier, or has some other type of job that requires precise use of a machine, this can translate into decreased typing speed or checkout speed, or an increased number of errors or even accidents. An occupational therapist can then do further testing to document these early changes; the measures used may include psychological tests, Parts A and B of the Trail Making Test, and the Digit Symbol subtest of the Wechsler Adult Intelligence Scale–Revised.

In regard to fine motor skills, the Purdue Grooved Pegboard, the Minnesota Rate of Manipulation, and the Rosenbusch Finger Dexterity Test are three tests designed specifically for testing hand and finger dexterity and speed of movement in patients. Another test that looks at fine motor functions often found in activities of daily living is the Jebsen–Taylor Hand Function Test, which examines the person's writing, card turning, picking up small objects, simulated feeding, stacking checkers, picking up large light objects, and picking up large heavy objects (Smith, 1978).

A test of hand and arm coordination designed for workers is the Pennsylvania Bi-Manual Work Sample; this test requires the assembly and disassembly of 100 nuts and bolts. The Crawford Small Parts Dexterity Test has the subject do two fine motor manipulations. The first is to pick up a pin with tweezers, insert it into a hole, and then place a collar over it with the preferred hand. The second is to pick up a screw, begin to thread it into a hole with the finger, and complete the task using a screwdriver (Smith, 1978).

Other tests that look at whole-body motor skills can also be used for assessment. However, none has been standardized for adults. Most clinicians who know normal developmental standards for adults can use these tests and identify problems by using the various subcomponents of the tests. One such test that can be used is the Purdue Perceptual–Motor Survey (Roach & Kephart, 1971; Clark, Allen, & Schanzenbacher, 1985). This survey looks at various perceptual–motor skills grouped into five main areas: form perception, ocular pursuits, posture and balance, body image and differentiation, and perceptual–motor matching. The survey can be done in about 30 minutes and requires a manual, rating sheet, and various types of equipment, including a balance beam, 4-foot pole, pillow, mat, and chalkboard. A final test is the Bruininks–Oseretsky Motor Development Scale, which looks at drawing, drawing between two lines, doing a maze, cutting paper on a line, jumping, walking a balance beam, and timed dots in a circle. This last test consists of a page printed with half-inch diameter circles in rows. The patients uses a pencil to make dots in the center of as many circles as possible in a specified time.

The observant occupational therapist will also look at how a person performs while doing various activities in a clinical or home setting. Examples may include cooking, shaving, putting on makeup or doing hair, dressing, playing a familiar game or learning a new game, gardening, or doing other housework. Some patients may also be evaluated at the work site for problems with clerical, construction, or mechanical skills.

Since psychomotor slowing is often an initial problem in HIV-associated dementia, care should be taken to identify whether the problem is predominantly cognitive or motor in each patient. This can be done by using the testing and observational techniques discussed above.

NOW WHAT?: HELPING THE PATIENT IN VARIOUS AREAS

Now that the occupational therapist has identified the patient's problems through patient/caregiver report, observation, interviews, and testing of the patient as appropriate, the next question is this: What can the clinician do to help? The answer is that a great many adaptations can be made to assist the patient in activities of daily living and at work. In addition, participating in recreational activities can be highly beneficial for the patient.

Adaptations for Activities of Daily Living

Cognitive changes such as forgetfulness can be compensated for by having the patient use calendars or organizers to keep track of information about appointments, phone numbers, names, and the like. Other important information can also be kept easily visible and accessible through this method. Patients and caregivers can also make checklists for performing all types of activities: how to use a particular appliance; what to gather and take when leaving the house for the day; how to take the bus to the store, work, or school; or what to pack for a vacation.

Remembering to take medications is often a problem. There are multiple ways to address this problem. Medications can be carried in a pill box that has a timer that rings to alert the person to take his or her medicine. Pill boxes that carry a week's worth of medications can be purchased; such a box allows the patient to see easily that all of the medication has been taken for the day. Timers on watches or alarm clocks can be set to remind the person to take his or her medicines. Charts can be made with the names and/or pictures of the medications and the times to take them. These can then be checked off by the patient each time they are taken. It is often beneficial to include possible side effects on the chart as well, to help remind the person to tell his or her physician if any of these are experienced. The chart method can also be used to remind the person to do tasks around the house or at work.

Another helpful idea is to set daily routines for the person to follow. Having a specific spot to keep keys, medications, phone numbers, or other important things can decrease the frustration of losing them, or of putting them somewhere and forgetting where they were left. Also, making a list of important information and posting it by the phone or a calendar can be helpful in emergencies. Finally, keeping a pen and paper handy in the car, in a pocket, or by the phone can allow the person to jot down questions, thoughts, or other information when the person thinks of it so that it, can be "recalled" at a later date.

A person who is having difficulty organizing his or her thoughts to complete daily tasks can be helped by making lists of what needs to be done during the day. This can be done either the evening before or early in the morning. These lists can be simple or complex, and either the patient or a caregiver may make them. The lists may break the tasks down into categories, such as self-care (shower, shave, makeup tooth care, etc.) and instrumental activities of daily living (shopping, meal planning and preparation, bill paying, running errands, etc.). Each task can also be broken down into smaller subsections (taking food from the freezer in the morning, taking the number 6 bus to the grocery store, etc.).

When a person has a problem with concentration, several things can be done to help. First, the client should decrease the distractions in the area. If the person is trying to read, write, type, or even have a conversation with someone, he or she shouldn't have the television or radio on. If the phone rings or someone comes to the door, the client should be instructed to turn off or turn down the volume of the radio or television.

When the person does tasks outside the home, he or she should be instructed to make lists and follow them. This is especially important for shopping, so that the person will remember to get all of the things that are needed and will not have to go back and forth to get things that were missed. To make activities such as shopping easier, the client might put a pad of paper and a pen or pencil on the refrigerator or some other handy place, so that a list can be made as the client thinks of items that are needed. Before leaving to go shopping, the client should be encouraged to check the list and look in the kitchen or other areas to be sure he or she hasn't missed something that is needed, or added things that are not needed. The client should also learn to remind himself or herself, "Make sure I take the checkbook and keys too!"

When the client gets to the store, he or she should shop in a routine manner, always beginning at one end of the store and going down each aisle. The client should take a pen/pencil and check off each item as it is found and placed in the basket. As the client is standing in the checkout line, he or she should look over the list to be sure everything has been found. The client can also use this time to begin writing a check if that is the method of payment.

Another area that can cause problems when concentration is decreased is meal preparation. To help in this area, advance menu planning can help. A client can decide from 1 to 7 days in advance what he or she will make on certain days, so that the recipes and ingredients will be on hand when needed. As he or she begins to cook a meal, the client should first gather all of the items needed and place them in a contained area. These will include the recipe, ingredients, containers, and utensils. If need be, someone can help with the gathering of the items, and with the timing of when various foods or courses should be started. Written instructions will help and should be followed carefully. Many cookbooks have instructions for and pictures of various foods at various stages of preparation. Timers are helpful for making sure things are not over- or undercooked. When ready to serve the meal, the client should check in the oven, in the microwave, in the refrigerator, and on the top of the stove where food may have been placed to keep warm or cool for the meal.

Slowed speech is another common area of frustration for some patients with HIV-associated dementia. Such patients should be encouraged to take time to collect their thoughts prior to engaging in conversations or answering questions. Patients should not allow people to rush them, and should give themselves permission to go slowly and carefully. They can also be encouraged to find friends who understand their slowness and who will keep talking to them on a regular basis; this will give them practice in talking to others. If their slow speech is too bothersome to others, a referral to a speech therapist may be helpful. Speech therapists can often give exercises and other hints such as singing, to help with any problems clients may be experiencing.

Many patients with HIV-associated dementia also begin having trouble following multistep commands, or following a sequence within a larger task. One easy way to check for this problem is to have a patient follow a multistep command in the office. An example of a three-step command is this one from the Mini-Mental State Examination (Folstein, Folstein, & McHugh, 1975): Take this paper in your right hand, fold it in half, and place it on the floor. If the patient cannot do this, he or she is unable to follow a three-step command and needs to have tasks simplified. It is also helpful to decrease the number of choices a person is given when he or she has difficulty following multistep commands. An example is to ask the person, "Would you like salad or a sandwich for lunch?", as opposed to "Would you like Italian, Chinese, or American food?" and all the choices those menus imply.

Most activities of daily living are multistep and sequential. Meal preparation, getting dressed, going to work, driving a car, and using a telephone are some general examples of such activities. For the patient to be able to do these activities for a longer period of time, they need to be simplified. Cooking can have written, step-by-step directions. Meal preparation can also be simplified by using healthy, good-quality, prepackaged meals that can be warmed in an oven or microwave or on the stovetop. Another option is to have someone prepare meals ahead of time that the person can take out of the freezer or refrigerator; these meals can then be warmed and eaten by the patient. The warming instructions can be simply written and taped to the meal. Finally, a caregiver can take over most of the meal preparation and have the patient help with simple tasks such as cleaning, cutting or stirring.

Dressing is yet another task that often becomes difficult. There are many ways to simplify this task, depending on what the person's problems are. For a person having difficulty choosing items that go together, the outfits can be stored in the closet or dresser as a set. Outfits can also be laid or hung out the night before to make the selection easier for the patient.

For the person having trouble with fasteners because of tremor, peripheral neuropathy, or other physical limitations, changing to larger buttons, snaps, large hooks, or Velcro can be helpful. Many items such as bras have front closures that make them easier to use. If tying shoes is a problem, tennis shoes with Velcro closures or elastic shoelaces can be used, or regular shoes that slip on can be worn instead of those with shoelaces that require tying.

Many clothes are available in special stores and catalogs for people with physical limitations. A general rule to tell patients is to choose clothes that are comfortable and slightly looser for ease of donning.

Telephone use may become a problem because of motor incoordination, visual problems, or cognitive difficulties. For patients with any of these problems, phones are available with large key pads and multinumber storage. Catalogs for health care professionals also have adaptive items that will hook on a phone pad to enlarge the dial area for people with tremor, weakness, or decreased vision. Finally, speaker phones are available that allow a person to use the phone without needing the handset; this feature is especially useful for the person with tremor or weakness in the upper extremities.

Adaptations for Work

What can be done for the person who is still working or wants to do something outside the home? If a patient has physical limitations because of tremors or balance, modifications can be made in the work station, depending on the type of work that the patient does. If this is the case, a trained occupational or physical therapist should be consulted. For patients who do primarily office or clerical work on computers but have tremor or other physical limitations, many simple adjustments can be made, such as changing the computer keyboard setting so that the keys must be struck more forcefully to register. Some people need 1- or 2-pound wrist weights to help control their tremor and enable them to type or write; such weights can also help with eating or other tasks. There are also weighted pens and other tools to assist a person with a tremor or other limitation in writing and other fine motor activities.

Additional ideas to help persons with clerical jobs include using a dictaphone and having someone else type information. Visually or physically impaired people can use voice recognition computers in a work situation.

For the person who has memory impairment that prevents him or her from working in a regular job, there are options of doing volunteer work or piece work that is simple and repetitive. Examples of the latter include stuffing envelopes, folding letters, or collating and stapling papers. Jobs involving such tasks can often be found in a sheltered workshop or day care program. These programs are available through St. Vincent de Paul, the Salvation Army, or other charitable organizations in many areas.

Participation in Recreation

Persons with HIV-associated dementia benefit a great deal from participating in recreation and leisure activities. Intrinsically, people benefit from exercise and participating in activities that they consider fun. Exercise can improve some mental abilities by 20–30% (Gordon, 1995).

It has been my own experience that many patients are able to engage in more activities that require concentration and memory when they exercise than when they do not exercise. This does not need to be anything strenuous. In most cases, a walk, general stretching, or games such as throwing and catching a ball for a few minutes are enough exercise. After this type of exercise, in my experience, the patients are then able to play other games that require more cognitive skills, such as Scrabble, various card games, or math and memory games.

It is also important to keep the patient interested in enjoyable activities such as games or hobbies. For many patients, participating in different leisure activities helps decrease depressive symptoms and improve self-esteem and self-efficacy, while maintaining cognitive function and helping with socialization. Participation in games or hobbies can also help with visual tracking skills, visual sequencing, visual–spatial relations, visual–motor skills, and visual recognition. Finally, these activities help patients maintain strength, endurance, and coordination.

Some of the activities most commonly used in group recreational settings for demented patients are card games, such as solitaire, spades, rummy, uno, hearts, old maid, and kings in the corner, to name a few. Various board games, such as Scrabble, Life, Monopoly, Sequence, and Memory, are also helpful in working on socialization and memory. Some games have been designed especially for use with patients with memory problems. Orientation, designed in England, is for lower-level patients. It asks questions about time, the number of players in the game, and simple math problems. Other games, such as Reminiscing and LifeStories, ask patients questions about their own past or historical information. This will often stimulate discussions among patients and staff members who remember these things happening when they were younger. Still other types of activities that are fun for patients include crossword and jigsaw puzzles.

Increasingly, many games and activities are available for use on the computer, as well as in the original versions. The benefit of the computerized versions in most cases is that the games can be modified to make them more or less challenging for patients, depending on their needs.

A final area of recreation is that of hobbies, such as sewing, knitting, painting, woodworking, or leather crafts. Many patients have enjoyed these activities in the past, and can continue to enjoy them with various adaptive aids available in catalogs (see below).

EQUIPMENT AND TRAINING

Once an occupational therapist has a firm idea of what a patient's problems are and what adaptations are needed for these, where does the clinician find the necessary equipment? What type of equipment will work? How much does it cost? Who will pay for it? How does the patient learn to use it?

The majority of the items that are described in this section can be obtained from medical supply companies, pharmacies, department stores such as Sears or Penney's, and office supply stores. The specialized items (e.g., walkers and wheelchairs) are available through companies such as Sammons™, North Coast Medical, Inc., Concepts ADL Inc.™, Smith Nephew Rolyan Rehabilitation Products, Enrichments, and adaptAbility. These companies have catalogs from which the therapist can purchase the items needed; the prices are usually included in the catalogs. Most of these companies have toll-free numbers to call or fax to order items. For most companies, credit cards can be used to pay for the things ordered.

Assistive Devices for Ambulation Problems

In the majority of patients who are diagnosed with HIV-associated dementia, the basic problem with ambulation is a difficulty with balance. Before any assistive device is prescribed or issued to help with balance or ambulation in general, a patient should be referred to a physical therapist. The physical therapist can perform a gait evaluation of the patient to determine what the problems are and what type of assistive device will be most helpful and safest for the patient. In some cases, strengthening and other exercises can help the patient improve his or mobility without the need of an assistive device.

If it is not possible to refer a patient to a physical therapist for evaluation, the patient may want to purchase an assistive device on his or her own. The most commonly used items are a single-point cane of wood or metal; a quad cane, which has four feet on the bottom (these are made of metal and are height-adjustable); and a pickup walker, front-wheeled walker, or four-wheeled walker. All of the walkers are metal and are height-adjustable. The walkers with four wheels generally have hand brakes to assist the person in stopping and to increase stability.

It is important to note that as patients' cognitive abilities decline, they will have more difficulty learning to use these devices safely. For patients to maintain their mobility, it is advisable for them to begin using the assistive devices before they really need them. In this way, they can get used to using the devices and will be able to use them safely when they really do need them.

Many of the ambulation aids described above can be purchased at pharmacies, at medical supply stores, or through catalogs. Cost of the items ranges from $7 for a wooden single-point cane to $400 for a deluxe four-wheeled walker with basket, tray, seat, and brakes. For people with health insurance, most of these items are covered when they are pre-scribed by a physician or physical therapist. As a safety precaution, small throw rugs should be removed or should have something placed under them to prevent slipping when patients use ambulation devices.

As the disease progresses, a patient's gait and balance problems may increase. Endurance and strength may also be affected. At this point it may be necessary to get the patient a wheelchair. The patient can be transported by a caregiver in the wheelchair or can wheel himself or herself. A patient who is able may walk behind the wheel-chair, using it to help with balance. It is important to provide safety training for the patient and caregiver who will be using the wheelchair. The brakes must be locked when the chair is stopped somewhere, such as at a table, or when the patient is getting into or out of the wheelchair. It is also important that the foot rests be raised when the patient enters or exits the wheelchair. However, if the patient is propelling himself or herself, the foot rests can stay up to allow the patient to use his or her feet to help propel the wheelchair.

If the patient is having difficulty with the wheelchair, such as sliding out of it, there are cushions and seat belts available to help keep the person in the chair. There are also cushions and other seating systems to make the chair more comfortable for the patient to use. If the patient is still at home and will be using the wheelchair in the community, there are different types of chairs available. Some chairs are very lightweight, which makes them easy to load or unload from a car. Other chairs are heavy, for patients who may have problems with severe tremor or myoclonic movements. This is important to note, because wheelchairs can tip over easily.

For a clinician to obtain an appropriate wheelchair for a patient, it is advisable to refer the patient to an occupational or physical therapist. The therapist will ask questions about the uses the patient will have for the wheelchair, observe any movement problems the patient may have, and measure the patient to get a chair that fits the patient correctly. The therapist can also order any special cushions, antitipping devices, or other safety items for the chair that the patient may need. As with the ambulation devices, the patient's health insurance will often pay at least partially for the wheelchair and any safety items needed if they are prescribed by a physician or therapist.

Memory Aids

The memory aids discussed earlier in the chapter include large calendars, day planners, and small notebooks. These can be found in catalogs, stationery stores, large discount stores, and specialty shops. Cost can range from a few dollars to over $100. It is advisable to keep calendars and planners simple and easy to use for the patient.

Items to help a patient remember to take pills come in many forms and can be found in the catalogs listed at the start of this section. They can also be found in drugstores, pharmacies, and discount stores, and at times in physicians' offices. A pill reminder box can be anything from a simple one-compartment box to a multicompartment box. The most common is the "mediplanner," which is a 28-compartment box that helps ensure correct medication dosage. There are often raised letters and Braille markings on each compartment. The mediaplanner allows for a four-time-per-day, 7-day schedule of medications. A "pill alert" has an easily programmable timer and alarm on a box that helps patients remember to take their medications. The timer and alarm use watch or AAA batteries, and the alarm resets automatically for the next scheduled time. This box is also small enough to fit easily in a patient's pocket. Some pill dispensers are very elaborate and expensive, costing up to $80. These can be mounted on the patient's refrigerator or wall. The patient simply pushes the appropriate buttons, and pills are released in a cup at the bottom. One such dispenser opens like a book, has 28 bins, and holds enough pills for four doses a day for a week, or one dose a day for a month. This device also has a childproof locking device if needed. If the patient is having difficulty with swallowing, there are also pill-crushing and pill-splitting devices available from the same places.

Adaptive Devices for Cooking and Eating

Many products are available to assist patients who have difficulty with cooking or eating because of tremor, decreased strength, loss of the use of a hand, and many other problems. Most commonly, the problems that patients with HIV-associated dementia will be experiencing will be fine motor problems. These can interfere with eating because the patient may drop food off utensils, push food off the edge of a plate, or splash liquids out of a cup or glass. In some cases, having the patient wear a 1- to 2-pound wrist weight will help resolve these problems; in other cases, adaptive equipment will need to be used. Some of the commonly available items include weighted utensils, which work on the same principle as the wrist weights, and plate guards, which fit the edge of a plate and help keep the food from being pushed off. Most people have seen and probably own a cup that has a lid and a hole to help keep coffee or other liquids from spilling out. These items were initially designed for patients with disabilities, but are handy also for use in the car or other places. The advantage of these items' becoming popular with the nondisabled is that they are acceptable for use by anyone at any time. One other handy item if the plate or other items skid around the table is a product called Dycem®. Dycem can be cut to size from a roll, or can be purchased as placemats or rounds. When Dycem is under a plate, it keeps the plate from slipping. Dycem can be purchased through the catalogs above; as an alternative, patients can use a rug gripper from Rubbermaid, cut to an appropriate size. This item is found in stores, usually near the shelf and contact paper, and is much less expensive. Instead of being solid, the Rubbermaid gripper is made of an open-weave material.

Adaptive Devices for Work

There are many types of adaptive devices for work, a few of which (e.g., special computers) have been mentioned earlier in the chapter. For patients who have jobs that require writing, there are weighted universal holders that hold pens, pencils, or even paintbrushes. The Steady Write® pen, grippers, "easy writers," and "easy typers" are all designed to help patients to continue doing clerical tasks even with tremors or other problems.

There are a number of writing and typing aids available, including "easy writer," "easy typer," "slip on writing aid," and "slip on typing keyboard aid," to name a few. The writing aids are similar in their ability to hold a pen or pencil in a plastic or metal device that is then strapped to the hand of the patient. The typing aids usually have a hard plastic rod with a rubber tip, which can be attached to a plastic or metal device and then strapped to either the patient's hand or, at times, their head using Velcro or other means. For many of these devices, the portion that fits in the palm area of the patient's hand can be molded by the occupational therapist in order to be more comfortable for the patient who uses it.

There are also "workmod" arm supports that help reduce the risk of repetitive injury, or assist those who have limited range of motion at the elbow or shoulder. There are also electric scissors, staplers, and pencil sharpeners for patients who need them. Many of these devices are available in large discount office supply stores. Adjustable tables are also important to help keep people working; many are available in the catalogs listed or at the office supply stores. These are especially helpful for a patient who may be using a wheelchair.

For those patients who have outdoor jobs in construction or gardening, or who simply enjoy these as hobbies, there are tool grips that are ergonomically designed to improve control and enhance strength. These fit on straight-shafted tools with a flexible split-screw. In addition, moldable tubing and self-adhesive nonslip strips can be used on hammers, saws, screwdrivers, or any other type of tool patients may use to help enhance the patients' grip.

Recreational Aids

One of the biggest areas of adaptive equipment is that of recreational aids. There are multiple types of card holders and even a card shuffler. Many different games have been adapted for patients who have tremors, weakness, decreased vision, or decreased motor dexterity. Some of the more common adaptations include jumbo and tactile dominoes, peg Chinese checkers, large and raised cards, peg checkers, giant scrabble with gridded and recessed surfaces, bowling ramps, and extra-large jigsaw and crossword puzzles.

Various items have also been adapted for the hobbyist, including knitting needle holders, book stands or holders, crafters' "extra hands," needle threaders, floor lamp magnifiers, and various types of scissors. Gardening tools have also been adapted, as have painting tools.

SUMMARY

This chapter has begun with a brief overview of the HIV-associated dementia patient's clinical presentation, including physical and cognitive changes an occupational therapist may find on evaluation. Various methods of evaluating patients' abilities and deficits have been explained. Specific ways to help a patient maintain or improve physical abilities and cognitive function in activities of daily living and at work have been described; the need for and benefits of evaluation by occupational, physical, and speech therapists for various problems have been stressed. Types of recreational activities and their benefits, including exercise, games, and hobbies, have also been discussed. Finally, various types of adaptive equipment have been described, including their use, cost, and availability.

REFERENCES

Buckingham, S. L., & van Gorp, W. (1994). HIV-associated dementia: A clinician's guide to early detection, diagnosis, and intervention. *Families in Society: The Journal of Contemporary Human Services, 75*(6), 333–345.

Clark, P. N., Allen, A. S., Clark, F., & Schanzenbacher, K. E. (1985). Instruments to evaluate component functions of behavior. In P. N. Clark & A. S. Allen (Eds.), *Occupational therapy for children* (pp. 163–190). St. Louis: Mosby.

Fernandez, F. (1989). Anxiety and the neuropsychiatry of AIDS. *Journal of Clinical Psychiatry, 50*(11, Suppl.), 9–14.

Folstein, M. F., Folstein, S. E., & McHugh, P. R. (1975). Mini-Mental State: A practical method for grading the cognitive state of patients for the clinician. *Journal of Psychiatric Research, 12,* 189–198.

Gordon, B. (1995). *Memory: Remembering and forgetting in everyday life.* New York: MasterMedia.

Maj, M. (1990). Psychiatric aspects of HIV-1 infection and AIDS. *Psychological Medicine, 20,* 547–563.

Mintz, M. (1996). Neurological and developmental problems in pediatric HIV infection. *Journal of Nutrition, 126*(Suppl. 10), 2663S–2673S.

Pulliam, L., Gascon, R., Stubblebine, M., McGuire, D., & McGrath, M. S. (1997). Unique monocyte subset in patients with AIDS dementia. *Lancet, 349*(9053), 692–695.

Roach, E. G., & Kephart, N. C. (1971). The Purdue Perceptual-Motor Survey. Columbus, OH: Charles E. Merrill.

Smith, H. D. (1978). Specific evaluation procedures. In H. L. Hopkins & H. D. Smith (Eds.), *Willard and Spackman's occupational therapy* (5th ed., pp. 158–183). Philadephia: Lippincott.

10

HIV/AIDS and Mental Capacity: Legal and Ethical Issues

ROBERT G. MEYER
SUSAN G. LEAVENWORTH

INTRODUCTION

Determination of mental capacity is critical when a client is infected with HIV/AIDS. From the time of HIV infection, the individual is at risk for decreasing mental capacity. However, deterioration of the brain can be confused with a myriad of other AIDS-related influences. This chapter addresses issues of legal and mental competence associated with HIV infection. First, we briefly discuss the types of psychological problems that are known to be associated with HIV infection. Second, the formal evaluation process is described. A brief description of involuntary commitment as it may pertain to those with HIV-infection comes next; this is followed by a thorough discussion of guardianship procedures and their appropriateness for individuals infected with HIV. Finally, we discuss two other legal issues related to HIV/AIDS and competence: employment discrimination and competence to make a will.

PSYCHOLOGICAL STRESSORS KNOWN
TO BE ASSOCIATED WITH HIV INFECTION

A wide variety of psychological issues may affect persons infected with HIV. Physical, psychological, and social influences interact to create unique potential stressors, such as physical changes, reduced cognitive skills, rejection by peers and family members, and serious socioeconomic pressures (Kyle & Sacha, 1994). Preexisting psychiatric conditions are often intensified; new psychological problems may be created; and self-esteem may be reduced. The infected individual may experience denial, shock, guilt, sadness, and rejection (Meyer & Deitsch, 1996; Riccio et al., 1993).

It is not surprising that these individuals, even those who are asymptomatic, may suffer from clinically significant levels of anxiety and depression. Sources of anxiety and depression surrounding HIV/AIDS include employment status, guilt, rejection, loss of bodily control, pain, and a high probability of a shortened life. Knowing that the virus is progressing is a continuous and increasing stress for many, especially as individuals experience loss of physical strength, weight, attractiveness, and problem-solving skills. Physical symptoms, which include oral thrush, sleep problems, rash, diarrhea, wasting, and musculoskeletal pain, are associated with AIDS-induced depression, which may also include suicidal ideation (Chesney & Folkman, 1994).

Adding to these problems can be cognitive decline, which results from central nervous system effects of HIV infection. Although the prevalence of this problem can be as high as 90% at autopsy, estimates of the timing and seriousness of earlier involvement vary widely. Many of those infected with HIV remain intellectually intact, although perhaps slower in speed of mental processing, at the end stages of the disease (Grant & Adams, 1996; Robertson & Hall, 1992; Egan, Brettle, & Goodwin, 1992).

Early cognitive changes associated with HIV infection include a gradual decline in intellectual functioning, impaired memory and concentration, and psychomotor slowing. Behaviorally, these individuals may exhibit apathy, social withdrawal, irritability, emotional lability, or psychosis. Riedel et al. (1992) reported that in a sample of 181 individuals with HIV infection, 20–30% of the individuals in stages prior to full-blown AIDS had these manifestations of central nervous system impairment. Among those who had reached full-blown AIDS, the percentage rose to 80%.

HIV may enter the central nervous system at the time of initial infection, but it is still unknown whether this occurs in all cases. Also, the precise mechanisms by which HIV affects the brain is still not known. The diagnosis of HIV-associated dementia (HAD) depends on the convergence of many factors. The effects of Treatable secondary infections are often confused with those of HAD. Medications intended to aid sleep or alleviate depression, which are frequently administered at later stages of the disease, may also impair cognitive and motor functioning in a manner that appears the same as HAD (Robertson & Hall, 1992).

Psychiatric illnesses may reveal causes other than HAD. Psychosis can result in cognitive debilitation similar to that seen in HAD. Depression and anxiety are common; approximately one-third of HIV-infected individuals have had at least one major depressive episode. Because of the nature of this disease, the risk of suicide is high at all stages. Misdiagnosis can result from the similarity between HAD and depression—namely, apathy, low energy, and slow responsiveness. Zidovudine is a drug known to improve intellectual function and to slow or halt the development of HAD (Grant & Adams, 1996; Robertson & Hall, 1992; Zegans, Gerhard, & Coates, 1994).

THE FORMAL EVALUATION PROCESS

An important issue to address is that of when a person infected with HIV should undergo a formal mental status evaluation. Since those with HIV disease often undergo a myriad of emotional and personality changes, an individual may become suicidal, impulsive, forgetful, suspicious, withdrawn, apathetic, angry, or emotionally labile. A history of substance abuse may make these symptoms more serious. These symptoms require collaborative work with other health care professionals for a neuropsychiatric evaluation (Kaplan & Saccuzzo, 1997; Zegans et al., 1994; Syndulko et al., 1994).

It is generally of limited use to perform detailed neuropsychological testing at the most advanced stages of HIV disease, since symptoms should be obvious. In less severe stages, formal testing may determine whether there is cognitive impairment and whether its etiology is HAD or other causes, such as psychosis or developmental disability. In early stages of HIV infection, there is usually no significant decline. When an individual begins experiencing symptoms related to HIV infection, cognitive decline may be mild to moderate. Further decline in cognitive functioning may occur as the infection progresses to later stages. Test results that confirm HAD indicate a pattern of affected motor control, concentration and processing speed, mental flexibility, visual–spatial skills, and memory. In later stages of HAD, virtually all of these areas will be affected (Kaplan & Saccuzzo, 1997; Robertson & Hall, 1992; Syndulko et al., 1994).

Determining when to refer a patient for a formal evaluation requires reviewing the multiple factors that can potentially affect the individual's cognitive status. Boccellari and Dilley (1992) developed a scale, the Neuropsychiatric AIDS Rating Scale (NARS), to increase accuracy in reporting the incidence and prevalence of the cognitive and behavioral changes occurring with HIV infection. Toward this end, the NARS describes six stages of HIV-related neuropsychiatric degeneration.

The first impairment stage of the NARS, which describes a normally functioning individual, is followed by "equivocal," which is characterized by complaints about memory problems, slightly slower motor and mental activity, and slight impairment in work-related matters. In order to have a baseline measure of the individual's cognitive status, it is wise to perform an evaluation of competence while the individual is still at least in one of the first two stages (Boccellari & Dilley, 1992; Walsh, Brown, Kaye, & Grigsby, 1994).

The third stage is marked by mild problems with memory, balance, and coordination, as well as by increasing irritability or withdrawal. The individual in this stage can perform simple daily activities, but has problems planning or completing work. The fourth stage, "moderate," is characterized by symptoms that are most often used to establish the dividing line between legal competence and incompetence. This stage includes disorientation and moderate memory problems, impulsivity or agitation, and severe impairment in the ability to solve problems. This stage is also characterized by poor social judgment and getting lost easily. The fifth stage, "severe," is marked by very poor judgment, severe memory loss, and inability to live on one's own. In the final stage, "end stage," the individual is almost completely vegetative and has virtually no memory (Grant & Adams, 1996; Boccellari & Dilley, 1992).

To the extent that information is available, the following areas should be addressed in a report: premorbid intelligence, attention, speed of processing, abstraction, language, visual–spatial skills, construction abilities, motor responses, memory, and mood. Since each of these factors constitutes a problem if it is different from the individual's normal daily functioning, comparison must be made if at all possible with the individual's level of baseline functioning (Meyer & Deitsch, 1996; Stern, 1994).

The mental health clinician's report should address the areas pertinent to the individual's needs. For example, if the person is interested in retaining employment in a specific job, the report should address the individual's ability to perform that job (Atkinson & Grant, 1994). Another area where specificity is important is designating whether past, present, or future functioning is the focus of evaluation. Unless it is relevant to the determination, reference to future functioning is usually not beneficial. This is because there is some variation in the progression through the stages of the HIV infection (Gitler & Rennert, 1992).

Mental status evaluations increasingly emphasize a person's ability to perform living skills. Basically, a functional evaluation avoids the traditional diagnosis/prognosis orientation and replaces it with a description of how well the person can manage on a normal day. This is especially true when the referring question is the need for appointing a guardian. Some states, such as New Hampshire, require a functional evaluation, and the petition must contain behavioral descriptions (N.H. Rev. Stat. Ann. § 464-A, 1979; Nolan, 1990).

A mental health practitioner may be called upon to evaluate an HIV-infected client for one of four types of legal proceedings: involuntary commitment decisions, guardianship procedures, discrimination proceedings, or testamentary capacity decisions. These are discussed below in turn.

INVOLUNTARY COMMITMENT

Involuntary commitment guidelines are fairly uniform among the states, because of decisions by the U.S. Supreme Court. This topic is relevant to those infected with HIV if they engage in behavior that is destructive to the self or to others. Because HIV can be transmitted sexually, an infected person expressing the intention to have unprotected sexual contact can place others at risk of contracting the virus (Garwood & Melnick, 1995). On the other hand, a person may have depression or suicidal tendencies exacerbated by knowledge of the HIV infection. Involuntary commitment requires a finding that persons in these situations are dangerous either to themselves or to others, and that they would benefit from hospitalization (Meyer & Deitsch, 1996; Bongar, Maris, Berman, & Litman, 1992; Nolan, 1990).

GUARDIANSHIP

This section reviews the alternatives available to a person with HIV who needs assistance in managing his or her affairs because of declining health or mental capacity. First, a general description of standard guardianship is provided. Next, public guardians and other alternatives to standard guardianship are described. Finally, advance directives are discussed; these include living wills, a durable power of attorney, and some trusts.

Standard Guardianship

"Guardianship" involves the decision to declare people incompetent to make decisions for themselves concerning financial and personal matters. The legal term for the individual who is declared incompetent is the "ward." Guardianship has the potential both for protecting and caring for those who cannot care for themselves, and for great abuse. In the most common type of guardianship, the authority for making all decisions is transferred from the ward to a guardian. The guardian takes control of the property and manages it; in addition, he or she makes personal care decisions, such as whether the ward will be placed in an institution, where the ward will live, and whether to consent to have the ward treated for physical and mental conditions. The ward may also lose a few rights that the guardian may not exercise, such as the right to vote (Peters, Schmidt, & Miller, 1995; *Archer v. Federal Deposit Ins. Corp.,* 1992; Uniform Guardianship and Protective Proceedings Act, 1982).

Upon learning that he or she has HIV, an individual should consider how to dispose of personal property, and how long he or she wishes to live with life support systems should he or she lose the ability to make decisions. Guardianship is a desirable alternative for a person with a significant other who can be trusted with personal and medical decisions. Courts give great weight to the stated preference of an individual while he or she is still competent as to who should be appointed the individual's guardian (Melton, Petrila, Poythress, & Slobogin, 1997).

Hearings and Process

A petition for guardianship will usually have to be filed in the state where the ward is a resident. Before a hearing, notice must be provided to family members and others. Problems occur when the notice does not adequately describe the legal implications of this determination (Peters et al., 1995). As noted above, a ward's preference for a guardian often prevails in the court's determination; this is especially true if the ward has expressed a preference in writing (Uniform Guardianship and Protective Proceedings Act, 1982; Nolan, 1990).

Under general guardianship law, the Uniform Guardianship and Protective Proceedings Act (1982) defines incapacity as "any person who is impaired by reason of mental illness, mental deficiency, physical illness or disability, advanced age, chronic use of drugs, chronic intoxication, or other cause (except minority) to the extent of lacking sufficient understanding or *capacity* [italics added] to make or communicate responsible decisions" (Part 2). The petition usually states that the proposed ward is unable to care for his or her person and/or property. In addition to a condition such as mental incapacity or old age, two inabilities usually must be proven: the inability (1) to care for person or property, and (2) to communicate or make decisions. Some states require either that the judge appoint a physician or psychologist, or that an affidavit by a physician and/or a psychologist be submitted with the petition. In the latter case, the petition should include a statement that the physician or psychologist examined the proposed ward within a period of time required by statute, the names of specific tests performed, the diagnosis resulting in the proposed ward's problem, and the proposed prognosis (American Bar Association, 1990).

Mental illness, "mental deficiency," or mental retardation may be the basis for incompetence in guardianship proceedings. Many states also include chronic intoxication, drug addiction, old age, or serious physical infirmity. In the past, being a spendthrift was also a basis for incompetence. Decline in brain functioning secondary to HIV infection is another example (Melton et al., 1997).

Guardianships are established following a judicial hearing, which may include a jury, depending on the jurisdiction.Evidence supporting the proposed ward's inability to manage his or her own affairs must be as concrete as possible. An example is evidence that facilities such as electricity or telephone service have been cut off while the proposed ward is accumulating uncashed paychecks. Witnesses may include friends, family members, or health care professionals. Most often, experts are appointed and called by the court; these are sometimes referred to as "impartial experts." States have recently begun to tighten the hearing procedures. Some now provide for the proposed ward's right to an attorney, his or her presence at the hearing, and his or her right to call and examine witnesses. In some states a person can be found incompetent only if incompetence is demonstrated through clear and convincing evidence (American Bar Association, 1990).

Determining the Proposed Ward's Incapacity

There is no clear-cut medical or psychological concept that corresponds directly to the legal concept of incompetence. A broad definition of the legal term "incompetent" is "lack of ability, legal qualification, or fitness to discharge the required duty" (Black, 1968, p. 906). Opinions among mental health professionals on what constitutes incapacity may vary widely. This is especially true of the multiple factors involved in HIV infection. Professional opinions can be supplemented by a showing of the ward's ability to function in daily life. The intervention of guardianship should be designed to meet the specific needs of the ward. The focus should be on the areas and degrees of the proposed ward's abilities, instead of a medical or psychological diagnosis. Three specific areas should be used to determine incapacity: (1) the proposed ward's disorder, (2) his or her ability to function, and (3) his or her ability to make decisions and communicate (Nolan, 1990).

1. With regard to the proposed ward's disorder, many states require a finding of mental deficiency in its various forms (e.g., mental retardation, mental illness, cognitive impairment). Cognitive impairment is a continuing concern to those with HIV. In this area, a professional's opinion is necessary. A report should include information concerning the amount of contact the professional had with the proposed ward; specific tests administered; any need for additional examination; whether environmental factors were taken into account; the effects of diet, drugs, depression, and/or disorientation; the stability of the proposed ward's symptoms; and the prognosis (Meyer & Deitsch, 1996; Roca, 1994).

2. The proposed ward's functional capacity is determined by his or her ability to care for self or property. Some states require that harm will result from the inability to manage self or affairs, such as being susceptible to fraud or manipulation. With regard to prognosis, HIV disease is unique because even though the disease itself is progressive, the dementia component may be resolvable with medication (Hollweg, Riedel, Goebel, Schick, & Naber, 1991; Nolan, 1990).

Information on functional capacity includes whether and how well the proposed ward maintains his or her responsibilities, and how much assistance he or she needs to make a decision in the following areas: nutrition, clothing, hygiene, health care, residence maintenance, and safety. Examples of indicators of functional incapacity in those with HIV/AIDS have included symptoms of dementia that affect the inability to run a household or to care for a pet; staying in bed all day; or having extreme suicidal ideation. The important point is that when the question of incapacity is approached from a functional perspective, the focus is on the person's behavior and not on the underlying diagnosis (Melton et al., 1997).

If a guardianship of the property is sought, the size, type, and complexity of the proposed ward's estate must be identified. The proposed ward's abilities in two areas will also provide support for the decision: ability (1) to collect benefits or money belonging to him or her, and (2) to manage money. In order to support a finding of incapacity, there must be a link between the proposed ward's condition and the problem behavior. For example, an individual with HIV may suffer from mild dementia, which affects his or her ability to communicate coherently some of the time. Despite this, he or she has continuously demonstrated the ability to manage finances and property. There should not be an appointment of a guardian over this person's property without more evidence of his or her inability to manage the property.

3. Some states require it to be shown that the proposed ward lacks the ability to evaluate information or to make or communicate decisions. The focus of this part of the inquiry is on the proposed ward's decision-making capacity. This can be shown by the proposed ward's awareness of unmet needs, awareness of alternatives available to meet the need, and understanding of his or her choices in terms of consequences. Presenting evidence concerning the ability to make decisions may be tricky. On the one hand, seeking assistance can be considered adaptive and responsible. On the other hand, the same evidence can be viewed as a sign of helplessness and need for ongoing assistance (Nolan, 1990).

An example of this dilemma is a widow who calls her daughter frequently and discusses her financial and property affairs. One argument would be that she is not able to think through situations without her daughter's assistance. Another view is that the woman needs only a small portion of her daughter's guidance (and that her ability is thus within the range of an average person's ability), but that she expands on these topics to meet her socialization and companionship needs.

Monitoring of Guardianship and Restoration of a Ward's Rights

Following a determination of incompetence and appointment of a guardian, the guardianship is largely unregulated. Ten states require regular court monitoring of guardianships. Reviews that do take place usually only include an accounting of the ward's financial affairs and do not report on any potential improvement in the ward's abilities (Peters et al., 1995).

Even though most guardianship proceedings are informal and brief, many significant issues can be raised, such as whether the condition is temporary or potentially reversible. This is an important fact for those infected with HIV, because there is evidence showing improvement of neuropsychiatric symptoms after an individual has taken zidovudine (Hollweg et al., 1991).

"Restoration" is the process of returning legal authority over a ward's affairs to the ward. This process can take place in any state through common law, which is based on former court decisions declaring an individual's rights. In addition, 46 states provide for restoration by statute. There is variability among the states as to who is allowed to initiate these proceedings. Even though there is a risk of too many lawsuits' being filed, many states permit the ward to initiate this proceeding.

Despite this, and even if an individual has regained the ability to manage his or her affairs, restoration of a ward's rights is unusual, rare, and extremely difficult. Some of the barriers inhibiting restoration are as follows: (1) Wards are typically removed from the rest of society, which increases their sense of helplessness in the process; (2) petitions written by wards are often not taken seriously by the courts; (3) costs of the proceeding are usually required to be paid from the ward's estate; (4) The burden of proof is usually on the ward to demonstrate that he or she is no longer incapacitated; (5) a ward whose property was managed by the guardian has no opportunity to show the court that he or she is capable of managing his or her property; (6) restoration proceedings, like the initial guardianship proceedings, require a medical or psychological evaluation and evidence that the ward is able to manage his or her affairs; and (7) an HIV-infected individual who is seeking restoration will have to convince the court that the effort is not futile, in view of the perception of inevitable physical and mental decline of persons with HIV/AIDS (Nolan, 1990; Hull, Holmes, & Karst, 1990). In a sample taken from six states, successful restoration to competence was determined to be so uncommon as to be virtually nonexistent (Schmidt, Miller, Bell, & New, 1995). Thus, an attempt at restoration can be an expensive, time-consuming, humiliating, and ultimately unsuccessful experience.

Legal Rights of Wards

A declaration of incompetence permits the state to severely limit a ward's personal liberty and property rights. Therefore, constitutional due process provisions apply to guardianship proceedings. Relatively little attention has been given to due process issues in these cases, compared with civil commitment and criminal incarceration. For example, in a year-long study reviewing 2,200 guardianship court files in all 50 states, one-fourth had no record of a hearing's having been held, and 44% indicated that the ward was not represented by an attorney (Walsh, 1992). These questions will undoubtedly be raised more frequently in the future, because of the increasing number of persons with HIV/AIDS and the aging population of the United States (Hull et al., 1990; Peters et al., 1995).

Duties of Guardians

Guardians are obligated to act as fiduciaries, making decisions that are in the best interests of their wards. Generally, guardians must periodically account to the court for their handling of the property of their wards. Less frequently, they are called to review for the court their actions to protect the physical and mental state of incompetents (Peters et al., 1995).

When making a life-threatening decision for the ward, the guardian may need special permission. The decision to terminate treatments instrumental to sustaining life is a critical area of the law. *In re Quinlan* (1976) allowed a guardian to terminate life-supporting treatments to a ward who, although not technically brain-dead, was terminally ill and in a permanent vegetative state. The guardian was required to show that the ward would have made the same decision if she could. The basis of this decision was a constitutional right to privacy, and the court reasoned that if an individual can refuse medical intervention, this right may be extended to those who can only act through a guardian (Winick, 1997).

Every state that has considered this issue (approximately 16 have done so to date) has allowed the guardian to make this type of decision under certain circumstances. After *Quinlan,* the issue became whether a guardian could authorize termination of life-sustaining care such as food and water. Whereas the courts of New Jersey and other states allowed this, the Supreme Court of Missouri did not. The only way this could be allowed in Missouri was if the proposed ward had executed a living will. When this case was appealed to the U.S. Supreme Court, it was upheld. This means that states are allowed to prohibit interrupting artificial life-sustaining equipment unless clear and convincing evidence shows that the proposed ward had a different desire (*Cruzan by Cruzan v. Director, Missouri Dept. of Health*, 110 S. Ct. 2841, 497 U.S. 261, 1990; see also Winick, 1997).

Public Guardians and Other Alternatives

Most states have now established a "public guardian," which is a public agency with the duty to exercise the powers of a guardian. Ordinarily public guardians act for those for whom a private guardian cannot be found. Most of the wards of public guardians are poor.

The major complaint about public guardians is that they are highly bureaucratized, with very heavy caseloads, and fail to provide personal relationships. It appears that public guardian offices have insufficient staffing and funding. Many wards of public guardians are seen only a few hours in an entire year. Even with this minimal amount of attention, many public guardians are reaching their maximum limit in numbers of wards (Walsh, 1992).

One alternative to this is a "limited guardianship." This type of guardianship recognizes that an individual has strengths in some areas. A limited guardianship removes decision-making authority only in specifically designated areas of functioning as determined by mental health experts. Unfortunately, this type of guardianship is not commonly used, possibly because of the difficulty encountered by mental health experts in determining precisely what areas of mental functioning are weak and strong. This may become even more challenging if a ward's areas of competence is subject to change (Smith & Meyer, 1987).

Other alternatives include the use of private nonprofit groups and public trusts to carry on the work of guardianship. When an estate has assets in the range of $50,000 or more, finding a guardian is much easier: Banking institutions are equipped to manage estates. A less desirable alternative to guardianship proceedings is benign neglect, in which individuals simply do not receive the required care. Another alternative is psychiatric hospitalization, which has been called "the poor man's guardianship" (Walsh, 1992).

"Conservatorships" involve court proceedings to protect a person who is not necessarily incapacitated but who is unable to manage his or her affairs properly. The court must determine that the individual cannot manage his or her property or affairs effectively, for reasons similar to those that must be given in a guardianship proceeding. An additional requirement is that "the person has property which will be wasted or dissipated unless proper management is provided, or that funds are needed for the support, care, and welfare of the person or those entitled to be supported by him and that protection is necessary or desirable to obtain or provide funds" (Uniform Probate Code, § 5-401(2), 1969).

A final alternative is the imposition of adult protective services (Nolan, 1990). This involves a community-based method to determine whether the survival needs of those who are believed to be incapacitated are being met. This procedure usually begins with a report by a professional or interested bystander. Investigators, usually social workers, usually visit the individual's home and interview the person who made the initial report. If the adult is determined to be at risk for abuse, neglect, or exploitation, and consents to the procedure, various services may be provided to him or her until the situation becomes stabilized and safe. The agency administering these services has various powers to enforce access to the individual or imposition of the services in case the individual does not consent (Winick, 1997). In conclusion, it seems probable that with an aging population and somewhat less cohesive family structures, the use of public guardians and adult protective services will continue to increase.

Advance Directives

There are other alternatives that help limit the uncertainty of substituted-judgment decision making or reduce the need for it. An "advance directive" is generally a legal document expressing one's desires for others to act upon the occurrence of a future circumstance. In order to be effective, these documents must be executed when the individual is deemed to have the requisite mental capacity (Walsh et al., 1994). Following are descriptions of the most commonly used types of advanced directives.

The first is the execution of "living wills" or "treatment wills," which are alternatives created to apply to a specific type of situation. An example is a living will requesting that no life support system be used in the event that the individual is determined to be brain-dead. Every state has now adopted laws for living wills; these usually state that the maker must be comatose for a certain period of time, the maker's health must be considered terminal, and the maker must be unable to express a decision regarding his or her health care (Walsh et al., 1994). The formal nature of these documents should help to ensure that people consider what they are signing, rather than making offhand comments. In addition, they give a relatively clear set of instructions concerning decisions that should be made (Cantor, 1992).

Other mechanisms, such as a durable power of attorney and some trusts, allow competent persons to appoint others to assume decision-making authority in the event that they become incompetent. A "durable power of attorney" gives legal decision-making authority to a specific, named individual. It is "durable" in that it is executed while the maker is competent, and allows the trusted person to make decisions on behalf of the maker in the event of mental incapacity. If there is doubt about the maker's mental abilities, he or she should have a psychiatric evaluation before giving a power of attorney, to avoid litigation. Most states provide that the durable power of attorney ends if there is a formal court proceeding to declare the maker incompetent. Thus, a durable power of attorney can begin to be effective when the maker in fact becomes incompetent, and then it ceases if the maker dies or if someone initiates a guardianship proceeding. As a practical matter, this arrangement is more effective than it may sound. So long as an individual is being cared for under the durable power of attorney, there is less chance that there will be others who are sufficiently concerned about the person's welfare to initiate a formal guardianship proceeding. Most states have adopted legislation allowing a durable power of attorney, and require that this document specifically note that the power of attorney is durable or should survive incompetence (Cantor, 1992). The durable power of attorney can be extremely helpful, and has been called "the cornerstone for planning for disability" (Walsh et al., 1994).

Finally, several types of legal trusts, such as revocable living trusts, convertible trusts, and protective trusts, may provide for the management of property. One creates a "trust" by turning over ownership of assets to the trust, to be managed by someone chosen by the owner, called a "trustee." The trustee is required to manage the property according to the wishes of the owner as he or she has written these into the trust document. When the trust is revocable, the owner/maker can terminate the trust at any time. The benefit of using this type of document is assurance of proper management of one's property, enduring after an owner/maker subsequently loses mental capacity. A lawyer is usually required to draft this document in a legally enforceable manner. A drawback is that these instruments do not provide for personal care decisions, but only financial decisions (Cantor, 1992; Goodart, 1995).

HIV/AIDS AND DISCRIMINATION

"Discrimination" is illegal treatment of persons based on protected classifications, such as race, national origin, gender, religion, or disability. In the past, those infected with HIV have been the subjects of discriminatory treatment. Unfair treatment also occurs against friends and relatives of individuals infected with HIV (Civil Rights Act of 1964, Supp. 1992; Rehabilitation Act of 1973, Supp. 1992; Americans with Disabilities Act [ADA] of 1990, Supp. 1992; Presidential Commission on the Human Immunodeficiency Virus Epidemic, 1988; U.S. Senate, Committee on Labor and Human Resources, 1989). Areas of discrimination against those infected with HIV include employment, education, health care, insurance coverage, housing, public accommodations, and treatment in commercial establishments (Gitler & Rennert, 1992).

In addition to state and local laws prohibiting discrimination against those with HIV/AIDS, there are two major federal laws that require minimum compliance with standards of nondiscrimination.

This means that if state or local laws are in conflict with the federal laws, the federal laws supersede the state or local laws to the extent that the latter have lower standards of protection. The ADA of 1990 (42 U.S.C.A. §§ 12101–12213, Supp. 1992) imposes requirements for nondiscrimination based upon disability. The Equal Employment Opportunity Commission (EEOC) and the U.S. Department of Justice, which are primarily responsible for enforcing the ADA, consider HIV infection as a disability even when an infected individual is asymptomatic (EEOC, § 163-.2(m), 1992).

Title I of the ADA, in addition to prohibiting employment discrimination against the disabled, prohibits discrimination against those who are related to or associated with an individual with a disability. Thus, those who care for individuals infected with HIV are also protected under the ADA (Mello, 1995).

In addition, an individual infected with HIV can invoke protection under the ADA against employment discrimination if the individual can prove that he or she is "qualified." This means that he or she must be capable of performing the essential functions of the position. The employer is required to make "reasonable accommodations" if such efforts will make it possible for the person to perform the essential functions of the job. It is generally accepted that early stages of HIV infection in which the individual is asymptomatic will not typically affect performance. When the HIV-infected individual becomes symptomatic, evaluations may become necessary to determine his or her ability to perform (Mello, 1995). Evaluations determining ability to perform job duties are required to be based on the individual's present skills and should not include opinions about future abilities (EEOC, § 1630.2(m), 1992). Thus, an individual with HIV infection cannot be refused employment or fired, merely on the basis of the employer's concerns about the person's ability to perform the job in the future (Mello, 1995).

An evaluation of an HIV-infected client wishing to retain or obtain employment can include opinions as to the client's abilities both in the job as described and in the job after an employer makes reasonable accommodations for the client. In addition, a professional's opinion can offer suggestions as to what those accommodations should be. Examples include allowing the use of accrued leave, advance leave, or leave without pay. However, the employer will not be required to provide additional leave with pay (EEOC, § 1630.2(o)(2)(ii), 1992). When an individual with HIV/AIDS is only capable of performing job duties if the employer makes reasonable accommodations, then the ADA requires the employer to make those accommodations (Mello, 1995).

Reasonable accommodations do not include any arrangements that could be construed as imposing "undue hardship" on the employer. In determining undue hardship, factors considered include the difficulty or expense of making the accommodation relative to the nature and size of the employer's business (ADA, 42 U.S.C.A. § 12111(10), 1992).

The professional making an evaluation is in a difficult position with regard to making recommendations for reasonable accommodations. On the one hand, the professional's opinion is required to support the client's interest in showing that he or she is able to work under specified conditions. On the other hand, if the suggested accommodations are determined by a court or administrative body as placing an undue hardship on the employer, the report will have the effect of supporting the employer's position in refusing employment to the client. Thus, if possible, suggestions should be made that are safely within the guidelines of reasonable accommodations. Title I sets forth some examples of reasonable accommodations:

> (A) making existing facilities used by employees readily accessible to and usable by individuals with disabilities; and
>
> (B) job restructuring, part-time or modified work schedule, reassignment to a vacant position, acquisition or modification of equipment or devices, appropriate adjustment or modifications of examinations, training materials or policies, the provision of qualified readers or interpreters and other similar accommodations for individuals with disabilities. (ADA, § 101(9), Supp. 1992)

Another area of the professional's opinion should address whether the client poses a threat to the health or safety of other employees. If it can be determined that others are so affected, and if the employer cannot make reasonable accommodations to prevent this, the employer is justified in refusing or terminating employment. EEOC regulations specifically require that expert opinions be used to determine whether a disability poses such a threat. Specifically, the regulations state:

> The determination that an individual poses a "direct threat" shall be based on an individualized assessment of the individual's present ability to safely perform the essential functions of the job. This assessment shall be based on a reasonable medical judgment that relies on the most current medical knowledge and/or the best available objective evidence. In determining whether an individual would pose a direct threat, the factors to be considered include:
> (1) The duration of the risk;
> (2) The nature and severity of the potential harm;
> (3) The likelihood that the potential harm will occur; and
> (4) The imminence of the potential harm. (EEOC, § 1630.2(r), 1992).

Another area of employment discrimination against those infected with AIDS has to do with automatically testing employees or prospective employees for HIV. This type of action is clearly prohibited unless all employees receive the same test and the employer can show that there is some relation between the testing and the job functions. Thus, an employer cannot single out one employee who is suspected of having the virus, and require him or her to be tested (Mello, 1995; ADA, § 102(c)(4), Supp. 1992). A problem with this arises when employers themselves insure the employees. Insurers generally make coverage limitations and exclusions based on HIV antibody test results. The insurance companies argue that HIV infection should be treated the same as all other infectious diseases, and that the companies would not be able to insure in large urban areas if they were not allowed to take this into consideration. Actual statistics about the cost of testing versus the cost of coverage do not entirely support this view. This is still an unprotected area under the ADA, which may allow the continuation of discrimination against those with HIV/AIDS. Thus, an employer who otherwise is not allowed to discriminate may do so in the capacity of a self-insurer (Mello, 1995).

There are other protections under the ADA. One area is discrimination by those in public and private accommodations, such as hospitals, day care centers, homeless shelters, food banks, and schools (ADA, 42 U.S.C.A., Subchapters II, III, & IV, Supp. 1992). Another is the delivery and funding of health services (ADA, § 301(7)(F), Supp. 1992). In addition, the Fair Housing Act (§§ 3601–3631, 1988) prohibits disability-based discrimination in selling or renting private housing and in residential real estate financing. Finally, the Individuals with Disabilities Education Act (§§ 1400–1485, 1988, Supp. 1992) supplements the ADA (which also prohibits discrimination in providing education) by requiring states that utilize federal funds for special education to accommodate the needs of children with disabilities (which include HIV infection).

TESTAMENTARY CAPACITY

The final area in which those infected with HIV may need to demonstrate competence is that of testamentary capacity. This usually becomes an issue after an individual's death, when others wish to challenge the property disposition designated in his or her will. This type of challenge is usually initiated by a relative who expected to be a beneficiary of the estate. The testator's decision in disinheriting a family member is not what is at issue; rather, it is the testator's thinking process that is being challenged (Melton et al., 1997). It should be emphasized that there are different legal standards of capacity, depending on the reason why capacity is being challenged. Thus, the level of capacity required to execute a will is different from that required to enter into a contract or make a gift. It is generally accepted that the least demanding standard of mental capacity involves testamentary capacity (Walsh et al., 1994).

The general rule in most states is that the maker of a valid will must be able to understand (1) the meaning of executing a will; (2) the nature and extent of his or her property; (3) the disposition of the estate; and (4) the natural objects of his or her bounty (Melton et al., 1997). In the administration of these requirements, courts have required the testator to have a minimum amount of intelligence (Melton et al., 1997; Bowle & Parker, 1960).

Capacity to understand a modest estate may not be sufficient to understand a large, diverse estate. Thus, some states have held that the amount of intelligence required varies with the size of the estate or complexity of the assets. Courts have been willing to overlook the fact that a testator does not know the value of his or her estate, so long as the testator knows generally what his or her assets are (*In re Will of Womack*, 1981).

When answering the question about understanding the disposition the testator wishes to make of the estate, the testator must know some of the consequences of the bequest. For example, the testator should know that transferring a majority of a corporation's stock will also give control of the corporation to that person. Outside factors can be indicative of capacity as well. For example, a court is likely to find a lack of capacity in a case where the testator lived in poverty while having millions of dollars.

On the other hand, capacity may be supported if it can be shown that the testator was able to conduct business affairs. As with the understanding of tax consequences, understanding business affairs may prove competence, but a lack of understanding of these affairs does not require a finding of incapacity.

With regard to understanding the natural objects of the testator's bounty, generally the testator must have an intelligent knowledge of his or her descendants; however, it is also possible that a court will only require the testator to be *able* to know this information (*In re Estate of Riley*, 1970). The mere fact that because one fails to provide for his or her descendants does not automatically invalidate a will.

Although attorneys generally apply the four-part test to determine testamentary capacity, they seek outside opinions when doubt remains. Some attorneys recommend the individual's personal physician; however, the ideal situation would be to obtain the opinion of a mental health professional (Smith & Meyer, 1987). The problem with outside mental health practitioners is that their testimony is of minor weight if the professionals never had any direct contact with the deceased (*In re Grahlman's Will*, 1957).

SUMMARY AND CONCLUSIONS

This chapter has provided an overview of the types of legal competence issues that may arise for individuals with HIV. Because there are several unique circumstances surrounding HIV, such as social stigma, unrealistic fears of others, difficulty of prediction, and possible mental deterioration, arranging one's affairs in advance can have important personal and legal consequences. This chapter has attempted to outline the issues and provide alternatives that may prove helpful in specific situations. An underlying theme is that planning ahead to provide for unforeseen circumstances may set one's mind at ease or prevent troublesome issues from occurring.

ACKNOWLEDGMENT

We would like to acknowledge contributions to this chapter made by Steve Smith, who made valuable suggestions and recommendations.

REFERENCES

American Bar Association. (1990). *Guardianship of the elderly: A primer for attorneys.* Washington, DC: Author.

Americans with Disabilities Act (ADA) of 1990, 42 U.S.C.A. §§ 101–102, 301–302; 12101–12213 (West Supp. 1992).

Archer v. Federal Deposit Ins. Corp. (Tex. App. Houston), 831 S.W.2d 483 (1992).

Atkinson, J. H., & Grant, I. (1994). Natural history of neuropsychiatric manifestation of HIV disease. *Psychiatric Clinics of North America, 17,* 17–32.

Black, H. C. (1968). *Black's law dictionary.* St. Paul, MN: West.

Boccellari, A. A., & Dilley, J. W. (1992). Management and residential placement problems of patients with HIV-related cognitive impairment. *Hospital and Community Psychiatry, 43,* 32–37.

Bongar, B., Maris, R. W., Berman, A. L., & Litman, R. E. (1992). Outpatient standards of care and the suicidal patient. *Suicide and Life-Threatening Behavior, 22*(4), 453–478.

Bowle, W. J., & Parker, O. H. (1960). *Page on wills*. Cincinnati, OH: Anderson.

Cantor, N. L. (1992). Prospective autonomy: On the limits of shaping one's postcompetence medical fate. *Journal of Contemporary Health Law and Policy, 8*, 13–48.

Chesney, M. A., & Folkman, S. (1994). Psychological impact of HIV disease and implications for intervention. *Psychiatric Clinics of North America, 17*, 163–182.

Civil Rights Act of 1964, 42 U.S.C.A. § 200 (West 1981, West Supp. 1992).

Cruzan by Cruzan v. Director, Missouri Dept. of Health, 110 S. Ct. 2841, 497 U.S. 261, 111 L.Ed.2d 224 (1990).

Egan, V., Brettle, R. P., & Goodwin, G. M. (1992). The Edinburgh cohort of HIV-positive drug users: Pattern of cognitive impairment in relation to progression of disease. *British Journal of Psychiatry, 161*, 522–531.

Equal Employment Opportunity Commission (EEOC), Equal Employment Opportunity for Individuals with Disabilities, Regulations to Implement the Equal Employment Provisions of the Americans with Disabilities Act, 29 C.F.R. Pt. 1630, § 1630.2(m–r) (1992).

Fair Housing Act, 42 U.S.C. §§ 3601–3631 (1988).

Garwood, A., & Melnick, B. (1995). *What everyone can do to fight AIDS*. San Francisco: Jossey-Bass.

Gitler, J., & Rennert, S. (1992). HIV infection among women and children and antidiscrimination laws: An overview. *Iowa Law Review, 77*, 1283–1312.

Goodart, N. L. (1995). *The truth about living trusts*. Dearborn, MI: Dearborn Financial.

Grant, I., & Adams, K. (Eds.). (1996). *Neuropsychological assessment of neuropsychiatric disorders*. New York: Oxford University Press.

Hollweg, M., Riedel, R. R., Goebel, F. D., Schick, U., & Naber, D. (1991). Remarkable improvement of neuropsychiatric symptoms in HIV-infected patients after AZT therapy. *Klinische Wochenschrift, 69*, 409–412.

Hull, L., Holmes, G. E., & Karst, R. H. (1990). Managing guardianships of the elderly: Protection and advocacy as public policy. In E. F. Dejorwki (Ed.), *Protecting judgment-impaired adults* (pp. 145–162). New York: Haworth Press.

Individuals with Disabilities Education Act, 20 U.S.C.A. §§ 1400–1485 (West 1988, West Supp. 1992).

In re Estate of Riley, 479 P.2d 1 (Wash. 1970).

In re Grahlman's Will, 81 N.W.2d 673 (Iowa 1957).

In re Quinlan, 70 N.J. 10, 335 A.2d 647 (1976), cert. denied, 429 U.S. 922, 97 S. Ct. 319 (1976).

In re Will of Womack, 280 S.E.2d 494 (N.C. Ct. App. 1981).

Kaplan, R. M., & Saccuzzo, D. (1997). *Psychological testing* (4th ed.). Pacific Grove, CA: Brooks/Cole.

Kyle, R. D., & Sachs, L. (1994). Perceptions of control and social support in relation to psychosocial adjustment to HIV/AIDS. *AIDS Patient Care, 8*, 322–327.

Mello, J. A. (1995). *AIDS and the law of workplace discrimination*. Boulder, CO: Westview Press.

Melton, G., Petrila, J., Poythress, N., & Slobogin, C. (1997). *Psychological evalu-*

ations for the courts: A handbook for mental health practitioners and lawyers (2nd ed.). New York: Guilford Press.

Meyer, R. G., & Deitsch, S. (1996). *The clinician's handbook: Integrated diagnostics, assessment and intervention in adult and adolescent psychopathology* (4th ed.). Boston: Allyn & Bacon.

N.H. Rev. Stat. Ann § 464-A (1979).

Nolan, B. S. (1990). A judicial menu: Selecting remedies for the incapacitated elder. In E. F. Dejorwki (Ed.), *Protecting judgment-impaired adults* (pp. 73–84). New York: Haworth Press.

Peters, R., Schmidt, W. C. Jr., & Miller, K. S. (1995). Guardianship of the elderly in Tallahassee, Florida. In *Guardianship* (pp. 91–106). Durham, NC: Carolina Academic Press.

Presidential Commission on the Human Immunodeficiency Virus Epidemic. (1988). *Report of the Presidential Commission on the Human Immunodeficiency Virus Epidemic.* Washington, DC: U.S. Government Printing Office.

Rehabilitation Act of 1973, 29 U.S.C.A. §§ 701–796 (West 1985, West Supp. 1992).

Riccio, M., Pugh, K., Jadresic, D., Burgess, A., Thompson, C., Wilson, B., Lovett, E., Baldeweg, T., Hawkins, D. A., & Catalan, J. (1993). Neuropsychiatric aspects of HIV-1 infection in gay men: Controlled investigation of psychiatric, neuropsychological and neurological status. *Journal of Psychosomatic Research, 37,* 819–830.

Riedel, R. R., Helmstaedter, C., Bulau, P., Durwen, H. F., Brackmann, H., Fimmers, R., Clarenbach, P., Miller, E. N., & Bottcher, M. (1992). Early signs of cognitive deficits among human immunodeficiency virus-positive hemophiliacs. *Acta Psychiatrica Scandinavica, 85,* 321–326.

Robertson, K. R., & Hall, C. D. (1992). Human immunodeficiency virus-related cognitive impairment and the acquired immunodeficiency syndrome dementia complex. *Seminars in Neurology, 12,* 18–27.

Roca, R. P. (1994). Determining decisional capacity: A medical perspective. *Fordham Law Review, 62,* 1178–1196.

Schmidt, W. C. Jr., Miller, K. S., Bell, W. G., & New, B. E. (1995). Summary and discussion of major findings from a national study of public guardianship and the elderly. In *Guardianship* (pp. 69–78). Durham, NC: Carolina Academic Press.

Smith, S. R., & Meyer, R. G. (1987). *Law, behavior, and mental health: Policy and practice.* New York: New York University Press.

Stern, Y. (1994). Neuropsychological evaluation of the HIV patient. *Psychiatric Clinics of North America, 17,* 125–134.

Syndulko, K., Singer, E. J., Nogales-Gaete, J., Conrad, A., Schmid, P., & Tourtellotte, W. W. (1994). Laboratory evaluations in HIV-1-associated cognitive/motor complex. *Psychiatric Clinics of North America, 17,* 91–123.

Uniform Guardianship and Protective Proceedings Act. (1982). *Uniform laws annotated: Vol. 8A.* St. Paul, MN: West.

Uniform Probate Code, § 5-401(2). (1969).

U.S. Senate, Committee on Labor and Human Resiurces. (1989). *Hearings on the Americans with Disabilities Act* (101st Congress, 1st Session). Washington, DC: U.S. Government Printing Office.

Walsh, A. C. (1992). *Mental capacity: December 1992 cumulative supplement.* Colorado Springs, CO: Shepard's/McGraw-Hill.

Walsh, A. C., Brown, B. B., Kaye, K., & Grigsby, J. (1994). Planning for incapacity. In *mental capacity: Legal and medical aspects of assessment and treatment* (2nd ed., pp. 4-1–4-16). Colorado Springs, CO: Shepard's/McGraw-Hill.

Winick, B. (1997). *The right to refuse mental health treatment.* Washington, DC: American Psychological Association.

Zegans, L. S., Gerhard, A. L., & Coates, T. J. (1994). Psychotherapies for the person with HIV disease. *Psychiatric Clinics of North America, 17,* 149–161.

Index

Abstraction ability, 18
Activities of daily living, 296
  adaptations for patients with de-
    mentia, 300–310
Adjustment disorders, 163–164, 214
  clinical course, 130–131
  diagnosis, 130
  epidemiology, 128–129
  etiology, 129–130
  treatment, 163–164
Advance directives, 323–324
Affect. *See* Mood; *specific affects*
Agitation, 18
Agraphia, 18
AIDS. *See specific topics*
Amantadine, 169
Ambulation problems
  assistive devices for, 305–307
American Academy of Neurology
  (AAN), diagnostic classification
  and criteria of, 5–8, 16, 75, 203
Amphetamines, 81, 160, 215
Amphotericin B, 85
Anticholinergic drugs, 81
Anticonvulsant drugs, 218
Antidepressants, 81, 161, 167, 215–
  216, 281. *See also specific drugs
  and drug classes*
  drug interactions of, 284

Antifungal drugs, 85
Antihistaminic drugs, 81
Anti-inflammatory therapy for dementia, 209
Antiretroviral therapy, 78–80, 167,
  208–210, 215, 219. *See also*
  Highly active antiretroviral therapy (HAART); Zidovudine (AZT)
  for children, 80, 210–212
Anxiety disorders, 18, 52, 162–163,
  216
  clinical course, 125
  diagnosis, 125
  epidemiology, 124–125
  etiology, 125
  neurobiological basis, 56
  treatment
    pharmacological, 162–163, 216–
      217
    psychological, 162–163, 216,
      236. *See also* Stress reduction
Apathy, 51, 56
Aphasia, 21
Aseptic meningitis, 73–75
Assessment, 251, 313–315. *See also
  specific tests*
  computerized tomography (CT),
    13, 14, 55, 78
  mental status evaluation, 313–315

Assessment *(continued)*
  neuroimaging, 13–15, 78–79
  neuropsychological, 298
    of cognitive/motor complex, 78–79
    computerized, 24–26
    indications for, 30–31
    test batteries, 31–33, 43–44
  of suicide risk, 278–279
Attention/concentration, 18–20, 32, 45–46
  practical considerations for dealing with impaired, 233
Auditory Consonant Trigrams (ACT), 19, 24
AZT. *See* Zidovudine

B

Basal ganglia dysfunction, 207
  hypermetabolism, 15–16
Beck Depression Inventory, 279
Beck Hopelessness Scale, 278
Behavioral disturbances. *See also specific disturbances*
  in cognitive/motor complex, 77–78
Benzodiazepines, 162, 165, 216
  drug interactions of, 284
  neurocognitive impairment due to, 216
Benztropine mesylate, 168, 169
Bereavement, complicated, 169–170. *See also* Depression; Grief reactions
  clinical course, 155–156
  diagnosis, 155
  epidemiology, 153
  etiology, 153–154
  treatment, 169–170
Bipolar disorders, 159–160. *See also* Depression; Mania; Mood disorders
  clinical course, 119–120
  diagnosis, 119
  epidemiology, 118
  etiology, 118
Blessed Dementia Rating Scale, 17
Borderline personality disorder, 163

Boston Naming Test, 20, 46
Bradykinesia, 214
Bradyphrenia, 24
Bromperidol, 168
Bruininks-Oseretsky Motor Development Scale, 299
Bupropion, 159
Burnout, in professional caregivers, 258–259
Buspirone, 162, 216–217

C

Calculation, 18
California Verbal Learning Test, 47
Carbamazepine, 217–218
Caregivers
  interventions of
    for mildly impaired patients, 250–251
    for patients with delirium, 252–254
    for patients with dementia, 251–254
  personal
    of hospital patients, support for, 254–255
    psychosocial issues of, 242–248
    reactions to cognitive impairment, 244–247, 257
    recommendations for, 255–258
  professional, 242
    burnout, 258–259
    psychosocial responses of, 248–249
    recommendations for, 258–259
Case management, 231–232, 234–238. *See also* Treatment, educational considerations
Case reports, 2–4, 24, 66, 72, 73, 83, 85–86, 88, 90, 92, 93, 229–231
Caudate nucleus dysfunction, 207
Centers for Disease Control (CDC), diagnostic classification and criteria of, 3–6, 201
Cerebral metabolic activity, 15
Cerebral toxoplasmosis, 12–13, 54, 86–88

Cerebrospinal fluid (CSF) abnormalities, 68, 71, 74, 78–79, 82–87, 91, 207
Children with AIDS/HIV
antiretroviral therapy for, 80, 210–212
L-dopa therapy for, 297
progressive encephalopathy in, 297
Chlorpromazine, 165, 217
Cidofovir, 94
Clonazepam, 217–218
Clozapine, 284
CMC. *See* Cognitive/motor complex
CMV encephalitis. *See* Cytomegalovirus encephalitis
Cognitive impairment, 2–3, 17–18, 32, 44–45, 203–205, 212, 233, 312–313. *See also* Delirium; Dementia; Intellectual functioning; Memory Dysfunction; Neurocognitive disorder; Neuropsychological functioning; Subcortical pathology
attention/concentration, 18–20, 32, 45–46, 233
benzodiazepines causing, 216
caregivers and, 244–247, 257
gross, 44–45
in HIV vs. normal aging process, 29–30
information processing speed, 45–46
language, 18, 20–21, 32, 46
learning, 47
naming, 18, 20
psychostimulants for, 215
psychotherapy for dealing with, 229–231
slowed cognition, 24
stages of, 16, 314–315
subjective complaints of and depression, 28–29
suicidal risk and, 279–280
Cognitive/motor complex, HIV (HIV CMC), 3, 72, 75–81
behavioral disturbances, 77–78
behavioral management, 81

clinical course, 15–16
diagnostic criteria, 7–8
evaluation, 78–79
neuroprotective treatment, 81
practical considerations for patients with, 230–236
symptomatic treatment, 81
Cognitive/motor disorder, minor, 203
Commitment, involuntary, 315
Computerized tomography (CT), 13, 14, 55, 78–79, 89, 91–93
Constructional ability, 18, 21, 46–47
Cooking and eating, adaptive devices for, 308
Coping skills, interventions to enhance, 214
Counseling, 231–232. *See also* Psychosocial interventions; Psychotherapy
Countertransference, 238–239
Crawford Small Parts Dexterity Test, 298
Cryptococcal meningitis, 12, 84–86
CSF. *See* Cerebrospinal fluid
CT. *See* Computerized tomography
Cytomegalovirus (CMV) encephalitis, 57, 92–94

D

Daily activities, 296
adaptations for patients with dementia, 300–310
Day treatment programs, 235
DdC. *See* Dideoxycytidine
DdI. *See* Dideoxyinosine
Delavirdine, 80
Delirium, 51, 78
caregiver interventions, 252–254
clinical course, 146, 296–297
diagnosis, 144, 146
epidemiology, 144
etiology, 144
suicide risk, 272–273
treatment, 164–165

Dementia, 56, 75–76, 203, 295–297.
    See also Cognitive impairment
  adaptive devices and training for
      patients with, 305
  ambulatory patients and, 305–
      307
  cooking and eating and, 308
  memory aids, 232, 250, 252,
      283, 300–301, 307–308
  recreational aids, 309–310
  work and, 303–304, 308–309
  caregiver interventions, 251–254
  clinical course, 143
  depression and, 237
  diagnosis, 140–143, 237
    diagnostic criteria, 5–6, 8, 9, 21, 43
  epidemiology, 137
  etiology, 137–140
  functional problems related to,
      296–303
    recreation, participation in, 304–
        305, 309–310
  practical considerations for pa-
      tients with, 232, 233
  subcortical, 49–50
  suicide risk, 237, 272–273
  treatment, 165–167
    anti-inflammatory, 209
Dementia complex, 2, 3, 78. *See also*
    Cognitive/motor complex
Dementia due to HIV Disease, 8–9,
    21, 43
2′-deoxy-3′-thiacytidine (3TC), 208
Depression, 18, 26–27, 51, 159–160,
    214–215, 237. *See also* Bereave-
    ment, complicated; Bipolar disor-
    ders; Mood disorders
  assessment, 27–28
  clinical course, 116–118
  dementia and, 237
  diagnosis, 115–116, 162
  epidemiology, 113–114
  etiology, 114–115
  HIV-related vs. major, 214–215
  neurobiological basis, 56
  practical considerations in dealing
      with, 233

  subjective complaints of cognitive
      decline, 28–29
  suicide risk, 273–274, 281
  treatment, 159–160, 215–216
Dextroamphetamine, 160, 215
*Diagnostic and Statistical Manual of
    Mental Disorders*, Fourth Edition
    (DSM-IV)
  HIV-related mental disorders, 111–
      112
    Dementia due to HIV Disease, 8–
        9, 21, 43
Didanosine (ddI). *See* Dideoxyinosine
Dideoxycytidine (ddc), 80, 212
Dideoxyinosine (ddI), 80, 167, 211
  IQ affected by, 212
Digit Span, 18, 20, 45
Discrimination, employment, 324–
    327
Dorsolateral prefrontal–subcortical
    dysfunction, 56
Drug abuse. *See* Substance abuse
Drug interactions, 284
Drug therapy. *See* Pharmacotherapy

E

Educational considerations, 236–
    237. *See also* Caregivers, personal
Electroconvulsive therapy (ECT),
    160, 215
Employment discrimination, 324–
    327
Encephalitis, cytomegalovirus
    (CMV), 57, 92–94
Encephalopathy, 3. *See also specific im-
    pairments*
  clinical–pathological correlations,
      55–56
  diagnostic criteria, 3–5
  neurobiological basis, 52–57
  prevalence, 50–52
  role of HIV in, 54–55
Evaluation. *See* Assessment
Executive functioning, 18, 21, 23,
    32, 47–48, 56

F

Family members, educational considerations for, 236–237
Fatigue, and mood disorder, 214
Finger Tapping Test, 23, 48
Fluconazole, 85
5-flucytosine, 85
Fluoxetine, 159, 215. *See also* Selective serotonin reuptake inhibitors
Fornix, structural abnormalities in, 202
Foscavir, 94
Frontal lobe functioning, 18, 21, 23, 32, 47–48, 56

G

Ganciclovir, 94
Geriatric Depression Scale, 28
Grief reactions. *See also* Bereavement
  dealing with, 284
  following HIV diagnosis, 213–214
  psychotherapy for, 156–159
Guardianship, 315–320
  determining incapacity and, 317–319
  guardian duties, 321
  hearings and process, 316–317
  monitoring of
    restoration of rights and, 319–320
  public guardians and other options, 321–323

H

Haloperidol, 165, 168
Halstead–Reitan Neuropsychological Test Battery, 43–44
Headaches, tricyclic antidepressants for, 216
Highly active antiretroviral therapy (HAART), 67, 70. *See also* Antiretroviral therapy; Zidovudine (AZT)

HIV-associated dementia (HAD). *See* Dementia
HIV central nervous system disease, differential diagnosis of, 71–72
HIV CMC. *See* Cognitive/motor complex
HIV diagnosis, grief reaction to, 213–214
HIV infection. *See also specific topics*
  as brain disease, 110–113
  incidence, 10
  stages of
    mental disorders and, 112
    neuropsychological functioning and, 17–18, 314–315
Home care, 255. *See also* Caregivers, personal
Home visits, 235–236
Hydroxyzine, 162
Hypomania, 160. *See also* Mania

I

ICD-10. *See* International Classification of Diseases
Incompetence (legal), determination of
  guardianship and, 317–319
Infections, CNS
  cryptococcal meningitis, 84–86
  cytomegalovirus encephalitis, 57, 92–94
  lymphoma, 54, 91–92
  neurosyphilis, 81–83
  progressive multifocal leukoencephalopathy, 12, 13, 54, 72, 86–88, 246
  secondary, 52–54, 57
  toxoplasmosis, 54, 86–88
Insomnia. *See also* Sleep disturbance
  mood disorders and, 214
  tricyclic antidepressants for, 216
Intellectual functioning, 44–45
  abstraction, 18
  calculation, 18
  effect of dideoxyinosine on, 212

Intellectual functioning *(continued)*
  judgment, 18
  sequential reasoning, dealing with
    impaired, 233, 302
International Classification of Diseases,
  10th revision (ICD-10), 44
Involuntary commitment, 315

J

Jebsen–Taylor Hand Function Test,
  298
John Cunningham virus (JCV), 88–89

L

Language functioning, 20–21, 32, 46
  expressive, 18
L-dopa therapy, for children, 297
Lesions (brain), focal, 53–54, 72, 87
Lithium, 160, 217–218
Lorazepam, 165
Lymphoma, CNS, 13, 54, 91–92

M

Magnetic resonance imaging (MRI),
  13–14, 55, 78–79, 89–91, 93
Magnetic resonance spectroscopy
  (MRS), 90
Mania, 18, 52, 160. *See also* Bipolar
  disorders; Mood disorders
  treatment, 217–218
MAO inhibitors. *See* Monoamine oxidase inhibitors
Memory aids, for patients with dementia, 232, 233, 235, 250, 252,
  283, 300–301, 307–308
Memory dysfunction, 18, 21–22, 47,
  202
  assessment of, 32, 47. *See also*
    Wechsler Memory Scale
  dementia and, 252
  drugs that exacerbate, 81, 216

Meningitis
  aseptic, 73–75
  cryptococcal, 84–86
Mental status, 17–18
Mental status evaluation, 313–315
Metabolic activity, cerebral, 14–15
Methadone maintenance, 162
Methylphenidate, 160, 167, 215
Mini-Mental State Exam, 17
Minnesota Rate of Manipulation,
  298
Molindone, 168
Monoamine oxidase (MAO) inhibi-
  tors, 160
Mood, 18, 32
Mood disorders, 159–160. *See also*
  Bipolar disorders; Depression;
  Mania
  fatigue and insomnia as symptoms
    of, 214
  pharmacotherapy for, 159–160
Motivation, initiative and, 234. *See
  also* Apathy
Motor/psychomotor functioning,
  18, 23–24, 32, 46, 48, 296, 298–
  299. *See also* Ambulation prob-
  lems; Cognitive/motor complex;
  Reaction time
  psychomotor slowing, 214, 298,
    299
Movement disorders, 168
MRS. *See* Magnetic resonance spec-
  troscopy
Multicenter AIDS Cohort Study
  (MACS), 32, 33, 204

N

Naming, impairment in, 18, 20
Nefazodone, 284
Neurobehavioral Cognitive Status Examination, 17
Neurocognitive disorder, mild
  clinical course, 135–137
  diagnosis, 133–135
  epidemiology, 131–132

etiology, 132–133
treatment, 165–167
Neuroimaging, 13–15, 78–79
Neuroleptic drugs, 81, 165, 168, 217, 284
side effects, 217
Neurological disease, 205–206. *See also specific impairments*
differential diagnosis, 71–72
focal vs. nonfocal presentation, 53, 72–73
host factors, 69
risk factors, 69–71
AIDS-defining illnesses, 70
immune status, 70
viral load, 70–71
secondary, 12–13
Neuropsychiatric AIDS Rating Scale, 314
Neuropsychiatric impairment, 106–110, 128–131. *See also specific impairments*
diagnostic issues, 110–113
stages of, 314–315
Neuropsychological functioning, 24, 33, 48–49. *See also* Cognitive impairment
agraphia, 18
etiology of impairment, 206–207
frontal lobe/executive ability, 18, 21, 23, 32, 47–48, 56
incidence of impairment, 10–12, 43–44
mental status, 17–18
motor/psychomotor, 18, 23–24, 48
reaction time, 25–26
sensory, 18
speech, 20–21, 233
stages of HIV infection and, 17–18
subcortical dementia, 49–50
visual–spatial–constructional, 18, 21, 46–47, 233
Neurosyphilis, 81–83
Neutropenia, 94
treatment of AZT-induced, 217
Nevirapine, 80

O

Obsessive-compulsive disorder, 162
Occupational therapy, 297–299, 305, 310
Olanzapine, 284

P

Paced Auditory Serial Addition Task (PASAT), 19, 45
Pain, 274–275
medications for, 216
psychological treatment for, 236
Panic disorder, 163
PCR. *See* Polymerase chain reaction
Personality disorders, 161, 163. *See also* Behavioral disturbances
clinical course, 128
diagnosis, 127–128
epidemiology, 125–127
etiology, 127
PET. *See* Positron emission tomography
Pharmacotherapy, 81, 85, 158–159, 207–209, 218–219. *See also specific disorders; specific drugs and drug classes*
drug interactions, 284
neuropsychiatric side effects, 144–145
nonretroviral, 212–213
Physical therapy, 305–306
Pimozide, 284
Polymerase chain reaction (PCR), 68, 79, 90
Positron emission tomography (PET), 14, 55–56
Progressive multifocal leukoencephalopathy (PML), 12, 13, 54, 72–73, 86–88, 246
Protease inhibitors, drug interaction with, 284
Psychomotor functioning. *See* Motor/psychomotor functioning

Psychosis, 51–52, 168–169, 217
  clinical course, 153
  diagnosis, 152
  epidemiology, 150–151
  etiology, 151–152
  treatment, 217
Psychosocial interventions, 229–231.
    See also Educational considerations
  to enhance coping skills, 214
Psychostimulants, 160, 166–167,
    215. *See also* amphetamines
Psychotherapy, 229–232, 236–238,
    283–284
  for adjustment disorder, 214
  countertransference, 238–239
  for dealing with cognitive changes,
    229–231
  for loss issues, 156–159, 169–170
Psychotic disorders. *See* Psychosis
Purdue Grooved Pegboard, 48, 298
Purdue Perceptual–Motor Survey, 299

R

Reaction time, 25–26
Recreation, dementia and participation in, 304–305
Recreational aids, 309
Rey Auditory Verbal Learning Test, 47
Rey-Osterrieth Complex Figure
    Test, 21, 30, 47
Risperidone, 284
Ritonavir, 80
  drug interactions of, 284
Rosenbusch Finger Dexterity Test, 298

S

Saquinivir, 80
Scale for Suicide Ideation, 278
Selective serotonin reuptake inhibitors (SSRIs), 215–216. *See also*
    Fluoxetine
  drug interactions of, 284

Sensory functions, 18
Sleep disturbance, 167–168. *See also*
    Insomnia
  course, 150
  diagnosis, 149–150
  epidemiology, 147
  etiology, 148–149
  treatment, 167–168
Social isolation and withdrawal
  practical considerations in dealing
    with, 233
  reduction of, 282–283
Speech impairment, 20–21
  practical considerations in dealing
    with, 233, 302
  slowed speech, 302
Speech therapy, 302
SSRIs. *See* Selective serotonin reuptake inhibitors
Stavudine (D4T), 80
Stimulants, 81. *See also* psychostimulants
Stressors, psychological, associated
    with HIV, 312–313
Stress reduction, methods of, 251
Stroop task, 20, 46
Subcortical pathology
  cognitive/emotional impact of, 56–
    57
  dementia, 49–50
Substance abuse, 111–112, 120, 162
  clinical course, 123–124
  diagnosis, 122–123
  epidemiology, 120–121
  etiology, 121–122
  suicide risk and, 272
  treatment, 160–162
Suicidal patients
  ethical issues with, 285–287
  management of, 280–284, 288–
    289
    establishing safety, 281–282
    grief work, 283
    no-suicide contracts, 282
    reducing isolation, 282–283
    reevaluating diagnoses, 281–282
  presentations of, 267

Suicide, 238, 263–267
  assessment of rationality of, 286–287
  assisted, 238
  prevalence, 267, 270
  research on, 267–271
  risk assessment, 237, 275–280, 288–289
    screening checklists, 278–279
  risk factors for, 264, 267, 271–275
    dementia and delirium, 272–273
    depression, 272–274, 281
    HIV-related stressors and perceived risk, 274–275
    pain syndromes, 274–275
    psychopathology, 237, 267, 272–274
    substance abuse, 272
  traditional and controversial views of, 265–266

T

3TC. *See* 2′-deoxy-3′-thiacytidine
Temporal lobe metabolism, decreased, 14
Testamentary capacity, 327–329
Testing. *See* Assessment
Thioridazine, 168
Thorazine. *See* Chlorpromazine
Toxoplasmosis, cerebral, 12–13, 54, 86–88
Trail Making Test, 24, 30, 45, 298
Trazodone, 167, 284
Treatment. *See also* Case management; Occupational therapy; Pharmacotherapy; Psychosocial interventions; Psychotherapy; *specific disorders and specific interventions*
  educational considerations, 236–237
  of symptoms of cognitive/motor complex, 81

Tricyclic antidepressants, 280
  drug interactions of, 284
  memory dysfunction exacerbated by, 216
Tumors, secondary, 52–57

V

Valproic acid, 217–218
Venlafaxine, 284
Verbal fluency, 18, 21, 46
Viramune. *See* Nevirapine
Visual scanning, 46
Visual–spatial–constructional functioning, 18, 21, 46–47
  practical considerations in dealing with impaired, 233
Vocabulary, 46

W

Wards, legal rights of, 320–323
  advance directives, 323–324
Wechsler Adult Intelligence Scale–Revised (WAIS-R), 2, 4, 17–18, 20, 21, 24, 30, 32, 45–47, 298
Wechsler Memory Scale, 30, 47. *See also* Digit Span
Wellbutrin. *See* Bupropion
Wisconsin Card Sorting Test, 23
Withdrawal, social. *See* Social isolation and withdrawal
Work
  adaptive devices for, 308–309
  problems related to, 303–304, 308–309
World Health Organization Auditory Verbal Learning Test, 47

Z

Zidovudine (AZT), 69, 79–80, 160, 167, 208–212
  treatment of neutropenia induced by, 217